11 MAR 2020

THE HANDBOOK OF MENTAL HEALTH AND SPACE

The Handbook of Mental Health and Space: Community and Clinical Applications brings together the psychosocial work on experiences of space and mental distress, and explores new links between the theoretical work in this field and clinical and community practice. In doing so, it provides a dialogue between academics, service users and practitioners, to provide potential ways of reconvening the spaces in which people experience distress.

This timely book works to stimulate discussion about mental health care spaces and their design. The volume is organised into three themed sections covering (a) institutional settings, (b) community spaces and (c) clinical and community interventions. It addresses both the experiences and needs of mental health service users at all stages of development, such as the provision made for children and the impact of social media, as well as the impact of other socio-demographic factors like gender and ethnicity.

With contributions from those involved in theorising space, those drawing on their own experiences of distress and space, as well as practitioners working on the ground, *Mental Distress and Space* will be of interest to mental health practitioners, people who experience distress and academics.

Laura McGrath is a Senior Lecturer in Psychology at the University of East London. She leads the undergraduate programme in Clinical and Community Psychology.

Paula Reavey is Professor of Psychology and Mental Health at London South Bank University. She is Director of Research and Education for the Design in Mental Health Network, UK.

THE HANDBOOK OF MENTAL HEALTH AND SPACE

Community and Clinical Applications

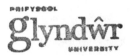

edited by
Laura McGrath and Paula Reavey

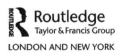

LONDON AND NEW YORK

First published 2019
by Routledge
2 Park Square, Milton Park, Abingdon, Oxon OX14 4RN

and by Routledge
711 Third Avenue, New York, NY 10017

Routledge is an imprint of the Taylor & Francis Group, an informa business

© 2019 selection and editorial matter, Laura McGrath and
Paula Reavey individual chapters, the contributors

The right of Laura McGrath and Paula Reavey to be identified
as authors of the editorial material, and of the authors for their
individual chapters, has been asserted in accordance with sections
77 and 78 of the Copyright, Designs and Patents Act 1988.

All rights reserved. No part of this book may be reprinted or
reproduced or utilised in any form or by any electronic, mechanical,
or other means, now known or hereafter invented, including
photocopying and recording, or in any information storage or
retrieval system, without permission in writing from the publishers.

Trademark notice: Product or corporate names may be trademarks
or registered trademarks, and are used only for identification and
explanation without intent to infringe.

British Library Cataloguing in Publication Data
A catalogue record for this book is available from the British Library

Library of Congress Cataloging in Publication Data
Names: McGrath, Laura, (Senior lecturer in psychology), editor |
    Reavey, Paula, editor.
Title: The handbook of mental health and space : community and
    clinical applications / Laura McGrath and Paula Reavey.
Description: New York, NY : Routledge, 2019.
Identifiers: LCCN 2018015373 | ISBN 9781138643932 (hardback)
    | ISBN 9781138643949 (pbk.) | ISBN 9781317216599 (epub)
    | ISBN 9781317216582 (mobipocket) | ISBN 9781315620312
    (Master) | ISBN 9781317216605 (Web)
Subjects: | MESH: Mentally Ill Persons—psychology | Facility
    Design and Construction—methods | Mental Disorders—
    therapy
Classification: LCC RC455 | NLM WM 29.5 | DDC 616.89–dc23
LC record available at https://lccn.loc.gov/2018015373

ISBN: 978-1-138-64393-2 (hbk)
ISBN: 978-1-138-64394-9 (pbk)
ISBN: 978-1-315-62031-2 (ebk)

Typeset in Bembo
by Swales & Willis Ltd, Exeter, Devon, UK

Printed and bound by CPI Group (UK) Ltd, Croydon, CR0 4YY

Laura: To Edward Lockhart. Without your extraordinary generosity, this book would never have existed.

Paula: Thanks to Jacqui Dillon, for her formidable strength, friendship and love of the Dawson.

CONTENTS

Notes on contributors   xii
Acknowledgements   xxi

    Introduction   1

PART I
Institutional spaces: containing distress in the
walls of the hospital   37

  1 Regulation and resistance in the smoking room at
     a mental health ward: struggles for a space 'in-between'   39
     Agnes Ringer and Mari Holen

  2 Madlove: a designer asylum   50
     Anna Zorwaska

  3 Children's spaces of mental health: users' experiences
     of two contrasting child and adolescent mental
     health outpatients in the UK   55
     Sarah Crafter

  4 Negotiating adult authority: young people's experience
     of adolescent mental health wards   74
     Jason Poole and Paula Reavey

5 Using experience-based co-design to improve inpatient
   mental health spaces　　　　　　　　　　　　　　　　　　88
   Zoë Boden, Michael Larkin and Neil Springham

6 Sensory space in child and adolescent mental
   health inpatient care　　　　　　　　　　　　　　　　　　102
   Nathan Parnell and Bernice Rooney

PART II
Community spaces: beyond the therapy room　　　　117

7 Sustaining spaces: community meal provision
   and mental well-being　　　　　　　　　　　　　　　　　119
   *Rebekah Graham, Darrin Hodgetts, Ottilie Stolte and
   Kerry Chamberlain*

8 Bursting bubbles of interiority: exploring space in
   experiences of distress and rough sleeping for
   newly homeless people　　　　　　　　　　　　　　　　135
   *Laura McGrath, Tassie Weaver, Paula Reavey and Steven
   D. Brown*

9 Caring spaces and practices: does social prescribing
   offer new possibilities for the fluid mess of 'mental health'?　149
   Carl Walker, Orly Klein, Nick Marks and Paul Hanna

10 Spaces of 'sanctuary': unfolding older mental health
   service users' experiences within the spaces of the home　163
   Lesley-Ann Smith

11 Spatial and social factors associated with community
   integration of individuals with psychiatric disabilities
   residing in supported and non-supported housing　　　180
   Greg Townley

12 Social media and mental health: a topological approach　200
   Lewis Goodings and Ian Tucker

13 Walking through and being with nature: meaning-making
   and the impact of being in UK wild places　　　　　　214
   Elizabeth Freeman and Jacqueline Akhurst

PART III
Interventions in space and place   235

14 *Geedka Shirka* (under the tree): cultural, migratory
    and community spaces for preventative interventions
    with Somali men and their families   237
    Amira Hassan, Iyabo Fatimilehin and Carolyn Kagan

15 Tea in the Pot, 'third place' or 'social prescription'?
    Exploring the positive impact on mental health
    of a voluntary women's group in Glasgow   250
    Maria Feeney

16 Institutionalising people in the community: a
    reflection on distress   263
    Vimala Uttarkar

17 Incorporating service user perspectives and the role
    of the home environment in mental health design   280
    Stephanie Liddicoat and Joe Forster

18 The Outsider Gallery: using art and music to open
    up mental health spaces   293
    Ben Wakeling and Jon Hall

Index   *308*

NOTES ON CONTRIBUTORS

Jacqueline Akhurst is a Professor in Community Psychology at Rhodes University. Her research focuses on community-based interventions, often utilising Action Research and Activity Theory. She is a Chartered Psychologist with the British Psychological Society (BPS), a Senior Fellow of the Higher Education Academy and registered with the Health Professions Council of South Africa (HPCSA) in both Counselling and Educational Psychology.

Zoë Boden is a Senior Lecturer in the Division of Psychology at London South Bank University. Her research focuses on emotional and relational experience in the context of mental health and distress. Zoë directs the Qualitative Approaches to Affect, Feelings and Emotions research network and is a member of the Experience-Based Co-Design in Mental Health research group. She has recently been funded by the Richard Benjamin Trust and the International Social Research Fund to undertake interdisciplinary research into the role of relationships in mental health. Her previous research has included exploring trust and suicidality, and the hospitalisation experiences of young people experiencing psychosis and their families. She undertook her PhD at Birkbeck University of London, exploring men's experiences of guilt in relationships. Methodologically, Zoë takes a phenomenological-hermeneutic perspective, incorporating visual and embodied data collection methods. She is currently also training as a psychotherapist at Gestalt Centre London.

Steven D. Brown is a Professor of Social and Organisational Psychology at the University of Leicester. His research interests are around social and collective remembering, particularly within 'vulnerable' groups. He is author of *The Social Psychology of Experience: Studies in Remembering and Forgetting* (with David Middleton, Sage, 2005); *Psychology without Foundations: History, Philosophy and*

Psychosocial Theory (with Paul Stenner Sage, 2009); and *Vital Memory and Affect: Living with a Difficult Past* (with Paula Reavey, Routledge, 2015).

Kerry Chamberlain is a Professor at Massey University, New Zealand. His current research interests focus on health in everyday life, with a particular interest in topics that advance understandings of disadvantage and provide assistance for disadvantaged peoples. He utilises mainly qualitative research methodologies in his research, predominantly critical discursive approaches, and innovative methods, such as photo-elicitation, diaries, maps and the use of material objects like personal possessions and photographs, to reveal the materiality and social practices of everyday life.

Sarah Crafter is a Senior Lecturer in the Department of Psychology at the Open University. She has a PhD in Cultural Psychology and Human Development and her theoretical and conceptual interests are grounded in sociocultural theory, transitions, critical or contested ideas of 'normative' development and cultural identity development. This includes the study of contested spaces in childhood. Her most recent work has focused on the practice of child language brokering (translating and interpreting for parents who do not speak the local language following migration) and the experiences of separated child refugees.

Iyabo Fatimilehin is a Consultant Clinical Psychologist and Director of Just Psychology CIC, a social enterprise that addresses the psychological and mental health needs of children, families and communities with a particular focus on cultural diversity, cultural competence and social justice. Previously, she worked in the National Health Service for over 20 years and was service lead for a specialist child and adolescent mental health service for Black and minority ethnic (BME) children and families for several years. She works as a trainer, therapist, supervisor and consultant and provides expert witness assessments for the courts. Iyabo's skills and experience include service development and management, facilitation of community participation and community development, research and evaluation. She has published journal articles and book chapters on issues of race, culture and ethnicity in relation to working with BME children and families. She has presented at national and international conferences on racial and ethnic identity development, community-based interventions, social exclusion, attachment, parenting and working with culture. Iyabo is an Associate Fellow and chartered member of the British Psychological Society and is a registered practitioner psychologist with the Health and Care Professions Council.

Maria Feeney was a Lecturer in Sociology at the University of the West of Scotland, where she researched and taught across a broad spectrum of sociology, social theory and cognate disciplines. Her primary research and teaching interests lie in interdisciplinary research and study across the fields of art and culture, the city and the experience of city life, place and space and the concept of third place. Maria has retired from the University but maintains contact with her key areas of research.

Joe Forster is a mental health practitioner with special interests in service user involvement and design. In person, through his own consultancy and as President of the charity Design in Mental Health Network he champions innovation and improvement in services and environments for mental health care. He is a frequent presenter at various events where he challenges audiences to set aside preconceptions and adopt new styles of partnership for innovation.

Elizabeth Freeman is a community-environmental eco-psychologist, who has recently formed a Nature Connections Research Network (NCRN) alongside colleagues at Derby University, which brings together people nationwide to explore nature connectedness and well-being. Elizabeth has an expertise in human–nature inter-relationships and meaning-/place-making and their role in engendering improved well-being. Her research has involved her working with military veterans and adults experiencing mental health issues, and her thesis investigated human–environment interaction and people's meaning-making and experience of a Walking and Solo Experience (WSE), employing a qualitative methodology.

Lewis Goodings is a Senior Lecturer in Psychology at Anglia Ruskin University. His research is dedicated to the intersections between social media and mental health and he applies theories from social psychology to the study of the everyday entanglements with social media. He is always looking to explore the broader social dynamics of technology, space, discourse and organisation.

Rebekah Graham is a recipient of the Massey University Vice Chancellor's Doctoral Scholarship and is completing her PhD in Societal Psychology. Her research considers the ways in which food-related traditions invoke connection and belonging, linking people to each other and to broader socio-cultural narratives. Specifically, her PhD considers wider social issues associated with ongoing precarity and food insecurity.

Jon Hall is a music therapist and founder of 'Outsider Music'. He has over 20 years experience in music production, songwriting and remixing. Jon re-trained as a music therapist in 2006 and now brings together his skills as music therapist, music producer and musician, working with clients with mental health issues, brain injury and learning disabilities. He now combines music therapy with elements of performance and recording, to promote greater engagement between clients, communities and families, as well as transforming perceptions of distress.

Paul Hanna is a Lecturer in Sustainable Tourism. Prior to joining the University of Surrey in 2014, Paul obtained a BA (Hons) in Applied Social Science (University of Brighton), an MSc Applied Social Psychology (University of Sussex) and in 2011 was successfully awarded his doctorate from the University of Brighton for his thesis 'Consuming Sustainable Tourism: Ethics, Identity, Practice'. From this research Paul has published theoretical and empirical insights into the experiences of engaging with and consuming sustainable tourism, alongside further developing understandings of the relationship between humans and the environment.

Amira Hassan is a Chartered Counselling Psychologist and currently Head of Psychology for a paediatric psychology service for children with developmental delay and social communication difficulties in Qatar. Previously, she worked in the UK National Health Service for over 10 years in child and adolescent mental health. The majority of her work in the UK was with Black and minority ethnic communities. She led innovative intergenerational work with Black and Muslim fathers and sons, which addressed issues of acculturation and relationships that are strained by migration and living between two cultures. Amira's skills and experiences include the provision of culturally appropriate psychological assessment and intervention, service development, supervision and training. She has presented at national and international conferences and published journal articles and book chapters on issues of race and culture. Amira is a chartered member of the British Psychological Society and is a registered practitioner psychologist with the Health and Care Professions Council.

Darrin Hodgetts is a Professor of Societal Psychology at Massey University, New Zealand. His research interests centre on urban poverty, the social determinants of health, everyday life, homelessness and the precariat. Darrin has an ongoing interest in indigenous psychologies and has worked on various community projects to address issues of Māori well-being, food insecurity and social justice. Darrin is currently a co-editor of the *Journal of Community and Applied Social Psychology* and the *Sage Handbook of Applied Social Psychology*. Darrin's recent publications include *Urban Poverty and Health Inequalities* (with Ottilie Stolte, Routledge, 2017).

Mari Holen is an Associate Professor at Roskilde University in Denmark. She researches in health policy and health strategies, and how welfare institutions translate dominant ideas of health. For example, she has been interested in the concepts of recovery and user involvement, which has been spread widely throughout the mental health system, and especially how these concepts are understood and what they do.

Orly Klein is a Senior Lecturer in Psychology at the University of Brighton, specialising in Critical Parental Studies. Her current research interests are focused on challenging the denigration of women who bottle-feed their infants, mothers' interactions with midwives and health visitors and the manufacture and management of risk with regards to parenting. Alongside this, Orly has a developing interest in the impact of welfare cuts and austerity measures on families, and identifying alternative ways of mitigating these effects.

Carolyn Kagan is a Professor Emerita of Community Social Psychology at Manchester Metropolitan University's Faculty of Health, Psychology and Social Care.

She was formerly the first Director of the Research Institute for Health and Social Change at the University. Carolyn has qualifications in academic social psychology, social work and counselling psychology. She has worked in partnership with public, community and voluntary sector organisations throughout her career, mostly on collaborative and sometimes participative action research projects concerned with well-being and social change. Her areas of expertise include working with marginalised social groups (including disabled people, migrants and people living poverty), organisational change and development, urban regeneration, sustainable development and social policy critique and development. She is widely published and her works include the textbook *Critical Community Psychology* (Wiley, 2011). She was a founding editor of the journal, *Community, Work and Family*. She was elected Honorary Fellow of the British Psychological Society in 2017 in recognition of her work 'giving psychology away' and was awarded the Society's award for promoting equal opportunity in 2005. She is a Director of *Just Psychology* and Chair of Trustees of *From Generation to Generation*.

Michael Larkin is a Reader in Psychology, at Aston University. He has a specific interest in phenomenological and experiential approaches to psychology, and particularly in qualitative methods. His research involves using these approaches to explore the relational experience and context of anomalous or distressing experiences.

Stephanie Liddicoat is a researcher and architectural design academic at the University of Melbourne, Australia. Stephanie's research interests are at the nexus of architecture and health, particularly in exploring service user perceptions of the built environment and the relationship between space and well-being within health care settings. Stephanie's PhD dissertation (completed in 2017) explored the mental health service user perceptions of built environments and implications for design. She is also interested in participatory research design methodologies and furthering the field of evidence-based design through such research projects. Stephanie has recently been involved in several master's design studios, conferences and research colloquia speaking about the built environment's role in mental health, and the implications for design practice and urban planning.

Laura McGrath is a Senior Lecturer at the University of East London. Laura's research focuses on the role of material context in experiences of mental distress, in community and inpatient settings, where she has helped develop new methodologies and theory within psychology that incorporate space into the research agenda. Her work hence draws on a variety of perspectives, including experts by experience, community psychology, human geography and social psychiatry. Her research is qualitative, with a particular expertise in using visual and creative methodologies, where she has sought to increase participant agency, in order to create a more democratic agenda for research more generally.

Laura directs and contributes to both undergraduate and postgraduate programmes on mental health and community psychology, and works closely with community groups and practitioners involved in the delivery of mental health services and social support networks.

Nick Marks is a PhD student in the School of Applied Social Sciences at the University of Brighton. He is interested in exploring 'recoveries' in mental health that take place in non-medical social environments, and in particular how technical proficiency in the refurbishment of mechanical devices can contribute to these 'recoveries' as part of a broader notion of 'relational citizenship'.

Nathan Parnell is a Trainee Clinical Psychologist. He studied at the University of the West of England to obtain a BSc (Hons) in Psychology, before going on to study for his MSc in Mental Health Studies at King's College London. He has worked for over 10 years in various areas of mental health and throughout the developmental lifespan in both NHS and private health care settings. His professional research positions prior to psychology training focused on family and young person well-being. His main interests, both research and clinically, lie with children, adolescents and families. Within these areas, at present, he aims to develop his research and clinical interests from both interventional and epistemological standpoints in the context of a changing NHS and society.

Jason Poole is a Trainee Clinical Psychologist, researcher and service user with professional experience in national and specialist child and adolescent mental health services. He is interested in spaces of detention and how these shape their residents' lived experiences of distress, both during and post-admission. Jason lectures as an Expert by Experience. His teaching is concerned with experiences of anxiety, unusual beliefs, embodied affect and ontological trauma. His work is further interested in issues of epistemic value in mental health research, socio-cultural conceptions of madness and social inequalities as a foundation of distress.

Paula Reavey is a Professor of Psychology and Mental Health at London South Bank University and the Director of Research and Education for the Design in Mental Health Network, UK. She has co-edited two volumes, *New Feminist Stories of Child Sexual Abuse: Sexual Scripts and Dangerous Dialogues* (with Sam Warner, Routledge, 2003) and *Memory Matters: Contexts for Understanding Sexual Abuse Recollections* (with Janice Haaken, Psychology Press, 2009), and a sole-edited volume, *Visual Methods in Psychology: Using and Interpreting Images in Qualitative Research* (Routledge, 2011). She has also published two monographs *Psychology, Mental Health and Distress* (with John Cromby and Dave Harper, Palgrave, 2013 – winner of the British Psychological Society Book Award, 2014) and *Vital Memory and Affect: Living with a Difficult Past* (with Steven D. Brown, Routledge, 2015). She has also published the Design with People in Mind book series for

Design in Mental Health, which aims to provide an evidence base for practitioners and academics seeking to understand the relationship between built environments and experiences of distress and care. Paula has also published numerous articles and book chapters on lived experiences of distress, social remembering and child sexual abuse, using qualitative and visual methodologies.

Agnes Ringer is a Clinical Psychologist working in adult mental health services and a part-time lecturer at the Centre for Health Promotion Research, Roskilde University, Denmark. Her research interests are in critical psychology and post-structural approaches to mental health, and she has written a number of articles that take a critical perspective on traditional psychiatric practice.

Bernice Rooney is currently undertaking a postgraduate diploma in Occupational Therapy at London Southbank University. She studied at the University of Lincoln to obtain a BSc (Hons) in Psychology with Clinical Psychology. After graduating, she worked for seven years in NHS child and adolescent mental health services, in a forensic medium-secure inpatient ward, and then moved to a community discharge service. Bernice is currently working on a role-emerging practice placement, developing and piloting an occupational therapy service within a homelessness charity. Once qualified Bernice would like to continue working within mental health services.

Lesley-Ann Smith is a Senior Lecturer in Psychology, Faculty of Health and Society at the University of Northampton. Lesley-Ann's teaching focuses on social psychology, qualitative methods and critical perspectives around gender, sexuality and ageing. Her doctoral research explored experiences around the spatial environments of older mental health service users within the home, day centre and psychiatric institutions. Currently, she has research projects encompassing the social perceptions and gendered behaviours of young females and intimate grooming practices. In addition, she has two ongoing projects exploring the lived experiences of users of psychedelics and ayahuasca, incorporating issues of transformative identity and the importance of spatial settings within altered states of consciousness.

Neil Springham is a consultant art therapist at Oxleas NHS foundation Trust in London where he is also Borough lead for psychological therapies and patient experience. He trained in art therapy in 1988 and has worked in adult mental health, addictions and now specialises in services for people diagnosed with personality disorder. He was a course leader at the Unit of Psychotherapeutic Studies, Goldsmiths College, co-founded the Art Therapy Practice Research Network and was twice elected chair of British Association of Art Therapists. He has a PhD in Psychology and founded ResearchNet, a service user and provider collaboration that develops co-produced research in mental health. He has published and lectured internationally on a wide range of issues in art therapy, mentalisation, co-production and experience-based co-design.

Ottilie Stolte is a Senior Lecturer in the School of Psychology at the University of Waikato. Ottilie completed a PhD in 2006 on training schemes for disadvantaged unemployed people. Since then she has taught social and community psychology, and has pursued research on homelessness, inequalities, poverty, health and everyday life. A key focus is understanding the lifeworlds of people who are 'disadvantaged' due to issues such as poverty, illness, disability, ethnicity or socio-economic status, in order to advance social change.

Greg Townley is an Assistant Professor in the Department of Psychology at Portland State University. He earned his PhD in Clinical-Community Psychology from the University of South Carolina, and BAs in Psychology and Africana Studies from NC State University. His research focuses primarily on community inclusion of individuals with psychiatric disabilities, homelessness and sense of community among marginalised groups. In his work, Dr Townley uses a variety of social-environmental research methods, including Geographic Information Systems (GIS), neighbourhood assessments and ethnographic approaches. He has extensive experience working with consumer-run organisations and community mental health centres to implement and evaluate supported housing and peer support programs. His experience with mental health service systems as a clinician, consultant and consumer provides him with an additional depth of understanding beyond his extensive research training.

Ian Tucker is a Reader in Social Psychology at the University of East London. He has a long-standing interest in the social-psychological aspects of emotion and affect, which has theoretically informed empirical work in the areas of mental distress, social media and surveillance. He has conducted research for the Mental Health Foundation and the EPSRC Communities and Culture Network+, and is currently working on a project exploring the impact of social media on psychological support in mental health communities. Ian has published numerous articles in the areas of mental health, social media, space and place and surveillance.

Vimala Uttarkar is the Director of a non-profit organisation working in the rehabilitation of people who have severe and enduring mental illness, forensic histories and challenging behaviours. She holds a doctorate from the University of East London and is a Visiting Lecturer for the Doctoral Programme at the Tavistock Centre, where she mentors and supervises research students. She is a reviewer for the *Journal of Social Work Practice* and a specialist mental health advisor to the Care Quality Commission. With extensive experience in the provision of mental health services, her wide-ranging interests include risk behaviours of service users and the coping strategies and group dynamics of teams who work with difficult to engage, high-risk people in the community.

Ben Wakeling is an artist based in London and founder of the Outsider Gallery, London. The Outsider Gallery engages clients, families, communities and the public in ideas and experiences around distress and madness, including through opening a space for art-making, workshops, exhibitions and guerrilla interruptions. Bringing community into healing and healing into community, street art into psych units and psych art into streets, the Outsider Gallery is committed to bringing the outside in and the inside out, to reshaping – or breaking – the borders of mental health.

Carl Walker is a Community Psychologist from the University of Brighton. He is on the British Psychological Society National Community Psychology section committee. His research interests include exploring the relations between debt, inequality and mental health and the use of community initiatives to work toward addressing mental health needs.

Tassie Weaver has spent many years working in client-facing roles supporting vulnerable adults experiencing multiple disadvantage. Soon after beginning her career in the homelessness sector, Tassie became interested in the lived experience of those accessing services and the ways in which support services could adopt more psychologically and specifically trauma-informed approaches to service delivery. In her current role as Local Networks Manager with the Making Every Adult Matter coalition, Tassie continues to promote trauma-informed care, supporting local areas to ensure that those with lived experience of multiple disadvantage and service use are placed at the heart of the design and delivery of interventions.

Anna Zorwaska is a former trainee of artists Hannah Hull and James Leadbitter (aka the vacuum cleaner), and "Madlove – A Designer Asylum" project assistant. Currently Anna is working as a producer in non-governmental theatre "Dirty Deal Teatro" in Riga, Latvia and freelance stage manager. Anna has studied Theory of Theatre and Audiovisual Arts at the Latvian Academy of Culture, had a study exchange semester in Inter-Faculty Individual Studies in the Humanities at Jagiellonian University, Krakow, Poland and post-graduate internship in Artsadmin, London, United Kingdom.

ACKNOWLEDGEMENTS

This book is the culmination of around a decade's work on mental distress and space, and there are many people who have helped and inspired us along the way. In particular, thank you to Steve Brown, John Cromby, Dave Harper, Alice Parshall, Ava Kanyeredzi, Jason Poole, Paul Stenner, Ian Tucker, Carly Guest, Zoe Boden and everyone at Psychologists for Social Change. Thanks to the Lived Experiences of Distress Research Group at London South Bank University and to Katharine Harding in particular for her humour and support. We have had the privilege of working alongside colleagues from St Andrew's Healthcare, the Maudsley and Bethlem hospitals and the Design in Mental Health Network, UK, in trying to find more effective ways to improve services environments. This gratitude further extends to colleagues and friends from key community and living expert groups for insightful discussion and ways of working: the Dragon Café, MadLove, the Hearing Voices Network, Camden MIND, Rethink and the Experts by Experience group in London who have helped us to think more sensitively, intelligently and creatively about the relationship between space, distress and togetherness. Brian Dawn, Seth Hunter, Jacqui Dillon, Dolly Sen, Rai Waddingham and Akiko Hart are just wonderful, and we want to thank you from the bottom of our hearts for your wisdom and insight.

Thanks especially go out to Alex, Oskar and Viktor for making the home space for PR so safe, joyous and lively. You are much loved and appreciated. And from LM to Dan and Ava Carney, for your general brilliance – thank you.

We have been so lucky to have a community of academic colleagues and collaborators who have helped in various ways to support, inspire and contribute to this work, and we really rather like each other, so have had a ball editing this book. We hope you enjoy reading it as much as we have enjoyed making it.

INTRODUCTION

The vivid, yet ethereal description of hospital life described here by Janet Frame, magically cleaves the world of supposed ordinary life, from that of the hospital for the mentally 'unwell'.

> I was put in hospital because a great gap opened in the ice floe between myself and the other people whom I watched, with their world, drifting away through a violet-coloured sea where hammerhead sharks in tropical ease swam side by side with the seals and the polar bears. I was alone on the ice. A blizzard came and I grew numb and wanted to lie down and sleep and I would have done so had not the strangers arrived with scissors and bottle of poison, and other dangers which I had not realised before-mirrors, cloaks, corridors, furniture, square inches, bolted lengths of silence – plain and patterned, free samples of voices. And the strangers, without speaking, put up circular calico tents and camped with me, surrounding me with their merchandise of peril.
>
> (Frame, 1961/1980, p. 10)

The ice floe, and violet-coloured sea beautifully depicts a physical and felt alienation, for those entering the clearly demarcated space of the asylum. For the renowned New Zealand scholar and novelist, whose life was marked by frequent and lengthy spells in asylums, the space of her confinement was one that clearly defined periods of distress and loss of a connection with others. These periods were in essence 'housed' by institutions, whose task it was to steer her through the murky terrain of her 'madness' on to the other 'side'.

The inclusion of rich details of that physical space and spatial metaphors in Frame's writing, via the corridors, the furniture, the mirrors, at once capture the tangible and physical presence of the place she enters when distressed, and the newly found fear she experienced, in navigating such frightening feelings in the rule-bound and regimented order of that alien place. Though alien, asylums were the allocated space where order and reason would supposedly be restored, or a space containing and disciplining those who failed.

Before the almost global termination of lengthy asylum provision, asylum spaces were thus clearly demarcated; they felt divorced from the world, partly because they physically were, from the point of industrialisation to the end of the twentieth century; the sequestering of distress, and a clear marker of otherness and illness, bound by the imposing hospital walls. As we will explore in this introductory chapter and throughout this book, distress is no longer so clearly spatially marked and delineated as it was during the asylum period. Many of those experiencing severe and intense periods of distress may never enter secure settings, but instead negotiate these experiences in and through the same spaces where they live and work. While spatial boundaries have become less clear, the experiences of alienation, separation, othering and objectification described here by Frame remain firmly threaded through the disparate spaces of community care.

The shift from asylums to community care is only one example of the mutating spatial practices that have historically been part of how distress has been delineated and defined. These spatial practices have been infused by differing theoretical frameworks, and their accompanying remedies. Until around 1700, for instance, distress was mainly, as Roy Porter (2004, p. 89) puts it, "a domestic responsibility". The Industrial Revolution, urbanisation, and the shift from feudal to governmental power structures led to the establishment and expansion of the asylum system (Foucault, 1965; Porter, 2004; Shorter, 1997; Warner, 2000). Industrialisation involved the sharper separation of work and home, as factories required workers to be out of the house for daily, 12-hour shifts. This lead to the expansion and formalisation of institutions for those who could not be accommodated within the new economic and spatial model: workhouses, asylums and prisons (Warner, 2000).

Developing in haphazard and localised ways in the UK, asylums became increasingly formalised throughout the eighteenth and nineteenth centuries, with provision eventually becoming an obligation of the state through the 1824 Poor Law. Asylums themselves changed in meaning and focus with the times. Moral management, prevalent in the mid-nineteenth century, saw madness as a moral failing and subsequently created peaceful, rural spaces where inmates could be taught how to be social and moral citizens. Late Victorian asylums, the crucible for modern biological psychiatry, were more characterised by overcrowding, restraint and physical treatments. Emergent genetic and evolutionary theories helped to fuel increasing pessimism over the possibility of recovery (Porter, 2004), as madness was increasingly seen as a pathology of individual biology. Spaces, treatments and theories of mental health hence have always mutually shaped each other, producing together the context in which people experience distress.

Contemporary mental health care in the UK is, at first glance, less easily identifiable by place. Large-scale asylums, situated out of town, where people lived for months or years at a time, are gone. Asylum closure attracted an unlikely coalition of left-wing human rights campaigners, fuelled by the nascent service user movement (Campbell, 1996, 2001), and individualistic right-wingers opposed to large-scale state solutions. Institutional spaces remain, but contemporary psychiatric wards are often seen, as Quirk, Lelliot, and Seale (2006) argue, as a failure of the system, rather than its focus (McGrath & Reavey, 2015). Instead, mental health services have tended increasingly to be focused on moving service users away from fixed institutional sites of mental health care, and into community spaces. Successions of UK policy buzzwords underline this trend: moving from 'mainstreaming' (DoH, 1999) through 'social inclusion' (DoH, 2006; ODPM, 2004), and finally, to 'freedom' (DoH, 2011). Sites of mental health care, therefore, have simultaneously expanded and contracted, becoming more numerous but less visible and differentiated.

As with the development of the asylum system, its demise contains a number of social, political and theoretical shifts. Porter (2008) argues that the twentieth century saw a blurring of the strict line between 'mad' and 'sane' drawn both conceptually and spatially. A century of war saw successive generations of young men visibly traumatised by their experiences, troubling the idea that madness was only emergent from faulty genes. In seeming contradiction, the scope of psychiatric practice also slowly expanded to include more 'everyday' experiences of depression and anxiety as well as psychosis. The development of psychiatric medication located the site of psychiatric practice in the individual and mobile body, less tied to institutional spaces. Post-war individualism, consumerism and civil rights, as well as contemporary models of recovery, have all contributed to the privileging of individual choice, agency and freedom, rendering the paternalism of the asylum redundant. In this introductory chapter, we will examine concepts and literature to help us navigate this complex terrain. We start with a look at contemporary institutional and community spaces of mental health, before introducing some key theoretical concepts to help navigate the chapters that follow. We then end with a summary of the book.

Contemporary contexts of space and distress: community and institutional settings

A contemporary picture of space in mental health care is complex. In the UK, mental health services have tended increasingly to be focussed on moving service users away from fixed institutional sites of mental health care, and into community spaces. The ultimate aim and purpose of mental health services is often seen as that of becoming absent from service users' lives, to 'empower', 'enable' and 'support' people to be able to carry out their everyday activities without interference. In practice, this trend has often lead to the closure of specific mental health service sites, especially day services (Pilgrim & Ramon, 2009), and a move to using psychiatric wards for short-term crisis care only (Keown, Mercer, & Scott, 2008). The 2006 Department of Health report, *From Segregation to Inclusion*, stands as a good example of the discourse of such policies, stating in the section of the report entitled 'Beyond Buildings':

> A day service does not necessarily require a dedicated building or centre. It is the function of day services in maintaining and extending social networks and access to mainstream roles and activities that is critical and there is a need to move from group-based to individualised support.
>
> *(DoH, 2006, p. 17)*

Implicit in the description here is a kind of service common in the early days of community care, and increasingly rare in the UK: a day centre providing some therapy and group activities, but also acting as more informal space for service users to use as a safe place away from home. Such places were designed to provide both respite from a difficult world, and the opportunity to gain support from others in the same situation (see Chase, 2011; Taylor, 2014). An idea of respite or peer support is, however, increasingly absent in contemporary services, as seen in the above quote. Instead, the focus is on more individualised 'bridging' than group-based 'bonding' activities (Chase, 2011). Implied here is that any long-term engagement with services (as opposed to 'mainstream activities'), or association primarily with other service users, constitutes 'dependency', and is a priori negative.

The focus on 'social inclusion' at the expense of institutional or ongoing care has been widely discussed. The affinity of these policies with an agenda of the individualisation of responsibility, state shrinkage and the primacy of economic productivity has been noted (Rogers & Pilgrim, 1996; Spandler, 2007; Symonds & Kelly, 1998; Taylor, 2014). Spandler (2007), for instance, points out that 'social inclusion' can have the effect of placing blame on individuals for the effects of structural inequalities that are beyond their control, thus playing down the role of structural factors such as poverty, oppression or racism in their experiences (see also Cromby, Harper, & Reavey, 2013; Johnstone, 2000; Rogers & Pilgrim, 2003; Smail, 2001). Symonds (1998, p. 3) also points out that we cannot talk about 'the community' without talking about specific places and spaces:

> Community as a site of delivery does not exist [. . .] Try a simple test: ask for a delivery of supplies to the community and the first question will be 'where'? This will lead you to name a specific and fixed site which will be another description: that of a hospital, a private home, an institution, a clinic, a community centre, but the phrase 'community' will be revealed as an empty and non-existent site.

Community care is not place-less, therefore, it is enacted across multiple, disparate and complex sites, threaded through people's everyday lives (see McGrath & Reavey, 2013, 2015, 2016). As fewer people are admitted to hospital, for shorter periods (Quirk et al., 2006), more people are instead asked to negotiate distress and recovery in the same everyday spaces where they also live, work and manage their ongoing relationships. An attendance to these spaces, whether of home, work or socialisation, is therefore increasingly critical. It is also worth noting that as spaces have become more disparate in contemporary services (Rose, 1998;

McGrath & Reavey, 2013), time has correspondingly become more hard edged and formalised; individual appointments and meetings have become the norm for a service user/professional interactions (Bloomfield & McLean, 2003). These features of the space-time of contemporary services can be seen as constituting a 'helicopter service' (McGrath & Reavey, 2015) where professionals drop down into service users' lives for short, often pre-determined bursts of time, but spend most of the time circling above their lives, attempting to manage and survey them from afar. In considering mental distress and space, therefore, we must also widen our view from service use, considering institutional spaces and interactions in tandem with everyday places, spaces and experiences, as well as the administrative systems that monitor service users from a distance (McGrath & Reavey, 2015).

The complexity of the relationships between space and mental health hence have a particular flavour for service users living in the community. A set of researchers, particularly those influenced by human geography, have examined the location of experiences of inclusion and exclusion, across the multitude of spaces that service users now occupy (Curtis, 2010; Davidson, 2003; Knowles, 2000a, 2000b; Parr, 1997, 2008; Pinfold, 2000). A key theme we wish to highlight here is that public space is often cited as particularly problematic for service users. Parr (1997), for instance, noted that behaviour indicating distress (such as shouting or crying) invited more notice and censure in the street, than in a mental health drop in service. Pinfold (2000) also found that the service users she interviewed tended to have a few 'safe havens', such as their homes and friends' houses, in which they spent the majority of their time, avoiding more difficult public spaces. Similar arguments have been made by research with people diagnosed with agoraphobia (Davidson, 2000a, 2000b, 2001, 2003) and our own research with people diagnosed with anxiety disorders (McGrath, Reavey, & Brown, 2008). In these studies, participants described retreating to the home: in an attempt to stabilise experiences of insecure bodily boundaries (Davidson, 2000b, 2001, 2003); and as a reaction to feeling that public spaces were hostile (McGrath et al., 2008). Knowles (2000a), furthermore, looked at homeless people experiencing distress, arguing that they were not welcome in the public spaces they had to occupy during the day, having to forge out 'nooks and crannies' (Estroff, 1981) where they could remain relatively invisible. One example of this practice was the habit of sitting in convenience food outlets, for several hours; in these places they were still insecure occupants, and were ejected if they made themselves visible, for instance through talking to other customers, or shouting (Knowles, 2000a).

A number of researchers have drawn on purity metaphors to explain the makeup of public space in ways that help to inform these findings. Hodgetts, Radley, Chamberlain, and Hodgetts (2007) argued that public spaces are 'purified' of people who display or signify difference; Hodgetts et al. (2007) similarly argue that homeless people are seen to "infect, spoil or taint" (p. 722) the purity of public spaces, while Dixon, Levine, and McAuley (2006) argue that dislocating behaviour that is seen as properly 'private' into public space can be viewed as "transgressing the moral geography of everyday behaviour" (p. 197). The use of purity metaphors recalls Mary Douglas' (1966/2001) classic text *Purity and Danger*, in which she argues, looking across multiple societies, that those objects, people or behaviours that are conceptualised as 'dirty', 'dangerous' or 'impure' are generally those that disrupt or trouble whichever order has been constructed by that society; she argues that order is constructed to create purity, and purity to maintain order. These authors seem to be arguing that stigmatised groups in society, including mental health service users (Link, Cullen, Struening, Shrout, & Dohrenwend, 1989; Scheff, 1974, 1999), are placed in this role, of symbolic 'dirt', in the sense of "matter out of place" (James, 1901, p. 129, cited in Douglas, 1966/2001) when in public spaces. Key here is the idea that people who display difference, such as the distress observed by Parr (1997), can disrupt the usual, or more precisely ideal, spatial order of society (see also Curtis, 2010).

In previous work, we have outlined the complexities of this spatial order for service users, when trying to find ways to manage and negotiate their distress. Some people when experiencing crisis, for instance, find movement and engagement in outside space a crucial strategy to dissipate and alleviate their distress (McGrath & Reavey, 2015). Due to the spatial ordering of public and private space, however, in many ways a hangover from the asylum, they are often left without safe spaces to practice movement and agency. Displaying behaviour seen as 'out of space' is often described as potentially leading to sectioning via the police. In our work, one participant described ending up in the grounds of the psychiatric hospital, seeking both safety and movement, welcome neither in the exposure of public space or the containment of the hospital. Other participants described using toilets as private spaces, as places to transition between their private therapeutic self and a self acceptable in public space (McGrath & Reavey, 2016). Within the shrunken spaces of community care, service users often seemed forced into the 'nooks and crannies' to express, experience and manage their distress.

Clear from these examples is the complexity of the relationship between mental health and space. While the physical asylums are gone, a legacy of sequestration remains embedded in the spatial practices of services and everyday community life. Both everyday community living and institutional practices are therefore crucial in exploring and understanding the relationship between space and mental health in contemporary practice.

Living in space: how environments relate to mental health

There has been a recent upsurge in interest in whole environment, space and planning approaches to enhancing and supporting good mental health. From 'happy cities' (Montgomery, 2015) to 'resilient places' (Jones & Mean, 2010), ideas of emotional well-being and mental health are increasingly embedded in environment and planning policy. The New Urban Agenda, adopted by the UN in 2016, for instance, highlights 'developing resilience' as an explicit aim of urban policy worldwide, alongside reducing inequalities and environmental sustainability. At the same time, there have been moves in global mental health policy that acknowledge the material antecedents of mental health experiences. Much of this work has focused on poverty and inequality, including key reports by Friedli (2009) and Marmot (2010). Overall, these studies find that mental health is distributed in much the same way as the distribution of resources across society; those with greater resources have, on average, better mental health (Friedli, 2009). There are also, however, resilient neighbourhoods, where residents are healthier and happier than those in other demographically similar areas (Tunstall, Mitchell, Gibbs, Platt, & Dorling, 2007).

Several aspects of community life predict good mental health and resilience, including equality, civic participation, social cohesion and political efficacy (see, McGrath, Griffin, & Mundy, 2015). Being valued, heard and feeling connected are threaded through these aspects of life. Similar patterns are also found on a micro scale; it has been consistently found that those living lower down in tower blocks have better mental health than those on higher floors (Freeman, 1984, 2008; Mitchell, 1971). Similarly, people in dwellings with closed corridors, rather than open deck access, have lower levels of depression (Weich et al., 2002). Even on the scale of buildings, settings that create social contact and create a feeling of agency and ownership over the environment are consistently found to be associated with better mental health (Evans, 2003). Built environment policies that aim to increase well-being and resilience hence often focus on ways to better facilitate cohesive and equitable communities. This might include making cities less car dependent and more walkable, therefore reducing social isolation (Montgomery, 2015).

Friedli (2009, p. 11) however offers an important caution in thinking about the protective power of good mental health and resilient places:

> Positive mental health does confer considerable protection and advantage, but it does so predominantly among those with equal levels of resources. In other words, among poor children, those with higher levels of emotional wellbeing have better educational outcomes than their equally poor peers. However, richer children generally do better still, regardless of emotional or cognitive capability. [. . .] Emerging evidence suggests that the same pattern may be true for resilient localities: high levels of social capital may help to explain why one poor neighbourhood has lower mortality than other equally deprived areas, but these poorer, resilient communities still tend to have higher mortality than affluent areas.

A potentially useful concept to understand these relationships is that of the capability approach. Nussbaum and Sen (1993) argue that the aim of development should be to support people's capability to live well, to give people: "the freedom to live a valued life" (Sen, 2009). Suggested capabilities include ensuring people have the capacity to be healthy; to think, feel and act freely; to have control over their environment; and to form communities. While strong communities, high social capital and well-designed, liveable places can all can enhance these capabilities, Friedli's point is that the impact of these enhanced environments is always limited by the material resources people have at their disposal.

Perhaps unsurprisingly from these findings, those places that are more toxic to mental health are often those with reduced resources, less social cohesion, higher levels of threat and disorganisation. Much of this research has focused on the elevated levels of mental health diagnoses in inner-city areas, first observed by Faris and Dunham (1939) in Chicago. For much of the twentieth century, as Boydell and McKenzie (2008) note, this pattern was explained as an outcome of the poverty experienced by many service users, either in terms of 'social drift', where service users were thought to be forced to move to poorer areas, or 'social residue', meaning they were unable to move out. Research in Sweden (Lewis, David, Andréassson, & Allebeck, 1992) and Denmark (Mortensen et al., 1999) has, however, found that being born in an urban environment increases adult diagnoses of schizophrenia, when controlled for both socio-economic status and family history. Multiple features of inner-city environments have been put forward as candidates to explain this pattern, including poverty (Rogers & Pilgrim, 2003); poor and multiple occupancy housing (Evans, 2003); social disorganisation (Silver, Mulvey, & Monahan, 1999); isolation (Van Os, Driessen, Gunther, & Delespaul, 2000); experiences of fear (Bentall, 2009); crime and vandalism (Ross, Mirowsky, & Pribesh, 2001); and inequality (Wilkinson & Pickett, 2009). In different spaces and settings, however, these different facets of the environment coalesce to shape experiences of those living there. One example is the relationship between proximity to wealth and the impact of poverty; one study in South Africa found that between two communities of comparable levels of deprivation there were higher levels of dissatisfaction and distress in the community that was located on a hill overlooking a rich neighbourhood as opposed to the other area surrounded by neighbourhoods of similar wealth (Rogers & Pilgrim, 2003). The same material circumstances given a different meaning, can be threaded through individual subjectivity in varying ways. This example highlights the need to also consider the individual-level experiences that help to mediate and modulate the context in which people are living, to shape experiences of mental health.

Subjectivity in the community: how environments get under the skin

The range of research that could be drawn on to understand the subjective experiences that mediate the relationship between environments and mental health is vast. Here we have drawn out some key themes in the literature, which nevertheless are not exhaustive. We aim, however, to examine how the complexity of people's environments, through the built environment, community relations, society and culture, might coalesce and emerge as felt experiences more usually seen within the remit of psychological research.

Status and value

One theme that can be found in the literature is that surrounding ideas of social status and value. Emotions connected to a lack of status or feeling undervalued are consistently linked with poor mental health, including humiliation, shame and status anxiety. These are all emotions that include a moral judgement, of being worthwhile and valued members of society. The classic work by George Brown and colleagues (e.g. Brown & Harris, 1978; Brown, Harris, & Hepworth, 1995; Finlay-Jones & Brown, 1981), for instance, found that women who experienced repeated experiences of humiliation combined with severe loss trebled their chance of being diagnosed with clinical depression. Similarly, feelings of shame are central to many mental health experiences, to the extent that it has been called 'the bedrock of psychopathology' (Miller, 1996, p. 151). Much of the literature discussing shame and mental health focuses on interpersonal experiences such as abuse and trauma. These are of course important, but also emergent here is that social status, material environments and access to resources are sources of shame. Chase and Bantebya-Kyomuhendo (2014) outline the ways in which shame is endemic to poverty, especially through contact with the benefits system. In addition, status anxiety has been posited as a potential psychological link between inequality and poorer mental health outcomes (Coburn, 2015; Marmot, 2004).

For those diagnosed with mental health conditions, these issues of status, utility and value are of course intensified. Mental health status is stigmatised, and there is some evidence that the shift from asylum to community care has increased, not decreased some forms of stigma. This issue has been captured in a large body of literature looking at service users' everyday experiences of stigma (Newnes, Holmes, & Dunn, 1999, 2001). Corker et al. (2013), for instance, report that in 2011, 88 per cent of surveyed service users reported experiencing direct discrimination. Phelan, Steuve, and Pescosolido (2000) found that people in 1996 were twice as likely to describe a service user as violent and dangerous than in 1955, despite no rise in violent offences. One aspect of living, and experiencing distress, in distributed community spaces, therefore, could be increased exposure to everyday stigma.

Added into this stigma are the ways in which people with diagnosed mental health problems can become disadvantaged in other routes to valued roles within society, namely employment and family life. Warner (2000) has documented the boredom and purposeless reported by many psychiatric service users in the United States, finding that days of half of people diagnosed with mental health problems in Colorado consisted of no more than one hour's structured activity. Employment in itself is not always the answer; low status and repetitive work is also associated with poor mental health outcomes (Stansfield, Fuhrer, Shipley, & Marmot, 1999). Warner et al. (1998) also found that Italian service users had a generally better quality of life than those in the United States, and were far more likely (73 per cent compared to 17 per cent) to be living with their families. It seems that the Italian culture emphasising family life was helpful in maintaining security and routine, while those who lived alone and independently, a sign of adulthood in the more individualistic United States (see Warner, 2000), in many ways fared worse, being less likely to be employed and more likely to have been accused of a crime. Remaining embedded in the social world it seems, in roles and relationships that are not wholly tied up with the position of being a service user, is central in the management of distress.

Trust and belonging

Related to these issues of status, equity and value are feeling and experiences of trust, connection and belonging. Being embedded in communities, is not enough without these feelings that bind people to each other, creating the cohesion found in resilient places. Closeness is not always the most desirable facet of a relationship, as can be seen in the literature on expressed emotion (EE), defined as being over-involved and critical (Vaughn & Leff, 1985). Families demonstrating high levels of this communication style have been consistently linked to increased likelihood of relapse (Barrowclough, Tarrier, & Johnston, 1996; Butzlaff & Hooley, 1998); a 15-year longitudinal study also found that high EE in families preceded the diagnosis of schizophrenia (Goldstein, 1985). Relationships characterised by a lack of trust have also been found to be toxic for mental health; low levels of trust can increase the chance of being diagnosed with depression by 50 per cent (Araya et al., 2006). People who live in neighbourhoods with high levels of distrust also have increased levels of all mental health problems; this relationship is particularly strong with psychosis. Cromby and Harper (2005) outline how paranoia can be understood as a response to social inequality and oppression, manifesting partly as a lack of trust in the world. Certainly those with less power, who are marginalised or poorer, have higher levels of paranoia diagnoses. Unequal societies overall are less trusting (Wilkinson & Pickett, 2009), and also have higher levels of mental health conditions; as people's lives become more differentiated and separate, then arguably the bonds between them become weaker and trust within and between communities begins to dissolve. The psychological importance of a built environment that facilitates connections and interactions between people, become clear here; one component of trust is interaction with others outside of our social and work circles.

Martin et al. (1957, cited in Halpern, 1995), for instance, studied the effects on communities of being moved to new suburbs as part of inner-city slum clearances in the 1950s. An initial boost in well-being was followed by increased reports of distress, particularly manifesting as depression, in the long term. This pattern was, as many as these place effects are, particularly prevalent among women. Although the new homes were improved on many 'poor-quality housing' indicators and so objectively 'better', the women reported finding suburban life isolating and missing the strong community of their previous home. The change in how these women's domestic and community spaces were laid out can be seen to have served to inhibit, or fail to facilitate, the kind of daily interaction with their neighbours that was a part of how their previous community had been built up and sustained. There is a wealth of evidence that both social (e.g. Warner, 2000) and cultural (e.g. Bhugra & Arya, 2005) isolation are central to the development of distress; what this research perhaps indicates is that these kinds of experiences are in part produced or mediated by the particular material environments in which social and cultural relationships take place; the social and material here collide in order to produce experiences of distress, and the two can exacerbate and feed into each other.

Power and agency

Another set of related experiences that research suggests fuel community experiences of mental health are those of agency, power and entrapment. Many aspects of people's lives, communities and environments feed into their level of felt agency. Living in poverty is a key circumstance that can reduce someone's capability to feel agency. Both living on a low income (Lefkowitz, Tesiny, & Gordon, 1980) and working in low-status, passive jobs (Landsbergis, Schnall, Deitz, Friedman, & Pickering, 1992), are related to a more external 'locus of control', a feeling that life is more controlled by others than yourself. These experiences are important, as Brown and Harris (1978) have highlighted the importance of feelings of entrapment in fuelling distress; long-term and repeated entrapping life experiences nearly treble the incidence of anxiety and depression. Power relations have also been argued to be central to structuring experiences of both voice hearing (Hayward, 2003; Romme & Escher, 1993) and unusual beliefs (Bullimore, 2012; Cromby & Harper, 2005), to the extent that therapeutic approaches have been developed to encourage voice hearers to develop more equitable, mutual dialogues with their voices (Romme, Escher, Dillon, Corstens, & Morris, 2009; Vaughan & Fowler, 2004). David Smail (2001) indeed has argued that all mental health problems are problems of power, from proximal power relations in relationships and everyday life, to distal societal power imbalances, oppression and injustice. Certainly, all oppressed groups in society have higher levels of mental health problems, including ethnic minorities, sexual minorities and women (Cromby et al., 2013). People are not, however, just passive recipients of power relations; our previous work has highlighted how people experiencing distress in the community use movement through their everyday spaces as a way to modulate agency and use different spaces to manage distress and crisis (McGrath & Reavey, 2015).

A further key site for the everyday enactment and negotiation of agency is that of home space. Home is often positioned as a private realm, identified with the self, emotion (Curtis, 2010; Mallet, 2004; Morley, 2000) and freedom from external surveillance (Saunders & Williams, 1988). This understanding is emergent from the Industrial Revolution, which entailed a clearer separation of home and (paid) workspaces than had existed previously, and the emergence of the nuclear family as the ideal domestic unit (Hareven, 1991). Prevalent conceptions of the meaning of 'home' therefore, can therefore be seen to identify this kind of space as (ideally) a private, domestic space identified with the self and family life. It would be simplistic, however, to conceive of the home as a universal 'safe haven' that is always characterised by agency and territory (Wardaugh, 1999). Wardhaugh (1999) points out that such arguments ignore both the violence and abuse that occurs within many homes, as well as implicitly excluding those who do not fit into the 'ideal home' being conjured, which she argues is assumed to contain a suburban, white, middle-class, heterosexual, nuclear family. As Julia Twigg (2000, p. 384) notes, the privacy of the home: "rests on a material affordance . . . the ability to shut the door on the outside world". Privacy can, after all, afford both agency and entrapment.

Safety, security and respite

A final set of spatialised experiences that are important in experiences of distress are those of safety, security, threat, fear and respite. Finlay-Jones and Brown (1981) identify that experiences of danger can precipitate anxiety, and experiences of loss often precipitate depression. Danger and threat do not have to be physical, but can also be thought of as insecurity or instability in a relational, social or economic sense. Brown, Lemyre, and Bilfulco (1992) further found that the best predictor of recovery was an experience of 'anchoring' – or finding a form of stability in previously unstable circumstances. Instability and trauma in early life are thought to shape our expectations of relationships, the future and the social world, as well as to some extent shaping our biological responses (Johnstone & Boyle, 2018). For instance, some people who experience trauma in early life develop hyper-sensitive stress systems, which mean they respond more readily to stress later on in life (Read, Fosse, Moscovitz, & Perry, 2014). These themes emerge across multiple levels of community living and the spaces that people occupy. People living in more visibly insecure neighbourhoods with higher levels of vandalism, litter or empty buildings have higher levels of mental health problems (Wanderman & Nation, 1998). These features of people's neighbourhoods can help fuel fear of crime, known to have detrimental effects on mental health and well-being (Green, Gilbertson, & Grimsley, 2002). A key route to security is also employment. As Standing (2011) outlines, however, that precarity is an increasingly common experience of those who are employed, through a combination of increasing insecurity in employment practices and, in the UK, expensive and insecure housing. Job insecurity is indeed related to poor mental health outcomes, independently of income or occupation level (De Witte, 1999).

There is also a related literature on the importance of green space in facilitating respite. Environmental psychologists have argued that views of, or proximity to nature plays a role in the 'restoration' of attention and cognitive capacity (Berg, Hartig, & Staats, 2007; Kaplan & Kaplan, 1989; Reavey, Harding, & Bartle, 2017). It has been found, for instance, that people who have a view of nature from their window recover more quickly from surgery (Ulrich, 1984) and that students who have a view of nature from their window perform better on tests of attention (Tennessen & Cimprich, 1995). Kuo (2001) compared groups of women living in a large high-rise housing estate in Chicago, of whom half had trees around their tower block and half did not. This natural experiment found that not only did those women living in the 'barren' areas perform worse on measures of attention, but also that women without immediate access to nature were found to be more likely to procrastinate in addressing major life issues, and reported these issues as more severe and more longstanding. It may be, therefore, that a lack of access to green space renders everyday life stresses more difficult to cope with and hence increases the impact that they have on residents' lives. It is noticeable that this pattern of attribution, of perceiving problems as more long term, or stable, bears some resemblance to the attribution pattern found in people diagnosed with depression (Bentall, 2003). To lend support to this idea, it has also been found that those areas of London with lessened access to private gardens have a higher incidence of depression, independently of socio-economic status (Weich et al., 2002).

These examples comprise only some of the ways in which we can understand environments as 'getting under the skin', or becoming embedded in subjective experience. They demonstrate the ways in which mental health is always an embedded phenomenon, lived through the settings, relationships, and structures through which people negotiate their lives. In this era of community care, those experiencing distress tend to remain located within the complex, multi-layered spaces where they also live and work, and so an understanding of the experience and meaning of such engagement with space is crucial. This is not to say, however, that institutional spaces have disappeared entirely. It is important to explore the role that institutional spaces still play in providing care in contemporary life; how individuals make sense and meaning from their time in them, and how they impact on life outside.

Contained in space: institutional spaces

Foucault (1977) considered institutions to be spatialised technologies of *disciplinary power*, which made subjects (people) objects of knowledge and power. Disciplinary power, which ordered and structured everyday life, worked by rendering observation and surveillance possible, literally as bodies could be located and ordered, in specific places – the hospital, school, the military, etc. Furthermore, he argues, this disciplinary power translates into a mode of reflection for the individual, who then turns the gaze upon themselves, monitoring and regulating their behaviour in reference to the norms of the institution. The institution need not discipline through outward aggression, it could discipline via the internalisation of its practices and procedures. In hospitals, this would include the internalisation of medical discourses, to make sense of, and manage distress.

In contemporary life, however, institutional spaces refer to a broader range of physical places, including hospitals (general and secure) but also outpatient clinics, as well as community places, such as crisis houses and supported accommodation. Disciplinary power works within all of these differing spaces in various ways, producing several possible subject positions for those who work and receive care (see McGrath & Reavey, 2015). In the main, hospital stays are shorter, more devoted to crisis, and often focused on risk reduction. Some scholars and service users argue that institutional spaces are now set up mainly to manage risk, as opposed to offering any form of meaningful treatment beyond medication (Bentall, 2004). The argument being that once stable, the person is better placed to receive long-term treatment outside of the hospital walls, where 'normal' life can be maintained. Given the vast majority of those entering inpatient settings are doing so while in 'crisis', the mental health system has gradually become one where crisis management now defines inpatient admissions (unless they enter via the forensic system).

Greatly reduced hospital stays indicate that individuals are discharged once they are stable, rather than 'well', or deemed no longer at risk, to self or the public more generally. The main objective of inpatient stay is thus stabilisation, followed by release and treatment, as an outpatient. While this is a positive shift towards greater freedom of movement for those who use services, it is still vital to understand people's experiences of inpatient spaces, as these spaces can be the first entry point into services, where building relationships with services is pivotal. Furthermore, inpatient settings still serve as a space for some, to retreat, and away from the demands of everyday life.

In the following section, we briefly outline some of the physical features of contemporary inpatient spaces, and importantly, the ways in which staff and patients make use of, and feel in these spaces. Running through this attempt to understand sense-making strategies, feelings and uses of space, we will explore various issues relating to how institutions invite and shape particular readings of these activities, affecting both patients and staff alike, and their emerging relationship to one another. Issues relating to power, choice, relations, emotions and risk are explored here, and throughout the book, because we would argue these are vital factors which impact on, and shape lived experiences of distress, as well as engagement with services (Cromby et al., 2013).

The built environment and institutional space

Now the Victorian asylums have closed down, institutional spaces of mental health provision are not immediately recognisable. The antiquated and imposing structures of the original mental hospitals, with their mean, dark rooms and long narrow corridors are beginning to be replaced with light, modern structures, which are designed with *healing* and *stabilisation* in mind (Reavey, Harding, & Bartle, 2017). Gesler, Bell, Curtis, Hubbard, and Francis (2004) note the influx of PFI money into the NHS around the turn of the twenty-first century increased interest in hospital design in general, with greater attention paid to health care environments, and their healing potential. Smaller 'unit-like' buildings have also now usurped the larger hospitals, which aim to blend into the broader cultural scene and create a more integrated environment for mental health provision. Some facilities are even nested neatly between other buildings in city centres, anonymous and generic. Many modern mental facilities are designed to resemble generic health facilities that emphasise the healing power of natural light and green spaces. Patients have private bedrooms, where they can retreat and recuperate, and have more freedom to move around as they wish. According to these principles, mental health should be no more stigmatised than any other health condition, and the space itself should reflect this emancipatory ethos, in providing sufficiently recovery focused 'therapeutic' spaces (Curtis, 2010).

Following this, there is now a move towards building facilities to resemble homes. The logic being that the more normalised the space is, the more likely service users are to recover and open up, and work positively with mental health and/ or social workers (Banks & Nissen, 2017). Such spaces are argued to offer greater hope of 'recovery', a sense of privacy and dignity, and de-stigmatised contact with the mental health system more generally. If the person's surroundings resemble a typical home and community space, the idea is the person will not feel so alienated, isolated, othered and hence stigmatised. Papoulias and colleagues' systematic review (2013) findings showed the provision of private spaces and homely design to be associated with such increased well-being and social interaction, due to a sense of belonging and being more normal.

The positive impact of a homely environment on well-being is also reported by Connellan et al. (2013) and Payne and May (2009), in an evaluation of a psychiatric intensive care unit refurbishment undertaken as part of the King's Fund grant supported 'Enhancing the Healing Environment' initiative (DoH, 2008). Within the new ward, patients perceived the experience of homeliness to be associated with a number of features, including the overall quality and cleanliness of the new environment as compared with the original ward, comfortable furniture, natural light, windows that can be opened to provide fresh air, indoor plants, private spaces for visitors, high-quality food and an increase in positive staff attitudes. The staff described the new environment as being calmer and having a greater sense of 'openness' and light than the original ward. The average length of patient stay also reduced by 20 per cent and a significant reduction in physical assaults on staff and other patients was reported.

Lawson, Phiri, and Wells-Thorpe (2003) also studied the effects of the architectural health care environment on well-being, comparing patient outcomes in an existing facility with a new-build medium-secure mental health environment. While the number of instances of physical and verbal aggression remained the same between the two sites, the severity of incidents was reduced in the new facility and there was also a two-thirds reduction in self-harm. Rates of seclusion were also reduced and there was a reduction in patient length of stay. Tactility and texture within environmental finishes and variation in lighting were reported to provide greater perceptions of homeliness in contrast to smooth clinical finishes and uniform lighting, which created a calmer atmosphere.

One of the principles behind this new era in health care provision is the acknowledgement that spaces can participate in the making (or breaking) of relationships. Stichler (2008) describes the holistic approach of the non-profit UK organisation 'Planetree' towards developing health care environments using a relationship-based philosophy that includes nine key considerations; human interaction; consumer and patient education; healing partnerships with patients' family and friends; food and nutritional nurturance; spirituality; human touch; healing arts and visual therapy; integration of complementary therapies; healing environments created in the architecture and design of the health care setting. Staff culture and attitudes are integral to the relationship-based approach and have been shown to have a positive effect on both patient and staff satisfaction. Particular environmental design recommendations also include natural lighting, natural finishes including timber and stone, water features, plants and 'homelike' interior features with the aim of creating calm environments.

While spatial tensions exist within mental health care settings between the mitigation of risk and the creation of de-institutionalised environments, the literature suggests that design creativity which facilitates a balance between achieving the required levels of safety and creating homely, non-sterile spaces should be a key consideration in mental health care design (Shepley et al., 2016). Part of this aim is to foster a sense of agency and choice among patients, rather than focusing on what can be done to contain them, as it is increasingly well known that containment and restraint can often lead to higher levels of distress, aggression and hostility. There is indeed evidence that this more liberal approach to the control of space in treatment spaces is beneficial for both staff and service users. Bowers et al. (2005) found that there were higher levels of self-harm and staff-directed violence in psychiatric wards where doors were locked. In general, they concluded that such restrictions put upon service users exacerbated problems of violence rather than contained them.

And yet, one of the remaining questions is how spatial configurations translate into experience, into feelings of distress and the interconnectedness of the space with the people living and working there. Much of the work that has looked more closely at the lived experiences of inpatients has concentrated on ward environments in hospitals, though of course there are many other spaces that warrant attention. And once again, there is recognition that spaces are much more than a physical container; they are experienced through relations, affecting how we feel. Part of this 'feeling' is conjured by the *atmospheres* or *climates* of the space. This meteorological metaphor speaks to the idea that the space signifies both an intensity and temperature, as well as a sense of changeability and unpredictability.

Ward environments and atmospheres

In the study of psychiatric wards, there is a large literature on 'ward atmosphere', 'ward climate' or 'milieu' and their evaluation with regards staff and patient wellbeing (Dickens, Suesse, Snyman, & Picchioni, 2014; Friis, 1986; Moos & Houts, 1968). Ward atmosphere, as the originators of the field first characterised it, is the study of both "perception of the socio-cultural environment [and the] prevailing philosophy and value system" (Moos & Houts, 1968, p. 604). These studies thus tap a mixture of affective, relational and cultural aspects of the psychiatric wards under study. The 'Ward Atmosphere Scale', for instance, focuses on the relationships between staff and patients, including levels of involvement, support, aggression and autonomy, as well as the organisation of the ward, such as how useful the activities provided are seen to be and the general orderliness and predictability of ward life (Friis, 1986). A more recent similar measure has categories of 'therapeutic hold', 'patient cohesion' and 'experienced safety' (Schalast, Redies, Collins, Stacey, & Howells, 2008). These studies have found that the ward climate, measured in this way, tends to remain stable over time, through staff and patient changes (Dickens et al., 2014; Jansson & Eklund, 2002; Kobos, Redmond, & Sterling, 1982). A better ward climate, meaning more interaction, cohesion and therapeutic focus, has been consistently linked to better recovery rates. There have also been consistent differences found in the way that staff and patients rate the environment of the wards. Studies have found that patients rate safety more highly than staff (Dickens et al., 2014), while staff rate the wards as being more therapeutic than patients do (Archer & Amuso, 1980; Dickens et al., 2014; Friis, 1986; Long et al., 2011). This difference would seem to fit with Curtis' (2010) argument that staff and patients on psychiatric wards have differing priorities, with staff being particularly preoccupied with risk; an emphasis on risk would logically include an inflated view of safety problems. The different experiences of staff and service users of the ward, has led some to describe a 'split milieu' (Nicholls, Kidd, Threader, & Hungerford, 2015), with patients and staff occupying the space in separate, and sometimes contradictory, ways.

It is, therefore, widely acknowledged, that the environment of the ward is important, and that the relationships, activities and culture afforded by different psychiatric ward environments help shape the experiences and recovery of patients. A large number of studies have also, however, found consistent problems on contemporary psychiatric wards with just these facets of the ward. A common complaint is the quality of the relationships afforded by this medicalised space. A lack of interaction has been widely noted in studies from the perspective of both service users (Ford, Durcan, & Warner, 1998; Reavey, Poole et al., 2017) and nurses (Bowers et al., 2005; Walton, 2000). Ford et al.'s (1998) study noted the increasing time spent by nurses in the ward office doing paperwork; administering the ward, rather than engaging with patients. The ward is often described as a reactive space, where staff observe service users passively, only engaging with them if there is 'trouble'. To this end, service users have been left to float, like spectres in a space; without much of an identity, a knowledge of why they are there or what the space is able to provide (see Reavey et al., forthcoming).

These patterns of feeling and behaving have been observed in other studies of psychiatric wards (Alexander & Bowers, 2004; Bowers et al., 2005; Quirk, 2002; Quirk & Lelliot, 2001; SCMH, 1998), where staff are increasingly concerned with controlling 'disruptive' behaviour. Encapsulating this relationship can be seen to be the 'goldfish bowl' set up on many wards, where the staff office is behind glass, where observation rather than interaction is prioritised (McGrath & Reavey, 2013; Schweitzer, Gilpin, & Frampton, 2004). Removal of this glass has been found to successfully increase staff/service user interaction, and to improve relationships, illustrating how the physical space of the ward impacts on relational ties and emotions.

A related complaint is that of a lack of activity on the wards. Some psychiatric wards have been described as a 'blank space' (McGrath & Reavey, 2013), lacking in meaningful activity or communal life. Farnworth, Nikitin, and Fossey (2004), for example, found that patients on a secure unit in Australia described their daily activities as 'killing time': the most common occupations described were personal care or leisure activities, individualised activities that filled time, rather than building either a sense of purpose or a meaningful experience of community. We have found this in our own work in adult, adolescent and forensic inpatient settings (McGrath, 2012; Reavey, Poole et al., 2017; Reavey et al., forthcoming). The picture that emerges here is that of environments that fail in many cases to afford either meaningful activity or satisfying relationships. A tension is also at play between staff and service user concerns; with staff prioritising risk and safety, while service users place greater importance on privacy and relationships. At the same time, however, there has been a surge in both research (Connellan et al., 2013) and investment in institutional settings in mental health, in line with a general pattern in health care (Gesler et al., 2004).

The newly stated priorities of this new wave of mental health facilities, which focus on well-being rather than containment, raise the question as to whether significant improvements in institutional life have been achieved. Indeed Nicholls et al. (2015), found that in a newly built facility in Australia, the change of building had only limited impact on 'ward atmosphere', with no overall improvement found. While the building had changed, they concluded, the culture and patterns of relating of the ward were transferred across into the new facility, almost unaltered. Attractive spaces are one thing, but when relations remain limited, it is important to ask whether more could be done to foster relational attunement and connection with others.

An alternative to institutions? A house rather than a hospital . . .

In contrast to the more typical institutional spaces described above, there have been limited examples of individuals being cared for outside of traditional medical settings; even those deemed to be severely and enduringly 'unwell'. One famous example is the Soteria project, set up in 1971 by Loren Mosher in California as an alternative to hospital treatment for acute psychosis (Bola & Mosher, 2003; Mosher, 1999; Mosher, Menn, & Matthews, 1975). Inspired by R. D. Laing's (1960, 1967) existential theories of psychosis, viewing madness as a meaningful journey through which people needed support rather than containment, Soteria was located in an ordinary suburban house, largely drug-free, and staffed by non-professionals offering non-medical psychosocial care (Bola & Mosher, 2003; Mosher, 1975, 1999). The project's ethos was compassion based, psycho-social, as opposed to biomedical, where consistent and constant care replaced surveillance and stabilisation. Comparisons with the local psychiatric ward, run on medical grounds, found that while there was no difference in levels of symptomatology (e.g. the presence of voices or unusual beliefs) after two years, the Soteria group performed significantly better on a series of psychosocial measures. They were more likely to be in work, to be living independently, and less likely to have accessed mental health services over the two years (Bola & Mosher, 2003; Mosher, 1999). If recovery is understood as a process of "recovering a new sense of self and of purpose within and beyond the limits of the disability" (Deegan, 1988, p. 11), rather than the 'removal' of 'symptoms', then Soteria can be seen to have succeeded in producing, to some extent, a better outcome for service users. Needless to say, Mosher created a storm in the North American psychiatric profession, resulting in his removal from the American Psychiatric Association in 1980. One does not dismantle, brick by brick, highly influential and profitable medical institutions, without consequence.

In describing a similar project in Colorado, Cedar House, Richard Warner (2000, p. 61) describes some benefits of such residential, but non-medicalised, environments:

> People receiving services in a non-institutional setting are called upon to use their own inner resources. They must exercise a degree of self-control and accept responsibility for their actions and for the preservation of their living environment. Consequently, clients retain more of their self-respect, their skills and their sense of mastery. The domestic and non-coercive nature of the alternatives described here makes human contact with the person in crisis easier than in hospital.

Warner (2000) argues that environments such as these are more conducive to recovery because they are less 'alienating' than hospitals; medicalised hospital environments have been argued to inculcate a passive 'patient role' in service users (Campbell, 1996b; Link et al., 1989; Scheff, 1974, 1999), removing agency through the inherent power inequalities between staff and service users, most clearly defined in the use of enforced restraint and seclusion. Warner's analysis is, however, far more extensive than examining treatment spaces alone. His approach situates institutionalised spaces in a much broader context of economic and cultural assemblages, which ascribe meaning and purpose to citizens who are more likely to be able to contribute to the creation and maintenance of capital. Mental health service users are not often deemed to be part of this assemblage, especially if unemployed, socially marginalised or living in institutions. Warner argued that bringing people back into the community, providing meaningful activities and pursuits and a safe and community-based environment to live in, would be a positive step towards recovery, acceptance and integration.

Theorising space

The evidence outlined above demonstrates a clear role for space in the experience, development and maintenance of mental distress. It is also apparent, however, that 'space' is a flexible term that can be used to describe physical and social environments on a number of scales, ranging from the particular arrangement of buildings to the make-up of people living in a similar area. These examples can be seen to demonstrate that 'space' is a nebulous concept; in its broadest sense, it can mean any form of dimensionality (Massey, 1994b), but it is also a term applied across a number of scales and modalities with similarly varying levels of specificity, from the general ('urban space', 'social space') to the specific (a particular psychiatric ward). It is also a term used metaphorically in terms such as 'head space' or needing 'space' in a relationship. In addition, the term 'place' is also used, sometimes interchangeably with space (e.g. Hubbard, Kitchin, & Valentine, 2004; Massey & Thrift, 2003; Relph, 1976; Tuan, 1977), to describe locality: again, places can range from a place set at a table up to a particular city, area or landscape (Massey, 1994a). The theoretical tools that can be brought to the problem of understanding space are varied and interdisciplinary. What is discussed below is far from exhaustive, yet nevertheless offers a range of potential approaches that are variously examined throughout the book.

A focus on the relationship between material space and experience has waxed and waned in popularity through the years, leaving a variety of theoretical approaches and tools to draw upon. Latour's (1996, 2005) observation that the social sciences ignore material space in favour of 'airy' (Serres, 1995) social and discursive practices was particularly accurate during the 1980s and 1990s, when discourse reigned supreme in social and critical psychological theory. Looking further back, there have been bursts of interest in theorising environmental relations. The 1920s and 1930s, for instance, featured a cluster of theories looking at the person within space, including ecological psychology (e.g. Lewin, 1935/2013), the holism of Gestalt psychology (Goldstein, 1985), Marxist socio-cultural psychology (Vygotsky, 1986), and the later phenomenology of Merleau-Ponty. Material and social context were often referred to during this period in 'the field', and these theories took various approaches to understanding the person as indivisible from their social and material context. A second important cluster of theorisation in this area centres around the 1970s, with the advent of community psychology (e.g. Rappaport, 1977) and a resurgence of research in environmental psychology (e.g. Proshansky, Ittelson, & Rivlin, 1976). Community psychology draws on an ecological framework and analyses of power inequalities to orientate psychology to the reshaping of material and social contexts rather than individual psychology (e.g. Kagan, Burton, Duckett, Lawthorn, & Siddiquee, 2011). Environmental psychology has taken a largely quantitative and cognitivist approach to understanding the impact of material environments on individual psychological processes (e.g. Kagan et al., 2011).

A key nexus in the more recent engagement with the relationship between space and experience has been, perhaps unsurprisingly, the field of human geography. Human geography has engaged with similar trends in theory and subject matter as the rest of the social sciences, including post-structuralism (e.g. Gregson & Rose, 2000; Murdoch, 2006; Rose, 1999), phenomenology (e.g. Davidson, 2001), actor-network theory (e.g. Bingham, 2000; Murdoch, 1998), embodiment (Hall, 2005; Teather, 1999), culture (Crang, 1998), emotion (e.g. Davidson, Bondi, & Smith, 2005), affect (e.g. Thrift, 2004, 2008), Marxism (e.g. Harvey, 1996, 2001, 2009;

Massey, 1984) and questions of globalisation (e.g. Amin, 2002; Brah, Hickman, & Mac, 1999). Due to the nature of the discipline, however, these different theoretical concerns have been consistently engaged with through a lens of theorising space, and the relations of people within space. This wide-ranging engagement with critical, social and political theory has produced, broadly, a view of space which posits that: "social, economic and political phenomena are the product of spatial-temporal locality, and that the articulation of inter-relations brings space into being" (Hubbard et al. 2004, p. 2). Space, or 'spatial-temporal locality' is hence seen as playing a central role in the production of all kinds of social and cultural phenomena, and the process by which space is produced is viewed as both relative and relational. As Massey (1994b, 1999) argues, this is contrasted to a view common in physical geography (and in many accounts of space outside the discipline of geography) positing space as 'absolute', a static landscape able to be objectively, definitively mapped. Human geographers have been highly critical of a static, cartographical view of space, and offer instead a complex, relational and dynamic view of space.

Relations in space

Highly influential in this strand of thinking is Lefebvre's (1991) argument that space is socially produced, defined by relationships. Lefebvre defined an idea of space as an abstract, static container of objects and people as "logico-mathematical space", differentiating this from the "practico-sensory realm of social space" (p. 15). The former, he argued, was an abstraction based on Euclidean geometry, and was not able to describe the differences between spaces or understand how they came into being. The theorisation of space, as it appears in the world, Lefebvre argued, therefore required an understanding of space as a form of practice:

> Everyone knows what is meant when we speak of a 'room' in an apartment the 'corner' of the street, a 'marketplace', a shopping or cultural 'centre', a public 'place' and so on. These terms of everyday discourse serve to distinguish, but not to isolate, particular spaces, and in general to describe a social space. They correspond to a specific use of space, and hence to a spatial practice that they express and constitute. Their interrelationships are ordered in a specific way.
>
> *(Lefebvre, 1991, p. 16)*

Lefebvre therefore argued that differences between spaces can be understood as differential "spatial practices", and hence are inherently active, productive and social. As the eminent geographer Doreen Massey (1994b) traces, a similarly relational view of space, building on Lefebvre's work, was expounded from the 1970s onwards through the twin development of Marxist and feminist geography. The spatial forms of capitalism, it was argued, had to be understood in terms of the social, economic and political processes that produced them; slums and factories were seen as produced, under this view, by capitalist economics. Once in place, however, as Massey argues, these spaces continue to produce future social processes and experiences; the communities of post-industrial Britain did not disappear, for instance, simply because the mines and factories that had initiated the towns closed down (Massey, 1994c). The continued presence of the material structures of the town can be seen as an anchoring presence, tying inhabitants to the area even after the activity that produced the spaces in question has desisted. Any study of space, therefore, necessarily required the study of social and political context. Space is here understood as not only produced by social relations, but also productive of social relations (Massey, 1994c; Lefebvre, 1991).

Also influential in Massey's work on the productive and relational nature of space is an engagement with the early twentieth-century paradigm shift from Newtonian to quantum physics. Quantum understandings of space, time and process are indeed a thread connecting early field theorists, such as Kurt Lewin (1936/2013), to the 'new materialisms' (Coole and Frost, 2010) which have become pervasive across social and critical theory in recent years. The shift from Newtonian to Quantum physics has constituted a fundamental disjunct in the understanding of the nature of space. The Newtonian world comprises static, passive objects waiting to be moved through the enactment of outside forces; think of a snooker table, a contained and static arena where objects are moved around according to stable laws and remain still in between being acted upon. It is a world of equilibrium, where both time and space are stable, and objects have stable, orderly properties that can be predicted.

Quantum theory, beginning with Einstein's theory of relativity and developing throughout the twentieth century has thoroughly disrupted this view. As Prigogine and Stengers (1984) state: "most of reality, instead of being orderly, stable, and equilibrial, is seething and bubbling with change, disorder, and process" (p. xv). Rather than stable, passive space and predictable, active time, Einstein proposed a four dimensional 'space-time', which is fundamentally relational (see Massey, 1994b). Space-time repositions relations, rather than objects as ontologically primary; time slows because of the speed at which an object is travelling or the density of the mass of a black hole. Study at both very small, or very large scales has made physics re-evaluate the nature of space from one of stable and predictable objects, to one of relationships, processes, events and potentialities. At the sub-atomic scale, for instance, quantum theory has established that electrons do not have stable positions in space, but instead exist as a cloud of probabilities, which become fixed only upon observation.

These ideas, of the unfixed and processual nature of the world, have been highly influential in thinking about how we understand people, society and experience (e.g. Whitehead 1926).

Living spaces

One example of this includes ecological approaches to understanding the relationship between space and experience (e.g. Bateson, 1972; Lewin, 1936/2013).

Central to these ideas is that life and living beings can be understood as intrinsically processual, as engaged in a process of 'becoming' rather than a static state of 'being'. Here we discuss two specific ideas, Ingold's (2000) 'meshwork' and 'dwelling', and Lewin's (1936/2013) 'life-space' as examples of ways to understand how people live in, occupy and experience space. As Ingold (2011, p. 91) says:

> The environment is, in the first place, a world we live in, and not a world we look at. We *inhabit* our environment: we are part of it; and through the practice of habitation it becomes part of us too.

Ecological thinkers see people as organisms, which are always and fundamentally embedded in context. It is not possible to meaningfully extract a person from their environment, as the context in which we are immersed is what gives shape to our lives, guiding our actions, forging relationships, affording or denying agency, opening up or shutting down future possibilities. Ingold (2000) points out that removing an organism from their environment means they die; as people, we can't breathe without air, and also we can't feel without relationships with the world, the things we affect and are affected by. When we live, we move through the world, forging experience from the substances of the world we are immersed in.

Ingold (2000, 2011) argues that organisms are characterised primarily by movement, becoming and growth, as well as being inseparable from their environment. Think of the difference between a photograph and a film; a photograph of a person looks static, and the relations that person has with their surroundings appear stable and fixed, but this is an illusion. A film reveals the photograph is only a still of an ever-changing, moving, evolving set of relations that that person has with their environment, pushing forward through time. In moving through the world, Ingold argues, we leave traces behind us; of relationships, of things that we have affected and have affected us; in living, we hence each carve a path through an ever-changing world:

> Proceeding along a path, every inhabitant lays out a trail. Where inhabitants meet, trails are entwined, as the life of each becomes bound up with each other. Every entwining is a knot, and the more lifelines are entwined, the greater the density of the knot. [. . .] Together they make up what I have called the meshwork.
>
> *(Ingold, 2007, p. 80)*

The 'meshwork' is here understood as the process of living with others, at once entangled together, located in particular, embodied, material locations, and yet still not wholly defined by that location, due to the unique paths which each person has forged through the world: "This tangle is the texture of world [. . .] beings do not simply occupy the world, they *inhabit* it, and in so doing – in threading their own paths through the meshwork – they contribute to the ever-evolving weave" (Ingold, 2000, pp. 66–67). Here Ingold captures a sense of inhabiting, rather than occupying, places. The way that buildings are inhabited is not a given; places are made and remade each day, through the activities, relationships and forms of life that are forged within them. Ingold (2000, 2011) names this process of living, making and remaking place, 'dwelling', defined as: "not the occupation of a world already built, but the very process of inhabiting the earth" (2011, p. 139). He contrasts the structure of a 'house', the building itself, with the experience of 'home', which is made daily, through the joint activities and relationships that make up domestic life. Dwelling, therefore, can be thought of as the holistic experience of living; the multiplicity of practices, experiences and actions that embed people into their living environments.

A similar concept is Kurt Lewin's (1936/2013) concept of life-space. Influenced by emergent quantum field theory, Lewin described life-space as the "totality of facts which determine the behaviour (B) of an individual at a certain moment. The life-space (L) represents the totality of possible events . . . It can be represented by a finitely structured space" (1936/2013, p. 216). A 'fact', for Lewin, is anything that is psychologically relevant, whether that is social, material, interpersonal or personal. Life-space 'facts' might be a memory that is particularly salient in a situation, a look from another person, an emotional reaction or a door, blocking someone's passage. Together these intertwine to afford, or block, action and possibilities for the person. Crucially, these possibilities are afforded by the relationship between the environment and the person, and are not intrinsic to either. Notable here is that these 'facts' do not have to be physically present. Life-space is instead topologically organised (see Brown, 2012; Brown & Reavey, 2015); what brings something into the 'region' of someone's life-space is the fact that they have a relationship to that thing, person, event, memory or other 'fact'. Life-spaces stretch through time and space, ordered by relationships, not metrical distance.

A working definition of agency can hence be formulated as the expansion and contraction of life-space (Brown & Reavey, 2015). If life-space is the psychological field of possibilities that exists at any given moment, then sensitivity to the range and extent of these possibilities is, for practical purposes, what constitutes agency. The more that a person feels connected to broader range of relationships, including those that are spatially remote, along with a stronger sense of the relevance of different aspects of the past and an enhanced capacity to anticipate different kinds of possible future, the greater their sense of agency is likely to be (Reavey et al., forthcoming). Lewin's work suggests that understanding any relationship between mental health and space, or any psychological experience, requires an analysis of the 'total situation' of the person. A concern with physical space alone is insufficient; attention needs to be paid instead to the relational space that people inhabit, whose boundaries extend spatially and temporally far beyond the present setting and moment. The life-space of a person, and their corresponding sense of agency, is expanded and contracted through psychological and not merely physical movement – that is, the ability to place oneself in relation to a broader trajectory of experience where the present moment is connected to a web of relationships that encompass past and future possibilities.

Together, these theoretical approaches all share an emphasis on the relational and dynamic nature of space. Far from a static container of objects and people, we can here understand space as a complex, shifting and dynamic assemblage. The social, relational and material can be seen here to be threaded together in dynamic relation with individual experience.

Aims of the book

This book aims to bring together the psychosocial work on experiences of space and mental distress, as well as make explicit the links between theoretical work and clinical and community practice. Our aim is to create a dialogue between academics, people who use services and practitioners, to provide potential ways of reconvening the spaces in which people experience distress. The scope of the book is thus far reaching, with contributions from those involved in theorising space, those drawing on their own experiences of distress and space, as well as practitioners working on the ground. The volume is organised into three themed sections covering (a) institutional settings, (b) community spaces and (c) clinical and community interventions.

Part I Institutional spaces: containing distress in the walls of the hospital

The authors in this section explore aspects of institutional spaces, drawing on themes of power, containment and regulation. In Chapter 1, Ringer and Holen discuss a case study of the regulation of smoking for one service user, Hanna, in a Danish psychiatric ward. They discuss how the smoking room may be regarded as a space 'in between' – simultaneously part of the institutional space and yet separate from it. Drawing on observational field notes from the professionals' discussions of the conflict and interviews with Hanna, the chapter analyses the professionals' ways of making sense of Hanna's resistance. In Chapter 2, Zorwaska describes the work of the Madlove project, a collaboration between the 'the vacuum cleaner' (James Leadbitter) and Hannah Hull. Madlove invites people with personal experience of mental health – plus carers, professionals, artists and campaigners – to redesign the 'asylum'. Two core messages of Madlove are that people should be given the option to accept their experience of 'madness'; and that the role of mental health care should be expanded to include making this experience safe. Chapter 3 by Crafter follows with a discussion of the space of outpatient services for children and young people. This chapter draws on research with staff, parents and children/young people attending two CAMHS (children and adolescent mental health services) outpatients about the built environment and space. Theoretical concepts from the sociology of childhood and critical-developmental studies are used to examine how child mental health settings contradict societal expectations of 'ideal' childhood. Thus, children who attend mental health spaces are constructed as both 'at risk' and 'risky', which is reflected in the materiality of the space in CAMHS. Such materiality manifests itself by CAMHS being a space that is materially neglected, materially 'risky' and largely adult-orientated. Notions of risk and power are further explored in Chapter 4 by Poole and Reavey, who explore the ways in which young people negotiate power and risk in their use of material spaces of a CAMHS inpatient ward. The authors explore a variety of spaces that represent the struggle for independence, agency and choice. Through their exploration of key ward sites, they examine how the material space participates in staff and patient negotiations of risk, autonomy, control and resistance. In Chapter 5, Boden, Larkin and Springham explore the possibilities of experience-based co-design as a way to combat experiences of inpatient mental health spaces as impermeable, separate and stigmatising and sometimes uncomfortable, chaotic and unsafe. Experience-based co-design is a participatory action research approach to service development, which has been used extensively in physical health care, but is only recently being used to improve mental health services. Bringing this section to a close are Parnell and Rooney (Chapter 6), who explore young people's experiences of using 'sensory spaces' within a traditional inpatient setting. Both Parnell and Rooney are practitioners who argue for sensory space as a means to explore young people's emotions and to encourage self-reflection and agency. They argue that the focus between the individual and the symbolic meaning of the space appears key to the young people's journey through the service, and that the flexibility of the space affords individuals' empowerment of choice to use the room, along with the potential for subsequent autonomy in their journey through services, and beyond.

Part II Community spaces: beyond the therapy room

In this section the authors explore the plethora of community spaces that are now sites for mental health care and practice, as well as those that fall outside service use. In Chapter 7, Graham, Hodgetts, Stolte and Chamberlain explore a community meal programme, approaching meal-sharing as a socialising force that can materialise networks of support, creating a sense of community, belonging, dignity, participation and inclusion. We situate the meal as a particular space for care within the broader landscape of despair that has been created by neoliberal austerity: a landscape that precariat families must navigate in their efforts to preserve their health. In Chapter 8, McGrath, Weaver, Reavey and Brown focus on newly homeless people with previous experiences of mental health problems. Drawing on Sloterdijk's theory of spheres, they explore the ways in which people make and recreate safety within exposing and stigmatising urban spaces. In Chapter 9, Walker, Klein, Marks and Hanna theoretically interrogate the idea of social prescribing, which distributes mental health care into disparate community spaces. Utilising the idea of the 'psycommons', they explore implications of these developments. Chapter 10 turns to the subject of the home, where Smith aims to gain a further insight into the strategies employed by older service users, arguing that pervasive notions of home can endorse a spatiality of sanctuary, while this analysis revealed more dichotomous expressions of security/relaxation and anxiety/isolation in the spatial negotiation of distress in the home. In Chapter 11, Townley continues on the theme of home and housing, utilising a mixture of geo-spatial analysis and qualitative data. Examples from research in the southeastern and north-western United States are used to illustrate strategies for siting supportive housing units, addressing barriers to community inclusion and assisting individuals as they navigate physical and social space. Extending beyond physical community spaces into virtual communities, in Chapter 12 Goodings and Tucker explore the complex terrain of this digital media space, to unearth the personal meanings underpinning this use of space, and the subsequent shifts in personhood and embodiment that ensue. Mental health dedicated social media sites are now recognised as legitimate forms of self-help, and statutory services have begun appropriating these spaces as a way to 'supplement' the ever decreasing levels of face-to-face contact with service users, in among increasing economic strain. The shift between such 'actual' and 'virtual' spaces, however, is not well understood. Goodings and Tucker (Chapter 12) unpick some of the theoretical and empirical challenges for understanding not only what it means when people are experiencing themselves through digital technology, but also how distress comes to be shaped by the characteristics of these forms of digital communication. In the final chapter of this section, Chapter 13, Freeman and Akhurst discuss the role of nature and in experiences of mental distress, drawing on insights from ecotherapy and theories of restoration.

Part III Interventions in space and place

The authors in this section discuss mental health interventions in which space plays a key role, in the experience of distress itself, as well as the utilisation of space to create more positive forms of expression and feeling. We start with Hassan, Fatimilehin and Kagan (Chapter 14), who discuss the intervention *Geedka Shirka* (meaning under the tree), which is a purpose-generated space for Somali men and their families to explore cultural, migratory and community issues affecting their mental health, including family tensions. The authors outline the participatory nature of the intervention and highlight the necessity of creating a community space that facilitates meal sharing and storytelling sessions, as a form of action research that unites generations of migrants. Chapter 15 continues the theme of community shared space, exploring some of the benefits and tensions that exist in providing a safe space for individuals with complex needs when statutory services appropriate these spaces under the remit of 'social prescribing'. Feeney describes Tea in the Pot, a women's group in Govan, Glasgow, which provides a safe environment for women to meet away from home and work, or 'third place'. Members report that attending the group helps to alleviate feelings of isolation and loneliness, builds confidence and a sense of belonging and connects them to their wider community. However, the growing use of the group by statutory services and the third sector to provide 'social prescriptions', particularly in the area of mental health, has created tensions and particular challenges for all who benefit from the informal and safe environment that Tea in the Pot provides. While volunteers are committed to supporting all disadvantaged women, they are often unable to meet the complex needs of those referred, creating anxiety in members and potentially undermining the good work of the group. Working tensions in the provision of community services is further explored by Uttarkar in Chapter 16, who describes the difficulties of reaching out to individuals with severe and enduring forms of distress in chaotic home spaces, which are not perhaps conducive to well-being and comfort. Uttarkar discusses the need to attend in clinical practice, to the function of the space on experiences of distress, including enabling clients to see a connection between their living arrangements, feelings and mental health. In Chapter 17, Liddicoat and Forster examine the role of the home space for those who self-harm and dissociate, and the influence of the spatial encounter in making sense of selfmanagement of distress and the therapeutic relationship. Their use of architectural theory, also informed by user-led initiatives, facilitates an analysis of user accounts of how they manage their distress at home, and how this could be mobilised in therapy to create a greater awareness of the link between spatial encounter, distress and practices of the self. The last chapter in the book, Chapter 18, discuses the Outsider Gallery, an art and music therapy project run by Wakeling and Hall. This chapter takes the form of an interview tour of the building, including the art studio, music studio and gallery space. Wakeling and Hall describe how this space affords more agentive forms of expression and understanding to emerge from these spaces, as the purpose is to hand authorship over to people and to explicitly invite moments of self-reflection and active participation.

References

Alexander, J., & Bowers, L. (2004). Acute psychiatric ward rules: A review of the literature. *Journal of Psychiatric and Mental Health Nursing, 11*(5), 623–631.
Amin, A. (2002). Spatialities of globalisation. *Environment and Planning A, 34*, 385–399.
Araya, R., Dunstan, F., Playle, R., Thomas, H., Palmer, S., & Lewis, G. (2006). Perceptions of social capital and the built environment and mental health. *Social Science and Medicine, 62*(12), 3072–3083.
Archer, R., & Amuso, K. (1980). Comparison of staff's and patients' perceptions of ward atmosphere. *Psychological Reports, 46*, 959–965.
Banks, M., & Nissen, M. (2017). Beyond spaces of counselling. *Qualitative Social Work, 15*, 225–247.
Barrowclough, C., Tarrier, N., & Johnston, M. (1996). Distress, expressed emotion, and attributions in relatives of schizophrenia patients. *Schizophrenia Bulletin, 22*(4), 691–701.
Bateson, G. (1972). *Steps to an ecology of mind: Collected essays in anthropology, psychiatry, evolution and epistemology*. Chicago, IL: University of Chicago Press.
Bentall, R. P. (2003). *Madness explained: Psychosis and human nature*. London: Penguin.
Bentall, R. P. (2004). *Madness explained: Psychosis and human nature* (2nd ed.). London: Penguin.
Bentall, R. P. (2009). *Doctoring the mind: Why psychiatric treatments fail*. London: Allen Lane.
Berg, A. E., Hartig, T., & Staats, H. (2007). Preference for nature in urbanized societies: Stress, restoration and the pursuit of sustainability. *Journal of Social Issues, 63*(1), 79–96.
Bhugra, D., & Arya, P. (2005). Ethnic density, cultural congruity and mental illness in migrants. *International Review of Psychiatry, 17*(2), 133–137.

Bingham, N. (2000). The geography of Bruno Latour and Michel Serres. In M. Crang & N. Thrift (Eds.), *Thinking space*. London: Routledge.
Bloomfield, B. P., & McLean, C. (2003). Beyond the walls of the asylum: Information and organization in the provision of community mental health services. *Information and Organisation, 13*(1), 53–84.
Bola, J. R., & Mosher, L. R. (2003). Treatment of acute psychosis without neuroleptics: Two-year outcomes from the Soteria project. *Journal of Nervous Mental Disease, 191*(4), 219–229.
Bowers, L., Simpson, A., Alexander, J., Hackney, D., Nijman, H., Grange, A., & Warren, J. (2005). The nature and purpose of acute psychiatric wards: The Tompkins Acute Ward Study. *Journal of Mental Health, 14*(6), 625–635.
Boydell, J., & McKenzie, K. (2008). Society, space and place. In C. Morgan, K. McKenzie, & P. Fearon (Eds.), *Society and psychosis*. Cambridge: Cambridge University Press.
Brah, A., Hickman, M. J., & Mac, M. (1999). *Global futures: Migration, environment and globalisation*. Basingstoke: Macmillan.
Brown, G. W., & Harris, T. O. (1978). *Social origins of depression: A study of psychiatric disorder in women*. London: Routledge.
Brown, G. W., Harris, T. O., & Hepworth, C. (1995). Loss, humiliation and entrapment among women developing depression: A patient and non-patient comparison. *Psychological Medicine, 25*(1), 7–21.
Brown, G. W., Lemyre, L., & Bilfulco, A. (1992). Social factors and recovery from anxiety and depressive disorders. A test of specificity. *British Journal of Psychiatry, 161*(1), 44–54.
Brown, S. D. (2002). Memory and mathesis: For a topological approach to psychology. *Theory, Culture & Society, 29*, 137–164.
Brown, S. D., & Reavey, P. (2015). *Vital memory and affect: Living with a difficult past*. London: Routledge.
Bullimore, P. (2012). The relationship between trauma and paranoia: Managing paranoia. In M. Romme & S. Escher, *Psychosis as personal crisis: An experiential approach*. Hove: Psychology Press.
Butzlaff, R., & Hooley, J. M. (1998). Expressed emotion and psychiatric relapse: A meta-analysis. *Archive of General Psychiatry, 55*(6), 547–552.
Campbell, P. (1996). The history of the user movement in the United Kingdom. In T. Heller, J. Reynolds, R. Gomm, R. Muston, & S. Pattison, (Eds.), *Mental health matters: A reader*. Basingstoke: Palgrave.
Campbell, P. (2001). The role of service users in service development: Influence not power. *The Psychiatrist, 25*, 87–88.
Chase, E., & Bantebya-Kyomuhendo, G. (2014). *Poverty and shame: Global experiences*. Oxford: Oxford University Press.
Chase, M. (2011). On being human in a depersonalised place: A critical analysis of community psychiatric practice (Unpublished PhD thesis). University of Portsmouth.
Coburn, D. (2015). Income inequality, welfare, class and health: A comment on Pickett and Wilkinson, 2015. *Social Science and Medicine, 146*, 228–232.
Connellan, K., Gaardboe, M., Riggs, D., Due, C., Reinschmidt, A., & Mustillo, L. (2013). Stressed spaces: Mental health and architecture. *HERD: Health Environments Research & Design Journal, 6*(4), 127–168.
Coole, D., & Frost, S. (2010). *New materialisms: Ontology, agency and politics*. Durham, MD: Duke University Press.
Corker, E., Hamilton, S., Henderson, C., Weeks, C., Pinfold, V., Rose, D., ... Thornicroft, G. (2013). Experiences of discrimination among people using mental health services in England 2008–2011. *British Journal of Psychiatry, 202*, 58–63.

Crang, M. (1998). *Cultural geography*. Abingdon: Routledge.
Cromby, J., & Harper, D. (2005). Paranoia and social inequality. *Clinical Psychology Forum, 153*, 17–21.
Cromby, J., Harper, D., & Reavey, P. (2013). *Psychology, mental health and distress*. Basingstoke: Palgrave Macmillan.
Curtis, S. (2010). *Space, place and mental health*. London: Ashgate.
Davidson, J. (2000a). A phenomenology of fear: Merleau-Ponty and agoraphobic lifeworlds. *Sociology of Health and Illness, 22*(5), 640–660.
Davidson, J. (2000b). '. . . the world was getting smaller': Women, agoraphobia and bodily boundaries. *Area, 32*(1), 31–40.
Davidson, J. (2001). Fear and trembling in the mall: Women, agoraphobia and body boundaries. In I. Dyck, N. Lewis, & S. McLafferty (Eds.), *Geographies of women's health*. London: Routledge.
Davidson, J. (2003). *Phobic geographies: The phenomenology and spatiality of identity*. Farnham, UK: Ashgate.
Davidson, J., Bondi, L., & Smith, M. (2005). *Emotional geographies*. Farnham, UK: Ashgate.
Deegan, P. E. (1988). Recovery: The lived experience of rehabilitation. *Psychosocial Rehabilitation Journal, 11*(4), 11–19.
Department of Health. (1999). *National service framework for mental health*. London: The Stationery Office.
Department of Health. (2006). *From segregation to inclusion: Commissioning guidance on day services for people with mental health problems*. London: Department of Health.
Department of Health. (2008). *Improving the patient experience: Sharing success in mental health and learning disabilities: The King's Fund's Enhancing the Healing Environment programme 2004–2008*. London: TSO.
Department of Health. (2011). *No health without mental health: A cross-governmental outcomes strategy for people of all ages*. London: Department of Health.
De Witte, H. D. (1999). Job insecurity and psychological well-being: Review of the literature and exploration of some unresolved issues. *European Journal of Work and Organizational Psychology, 8*, 155–177.
Dickens, G. L., Suesse, M., Snyman, P., & Picchioni, M. (2014). Associations between ward climate and patient characteristics in a secure forensic mental health service. *Journal of Forensic Psychiatry & Psychology, 25*(2), 195–211.
Dixon, J., Levine, M., & McAuley, R. (2006). Locating impropriety: Street drinking, moral order and the ideological dilemma of public space. *Political Psychology, 27*(2), 187–206.
Douglas, M. (1966/2001). *Purity and danger: An analysis of concepts of pollution and taboo*. Abingdon: Routledge. (Original work published 1966.)
Estroff, S. (1981). *Making it crazy: An ethnography of psychiatric clients in an American community*. Berkeley, CA: University of California Press.
Evans, G. W. (2003). The built environment and mental health. *Journal of Urban Mental Health, 80*(4), 536–555.
Faris, R. E. L., & Dunham, H. W. (1939). *Mental disorders in urban areas: An ecological study of schizophrenia and other psychoses*. Chicago, IL: University of Chicago Press.
Farnworth, L., Nikitin, L., & Fossey, E. (2004). Being in a secure forensic psychiatric unit: every day is the same, killing time or making the most of it. *British Journal of Occupational Therapy, 67*(10), 430–438.
Finlay-Jones, R., & Brown, G. (1981). Types of stressful life event and the onset of anxiety and depressive disorders. *Psychological Medicine, 11*(4), 803–815.
Foucault, M. (1965). *Madness and civilisation*. New York, NY: Vintage.

Foucault, M. (1977). *Discipline and Punish*. New York, NY: Pantheon.
Ford R., Durcan G., & Warner, L. (1998). One day survey by the Mental Health Act Commission of acute adult psychiatric inpatient wards in England and Wales. *British Medical Journal, 317*, 1279–1283.
Frame, J. (1980). *Faces in the water*. London: The Women's Press. (Original work published 1961.)
Freeman, H. L. (1984). *Mental health and the environment*. London: Churchill Livingstone.
Freeman, H. L. (2008). Housing and mental health. In H. L. Freeman & S. Stansfield (Eds.), *The impact of the environment on psychiatric disorder*. London: Routledge.
Friedli, L. (2009). *Mental health, resilience and inequalities*. Copenhagen: WHO.
Friis, S. (1986). Characteristics of a good ward atmosphere. *Acta Psychiatrica Scandinavica, 74*(5), 469–473.
Gesler, W., Bell, M., Curtis, S., Hubbard, P., & Francis, S. (2004). Therapy by design: Evaluating the UK hospital building program. *Health & Place, 10*(2), 117–128.
Goldstein, M. J. (1985). Family factors that antedate the onset of schizophrenia and related disorders: The results of a fifteen-year prospective longitudinal study. *Acta Psychiatra Scandinavica, 71*(319), 7–18.
Green, G., Gilbertson, J. M., & Grimsley, M. F. (2002). Fear of crime and health in residential tower blocks: A case study in Liverpool, UK. *European Journal of Public Health, 12*(1), 10–15.
Gregson, N., & Rose, G. (2000). Taking Butler elsewhere: Performativities, spatialities and subjectivities. *Environment and Planning D: Society and Space, 18*, 433–452.
Hall, E. (2005). 'Blood, brain and bones': Taking the body seriously in the geography of health and impairment. *Area, 32*(1), 21–29.
Halpern, D. (1995). *Mental health and the built environment: More than bricks and mortar?* Abingdon: Taylor & Francis.
Hareven, T. K. (1991). The home and family in historical perspective. *Social Research, 58*, 253–285.
Harvey, D. (1996). *Justice, nature and the geography of difference*. Malden, MA: Blackwell.
Harvey, D. (2001). *Spaces of capital*. Edinburgh: Edinburgh University Press.
Harvey D. (2007). *A brief history of neoliberalism*. Oxford: Oxford University Press.
Hayward, M. (2003). Interpersonal relating and voice hearing: To what extent does relating to the voice reflect social relating? *Psychological Psychotherapy, 76*(4), 369–383.
Hodgetts, D., Radley, A., Chamberlain, K., & Hodgetts, A. (2007). Health inequalities and homelessness: Considering material, relational and spatial dimensions. *Journal of Health Psychology, 12*(5), 708–725.
Hubbard, P., Kitchin, R., & Valentine, G. (2004). *Key thinkers on space and place*. London: Sage.
Ingold, T. (2000). *The perception of the environment*. London: Routledge.
Ingold, T. (2011). *Being alive: Essays on movement, knowledge and description*. London: Routledge.
Jansson, J., & Eklund, M. (2002). Stability of perceived ward atmosphere over time, diagnosis and gender for patients with psychosis. *Nordic Journal of Psychiatry, 56*, 407–412.
Johnstone, L. (2000). *Users and abusers of psychiatry*. London: Routledge.
Johnstone, L. & Boyle, M. (2018). *The power threat meaning framework: Towards the identification of patterns in emotional distress, unusual experiences and troubled or troubling behaviour as an alternative to functional psychiatric diagnosis*. Leicester: British Psychological Society.
Jones, S., & Mean, M. (2010). *Resilient places: Character and community in everyday language*. London: Demos.

Kagan, C., Burton, M., Duckett, P., Lawthorn, R., & Siddiquee, A. (2011). *Critical community psychology: Critical action and social change*. Leicester, UK: BPS Books.

Kaplan, R., & Kaplan, S. (1989). *The experience of nature: A psychological perspective*. New York, NY: Cambridge University Press.

Keown, P., Mercer, G., & Scott, J. (2008). Retrospective analysis of hospital episode statistics, involuntary admissions under the Mental Health Act 1983, and number of psychiatric beds in England 1996–2006. *British Medical Journal*, *337*, 1837.

Knowles, C. (2000a). *Bedlam on the streets*. London: Routledge.

Knowles, C. (2000b). Burger King, Dunkin Donuts and community mental health care. *Health & Place*, *6*(3), 213–224.

Kobos, J., Redmond, F., & Sterling, J. (1982). Measuring ward milieu and the impact of staff turnover on a psychiatry unit. *Psychological Reports*, *50*, 879–885.

Kuo, F. E. (2001). Coping with poverty: Impacts of environment and attention in the inner city. *Environment and Behaviour*, *33*(5), 5–34.

Laing, R. D. (1960). *The divided self: An existential study in sanity and madness*. Harmondsworth: Penguin.

Laing, R. D. (1967). *The politics of experience and the bird of paradise*. Harmondsworth: Penguin.

Landsbergis, P. A., Schnall, P. L., Deitz, D., Friedman, R., & Pickering, T. (1992). The patterning of psychological attributes and distress by 'job strain' and social support in a sample of working men. *Journal of Behavioural Medicine*, *15*(4), 379–405.

Latour, B. (1996). On interobjectivity. *Mind, Culture and Activity*, *3*(4), 228–245.

Latour, B. (2005). *Reassembling the social: An introduction to actor-network theory*. Oxford: Oxford University Press.

Lawson, B., Phiri, M., & Wells-Thorpe, J. (2003). *The architectural health care environment and its effects on patient health outcomes: A report on an NHS Estates Funded Research Project*. London: Stationery Office.

Lefebvre, H. (1991). *The production of space*. Malden, MA: Blackwell.

Lefkowitz, M., Tesiny, E., & Gordon, N. (1980). Childhood depression, family income, and locus of control. *Journal of Nervous & Mental disease*, *168*(12), 732–735.

Lewin, K. (2013). *Principles of topological psychology*. Redditch, UK: Read Books. (Original work published 1936.)

Lewis, G., David, A., Andréassson, S., & Allebeck, P. (1992). Schizophrenia and city life. *Lancet*, *340*(8812), 137–140.

Link, B. G., Cullen, F. T., Struening, E., Shrout, P. E., & Dohrenwend, B. P. (1989). A modified labelling theory approach to mental disorders: An empirical account. *American Sociological Review*, *54*(3), 400–423.

Long, C. G., Anagnostakis, K., Fox, E., Silaule, P., Somers, J., West, R., & Webster, A. (2011). Social climate along the pathway of care in women's secure mental health service: Variation with level of security, patient motivation, therapeutic alliance and level of disturbance. *Criminal Behaviour and Mental Health*, *21*, 202–214.

McGrath, L. (2012). *Heterotopias of mental health care: The role of space in experiences of distress, madness and mental health service use* (Unpublished PhD). London South Bank University.

McGrath, L., Griffin, V., & Mundy, E. (2015). *Psychological impact of austerity: A briefing paper*. London: Psychologists Against Austerity.

McGrath, L., & Reavey, P. (2013). Heterotopias of control: Placing the material in experiences of mental health service use and community living. *Health & Place*, *22*, 123–131.

McGrath, L., & Reavey, P. (2015). Seeking fluid possibility and solid ground: Space and movement in mental health service users' experiences of 'crisis'. *Social Science & Medicine, 128*, 115–125.

McGrath, L., & Reavey, P. (2016). 'Zip me up, and cool me down': Molar narratives and molecular intensities in 'helicopter' mental health services. *Health and Place, 38*, 61–69.

McGrath, L., Reavey, P., & Brown, S. D. (2008). The spaces and scenes of anxiety: Embodied expressions of distress in public and private fora. *Emotion, Space and Society, 1*, 56–64.

Mallet, S. (2004). Understanding home: A critical review of the literature. *Sociological Review, 52*(1), 62–89.

Marmot, M. (2004). *Status syndrome*. London: Bloomsbury.

Marmot, M. (2010). *Fair society healthy lives*. London: The Marmot Review.

Martin, W. T. (1957). Ecological change in satellite rural areas. *American Sociological Review, 22*(2), 173–183.

Massey, D. (1984). *Spatial divisions of labour: Social structures and the geography of production*. New York, NY: Methuen.

Massey, D. (1994a). A global sense of place. In D. Massey, *Space, place and gender*. Cambridge & Oxford: Polity Press.

Massey, D. (1994b). Politics and space-time. In D. Massey, *Space, place and gender*. Cambridge & Oxford: Polity Press.

Massey, D. (1994c). *Space, place, and gender*. Minneapolis, MN: University of Minnesota Press.

Massey, D. (1999). Space-time, science and the relationship between physical and human geography. *Transactions, Institute of British Geographers, 24*, 261–276.

Massey, D., & Thrift, N. (2003). The passion of place. In R. Johnston & M. Williams (Eds.), *A century of British geography*. London: British Academy.

Miller, R. S. (1996). *Embarrassment: Poise and peril in everyday life*. New York, NY: Guilford Press.

Mitchell, R. E. (1971). Some social implications of high-density housing. *American Sociological Review, 36*(1), 18–29.

Montgomery, C. (2015). *Happy city: Transforming our lives through urban design*. London: Penguin.

Moos, R. H., & Houts, P. S. (1968). Assessment of the social atmospheres of psychiatric wards. *Journal of Abnormal Psychology, 73*, 595–604.

Morley, D. (2000). *Home territories: Media, mobility and identity*. London: Routledge.

Mortensen, P. B., Pederson, C. B., Westergaard, T., Wohlfahrt, J., Ewald, H., Mors, O., . . . Melbye, M. (1999). Effects of family history and place and season of birth on the risk of schizophrenia. *New England Journal of Medicine, 340*(8), 603–608.

Mosher, M. D. (1999). Soteria and other alternatives to acute psychiatric hospitalization: A personal and professional review. *Journal of Nervous Mental Disease, 187*(3), 142–149.

Mosher, M. D., Menn, A., & Matthews, S. (1975). Soteria: Evaluation of a home-based treatment for schizophrenia. *Orthopsychiatry, 45*, 455–467.

Murdoch, J. (1998). The spaces of actor-network theory, *Geoform, 29*(4), 357–374.

Murdoch, J. (2006). *Post-structuralist geography: A guide to relational space*. London: Sage.

Newnes, C., Holmes, G., & Dunn, C. (1999). *This is madness: Critical perspectives on mental health services*. London: PCCS Books.

Newnes, C., Holmes, G., & Dunn, C. (2001). *This is madness too: Critical perspectives on mental health services*. London: PCCS Books.

Nicholls, D., Kidd, K., Threader, J., & Hungerford, C. (2015). The value of purpose built mental health facilities: Use of the Ward Atmosphere Scale to gauge the link between milieu and physical environment. *International Journal of Mental Health Nursing, 24*(4), 286–294.

Nussbaum, M., & Sen, A. (1993). *The quality of life*. Oxford: Oxford University Press.
Office of the Deputy Prime Minister. (2004). *Mental health and social exclusion: Social exclusion report*. London: Office of the Deputy Prime Minister.
Papoulias C., Csipke E., McKellar, S., Rose, D., & Wykes, T. Design in mind: The psychiatric ward as therapeutic space – a systematic review. *British Journal of Psychiatry, 205*, 171–176.
Parr, H. (1997). Mental health, public space, and the city: Questions of individual and collective access. *Environment and Planning D: Society and Space, 15*, 435–454.
Parr, H. (2008). *Mental health and social space: Towards inclusive geographies?* Malden, MA: Blackwell.
Payne, H., & May, D. (2009). Evaluation of a refurbishment scheme incorporating the King's Fund 'Enhancing the Healing Environment' design principles. *Journal of Facilities Management, 7*(1), 74–89.
Phelan, J., Link, B., Steuve, A., & Pescosolido, B. (2000). Public conceptions of mental illness in 1950 and 1996: What is mental illness and is it to be feared? *Journal of Health and Social Behaviour, 41*(2), 188–207.
Pilgrim, D., & Ramon, S. (2009). English mental health policy under New Labour, *Policy and Politics, 37*(2), 273–288.
Pinfold, V. (2000). 'Building up safe havens . . . all around the world': Users' experiences of living in the community with mental health problems. *Health & Place, 6*(3), 201–212.
Porter, R. (2004). *Madmen: A social history of madhouses, mad-doctors and lunatics*. London: Tempus.
Porter, R. (2008). *Madness: A short history*. Oxford: Oxford University Press.
Prigogine, I., & Stengers, I. (1984). *Order out of chaos: Man's new dialogue with nature*. New York, NY: A Bantom Books
Proshansky, H. M., Ittelson, W. H., & Rivlin, L. G. (1976). *Environmental psychology: People and their physical settings*. Oxford: Holt.
Quirk, A. (2002). Acute wards – problems and solutions: A participant observation study of life on an acute psychiatric ward. *Psychiatric Bulletin, 26*(9), 344–345.
Quirk, A., & Lelliott, P. (2001). What do we know about life on acute psychiatric wards in the UK? A review of the research evidence. *Social Science & Medicine, 53*(12), 1565–1574.
Quirk, A., Lelliott, P., & Seale, C. (2006). The permeable institution: An ethnographic study of three acute psychiatric wards in London. *Social Science & Medicine, 63*(8), 2105–2117.
Rappaport, J. (1977). *Community psychology: Values, research and action*. New York, NY: Holt, Rinehart, & Winston.
Read, J., Fosse, R., Moscovitz, A., & Perry, B. (2014). The traumagenic neurodevelopmental model of psychosis revisited. *Neuropsychiatry, 4*(1), 65–79.
Reavey, P., Brown, S. D., Kanyeredzi, A., Mcgrath, L., & Tucker, I. (Forthcoming). Spectres and agents: Life-space on a medium secure forensic mental health unit. *Social Science and Medicine*.
Reavey, P., Harding, K., & Bartle, J. (2017). *Design with people in mind*. London: Design in Mental Health Network.
Reavey, P., Poole, J., Corrigall, R., Zundel, T., Byford, D., Sarhane, S., . . . Ougrin, D. (2017). The ward as emotional ecology: Adolescent experiences of managing mental health and distress in psychiatric inpatient settings. *Health and Place, 48*, 210–218.
Relph, E. (1976). *Place and placelessness*. London: Pion.
Rogers, A., & Pilgrim, D. (1996). *Mental health policy in Britain*. London: Palgrave Macmillan.
Rogers, A., & Pilgrim, D. (2003). *Mental health and inequality*. London: Palgrave Macmillan.

Romme, M., & Escher, S. (1993). *Accepting voices*. London: Mind.
Romme, M., Escher, S., Dillon, J., Corstens, D., & Morris, M. (2009). *Living with voices: An anthology of 50 voice hearers' stories of recovery*. London: PCCS Books.
Rose, G. (1999). Performing space. In D. B. Massey, J. Allen, & P. Sarre (Eds.) *Human geography today*. Cambridge: Polity Press.
Rose, N. (1998). Governing risky individuals: The role of psychiatry in new regimes of control. *Psychiatry, Psychology and Law*, 5(2), 177–195.
Ross, S., Mirowsky, J., & Pribesh, S. (2001). Powerlessness and the amplification of threat: Neighborhood disadvantage, disorder, and mistrust. *American Sociological Review*, 66(4), 568–591.
Sainsbury Centre for Mental Health. (1998). *Acute problems: A survey of the quality of care in acute psychiatric wards*. London: Sainsbury Centre for Mental Health.
Saunders, P., & Williams, P. (1988). The constitution of home: Towards a research agenda. *Housing Studies*, 3(2), 83–93.
Schalast, N., Redies, M., Collins, M., Stacey, J., & Howells, K. (2008). EssenCES: A short questionnaire for assessing the social climate of forensic psychiatric wards. *Criminal Behaviour and Mental Health*, 18, 49–58. doi:10.1002/cbm.677.
Scheff, T. (1974). The labelling theory of mental illness. *American Sociological Review*, 39(3), 444–452.
Scheff, T. (1999). *Being mentally ill: A sociological theory* (3rd ed.). Princeton, NJ: Rutgers.
Schweitzer, M., Gilpin, L., & Frampton, S. (2004). Healing spaces: Elements of environmental design that make an impact on health. *Journal of Alternative and Complementary Medicine*, 10(Suppl.1), S–71.
Sen, A. (2009). *The idea of justice*. Cambridge, MA: Belknap Press/Harvard University Press.
Serres, M. (1995). *Genesis*. Ann Arbour, MI: Michigan University Press.
Shepley, M. M., Watson, A., Pitts, F., Garrity, A., Spelman, E., Fronsman, A., & Kelkar, J. (2017). Mental and behavioral health settings: Importance & effectiveness of environmental qualities and features as perceived by staff. *Journal of Environmental Psychology*, 50, 37–50. doi:10.1016/j.jenvp.2017.01.005.
Shorter, E. (1997). *A history of psychiatry: From the age of the asylum to the era of Prozac*. Washington, DC: John Wiley & Sons.
Silver, E., Mulvey, E. P., & Monahan, J. (1999). Assessing violence risk among discharged psychiatric patients: Toward an ecological approach. *Law and Human Behavior*, 23(2), 235–255.
Smail, D. (2001). *The nature of unhappiness*. London: Constable.
Spandler, H. (2007). From social exclusion to inclusion? A critique of the inclusion imperative in mental health, *Medical Sociology Online*, 2(2), 3–16.
Standing, G. (2011). *The precariat: The new dangerous class*. London: Bloomsbury.
Stansfield, S. A., Fuhrer, R., Shipley, M. J., & Marmot, M. G. (1999). Work characteristics predict psychiatric disorder. *Occupational and Environmental Medicine*, 56, 302–307.
Stichler, J. F. (2008). Healing by design. *Journal of Nursing Administration*, 38(12), 505–509. doi:10.1097/NNA.0b013e31818ebfa6.
Symonds, A. (1998). Social construction and the concept of 'community'. In A. Symonds & A. Kelly (Eds.), *The social construction of community care*. London: Palgrave Macmillan.
Symonds, A., & Kelly, A. (1998). *The social construction of community care*. London: Palgrave Macmillan.
Taylor, B. (2014). *The last asylum*. London: Penguin.
Teather, E. K. (1999). *Embodied geographies: Space, bodies and rites of passage*. London: Routledge.

Tennessen, C. M., & Cimprich, B. (1995). Views to nature: Effect on attention. *Journal of Environmental Psychology, 15*(1), 77–85.

Thrift, N. (2004). Intensities of feeling: Towards a spatial politics of affect. *Geographical Analysis, 86*(1), 57–78.

Thrift, N. (2008). *Non-representational theory: Space, politics, affect*. Abingdon: Routledge.

Twigg, J. (2000). *Bathing: The body and social care*. London: Routledge.

Tuan, Y.-F. (1977). *Space and place: The perspective of experience*. Minneapolis, MN: University of Minnesota Press.

Tunstall, H., Mitchell, R., Gibbs, J., Platt, S., & Dorling, D. (2007). Is economic adversity always a killer? Disadvantaged areas with relatively low mortality rates, *Journal of Epidemiology and Community Health, 61*, 337–343.

Ulrich, R. S. (1984). View through a window may influence recovery from surgery. *Science, 224*, 420–421.

Van Os, J., Driessen, G., Gunther, N., & Delespaul, P. (2000). Neighbourhood variation in incidence of schizophrenia: Evidence for person-environment interaction. *British Journal of Psychiatry, 176*, 243–248.

Vaughan, S., & Fowler, D. (2004). The distress experienced by voice hearing is associated with the perceived relationship between the voice hearer and the voice, *British Journal of Clinical Psychology, 43*(2), 143–153.

Vaughn, C., & Leff, J. (1985). *Expressed emotion in families: Its significance for mental illness*. New York, NY: Guilford Press.

Vygotsky, L. S. (1986). *Thought and language* (rev. ed.). Cambridge, MA: MIT Press.

Walton P. (2000). Psychiatric hospital care: A case of the more things change, the more they stay the same. *Journal of Mental Health, 9*, 77–88.

Wanderman, A., & Nation, M. (1998). Urban neighbourhoods and mental health: Psychological contributions to understanding toxicity, resilience and interventions. *American Psychologist, 53*(6), 647–656.

Wardhaugh, J. (1999). The unaccommodated woman: Home, homelessness and identity. *Sociological Review, 47*(1), 91–109.

Warner, R. (2000). *The environment of schizophrenia*. London: Brunner-Routledge.

Warner, R., de Girolamo, G., Belelli, G., Bologna, C., Fioretti, A., & Rosini, G. (1998). The quality of life of people with schizophrenia in Boulder, Colorado, and Bologna, Italy. *Schizophrenia Bulletin, 24*(4), 559–568.

Weich, S., Blanchard, M., Prince, M., Burton, E., Erens, B., & Sproston, K. (2002). Mental health and the built environment: Cross-sectional survey of individual and contextual risk factors for depression. *British Journal of Psychiatry, 176*, 428–433.

Whitehead, A. N. (1926). *Religion in the making: Lowell lectures*. New York, NY: Fordham University Press.

Wilkinson, R., & Pickett, K. (2009). *The spirit level: Why greater equality makes societies stronger*. London: Penguin.

PART I
Institutional spaces
Containing distress in the walls of the hospital

1
REGULATION AND RESISTANCE IN THE SMOKING ROOM AT A MENTAL HEALTH WARD

Struggles for a space 'in-between'

Agnes Ringer and Mari Holen

Introduction

This chapter explores the significance of the smoking room in a mental health ward in Denmark – as a place of struggle, regulation and resistance. Our data, produced by participant observation and interviews at an acute locked ward, indicate that the smoking room was an important place for service users. Many users stayed for hours at a time in the smoking room and reported that the relative privacy of the room and the company and open conversations with other users provided crucial support during their stay at the ward. This was in contrast to the other spaces of the ward, which were construed as belonging more to staff (Ringer, 2013b). This is in line with other ethnographic studies on psychiatric wards, which have noticed a symbolic meaning of the smoking room as an often 'staff-free' and special place for users. Ethnographies have alternately characterised the smoking room at mental health wards as a 'free area' for users (Terkelsen, 2009, p. 207), as a 'patients' arena' (Skorpen, Anderssen, Oeye, & Bjelland, 2008, p. 731) and as an 'inner sanctuary, a world within a world' (Thomas, Shattell, & Martin, 2002, p. 102). The smoking room has been described as a place where users can engage in an activity not related to 'being treated' and hence a space that may temporarily destabilise a position as 'psychiatric patient' (McGrath, 2012; Ringer, 2013b). In their study of the smoking room at a psychiatric ward in Norway, Skorpen et al. (2008) note that the smoking room became an arena for strategic resistance for users in that it provided 'a space and opportunity to retain parts of their civil life and dignity' (p. 733).

Our fieldwork reproduces many of the findings of other studies on the importance of the smoking room for service users. The present chapter, however, goes beyond an analysis of the significance of the smoking room for service users. Instead, we explore the smoking room as a space, whose status remained unresolved – and hence as an area of negotiations and struggles between users and professionals.

The smoking room in our study constitutes space at once produced as 'other' (Foucault, 1986) and subject to discipline and regulation. From this perspective, rather than it being a sanctuary or 'free space', we will argue that the smoking room at a mental health ward may be understood as having a complicated status as a space 'in-between': simultaneously part of the institution and yet different from it.

In 2007, it became illegal to smoke in public places in Denmark, including hospitals and psychiatric institutions. The introduction of the smoking law brought with it changes to the daily practices of psychiatric wards and new smoking rooms were arranged. Meanwhile, hospital employees were banned from smoking in the area of the hospital and were to be shielded from entering areas with cigarette smoke. This was in contrast to earlier practices, where users and staff could drink coffee and have a cigarette together in the same space (Skorpen et al., 2008). The smoking room now constitutes the one room at mental health wards in Denmark that does not have any clinical function, and where the professionals' presence is largely unwarranted. Since the professionals are responsible for the order of the ward and for treatment, finding an appropriate way of relating to such a space may become difficult. The chapter specifically analyses the course of events during a conflict on regulations of the ward's smoking room. Data are derived from an ethnographic study conducted by the first author (AR) involving participant observation, informal conversations and formal interviews at a locked acute psychiatric ward – here called ward D.[1] The fieldwork lasted six weeks and was conducted in 2011. The data selected for presentation primarily come from the first author's presence in the smoking room and the staff room, as well as interviews with users and professionals.

Based on Foucauldian perspectives on space and discipline, the analysis examines how negotiations about the smoking room connect to larger issues concerning the production of space, time and bodies at a mental health ward. The time at the ward and the time spent in the smoking room are separate, but interconnected. The disciplining of bodies, present in other spaces of the ward, becomes differently magnified and tangible in the smoking room. Thus, we argue, the 'in-between' status of the smoking room provides a 'mirror' for specific tensions and problems that epitomise fundamental issues concerning space and discipline in psychiatric hospitals in general.

Space and discipline in mental health practice

There is a growing interest in the importance of space and matter in mental health care, as evidenced by this book. Social constructionist accounts have traditionally placed a great emphasis on language in mental health practice and user experience, often neglecting to incorporate an analysis of the material and spatial aspects of the world. Yet, as Latour (2005) has argued, material objects are inherent to the social world of humans; objects mediate and transform interactions and experience and hence cannot be seen as either ontologically separate or only made meaningful through discourse (McGrath, 2012). From this perspective, space and the material participate in the production of social life and human experience and – conversely – the meaning of a particular space is emergent from the social interactions that take place in the space (McGrath, 2012).

Mental health wards are not just 'clinical spaces' or places for treatment. They are also juridical spaces, whose function is to separate and to attempt to 'same' individuals who have been rendered 'different' (Parr, 2008). Mental health wards have been argued to be spaces whose material makeup is permeated by a concern with risk, monitoring and observation (McGrath & Reavey, 2013; Rose, 1998) contributing to positioning users as 'risky' individuals in need of surveillance. The material and spatial make up of a mental health ward thus may be said to shape the experience of service use and the types of interactions that may take place in a ward.

In this chapter we draw on Michel Foucault's (1986, 1991) work on discipline and space to analyse the production of time, bodies and space in the smoking room. Fundamental to Foucault's argument is that discursive and non-discursive elements are intimately linked – and that the material and spatial context as well as a person's embodiment participate in the production of disciplinary power (McGrath & Reavey, 2013). Space plays a fundamental role in regulating and disciplining bodies (Foucault, 1991) and Foucault's analysis of the history of madness may essentially be read as a history of unreason being disciplined by reason through regulation of space, bodies and time (Parr, 2008).

Foucault's genealogical analyses have sometimes been interpreted as presenting a full picture of mental health care (Parr, 2008). Meanwhile, a 'totalising' application of Foucault's theories runs the risk of reducing the complexities of mental health practice to great unspecified patterns of domination (Barrett, 1996; Parr, 2008; Ringer, 2013a). Instead, as Parr (2008, p. 14) puts it, a Foucauldian analysis of mental health space must also make efforts to: 'rescue the mental patient from being an unreachable "other" in the history of the asylum, an "other" merely subjected and silenced into a docile body'. This provides an argument to select as our case the smoking room – a space produced as 'other', and not entirely 'institutional' by both professionals and users. By analysing a conflict between some users and professionals, we catch sight of how the smoking room exists by virtue of specific ways of disciplining time and bodies. At the same time the smoking room also becomes a platform for resistance, which allows for struggles to emerge for the right of access, ownership and self-determination.

The trouble in ward D

Ward D occupied one floor in a building surrounded by other mental health wards, next to a middle-sized town in Denmark. The ward had recently been refurbished and with its sparsely – but expensively – furnished clear spaces, it gave the impression of a modern clinic. It contained 14 single bedrooms for users, a staff room, a television room, a dining room, two rooms for conferences and conversations and an activity room with a table-tennis table, which usually stood folded by the door. The ward was a locked acute ward and the users were both voluntary users and users who were treated involuntarily. Individual user privileges, such as leave, no leave or assisted leave and the right to hold cigarettes were meticulously registered on a whiteboard in the staff room.

The smoking room was a glass booth adjacent to the outer wall of the ward, with grid flooring so smoke could escape. It did not contain any furniture, but the users would often sit directly on the grid-floor to smoke. Physically at once part of the ward and outside its walls, the entrance to the smoking room was located by the television room, with a glass door leading to it from the inside. As it was intended for users, and almost always remained 'staff-free' due to non-smoking workplace health regulations, many users would gather in the smoking room and sit for hours on the grid floor. The rules of the ward were many and included a ban on talking about distress, illness and medication, as the professionals believed this would confuse and worsen the users' condition. While the users therefore learned to regulate their topics of conversation in the other places of the ward, in the smoking room they could cover a range of 'forbidden' topics. They shared experiences of distress, discussed worries and thoughts about being at the ward, comforted each other, had disagreements and laughed together. Many users said they used the smoking room therapeutically to get 'peer-therapy' (Skorpen et al., 2008). One user said about the talks in the smoking room: 'We're not allowed to talk about each other's illnesses, but I've gotten more out of talking with the patients than with the staff [. . .] so we've really helped each other a lot'. Consequentially the smoking room played a symbolic role for many users, and it was produced as a 'private space' (McGrath, 2012; Ringer, 2013a) where they could negotiate topics of conversation without the influence of professionals.

The trouble in ward D began when the professionals attempted to introduce a ban on sitting down in the smoking room. The reason for enforcing the ban, they explained to me (AR), was that they wished to reduce the amount of time spent in the smoking room and prevent the formation of cliques among users. This rule was subject to debates both within the user group and during joint meetings between users and professionals. Two of the users who attended the smoking room frequently included a woman in her twenties, Hanna, and a man in his mid-thirties, Emil. We will explore the unfolding of events surrounding the smoking room by focusing on them.

During a staff morning meeting in the staff room, shortly after the introduction of the rule, the nurse, Amy, who had been away for some time, came back. She seemed upset and said that she had just been to the smoking room where she asked David, a service user and a friend of Hanna's, to stand up and not sit down. David got on his feet, but then Hanna, who had previously been standing in the smoking room, sat down right in front of the nurse. The nurse explained that she had asked Hanna to stand up, but Hanna had just replied calmly 'What's that to you?' Nothing like it had ever happened before and the nurses started discussing what to do. They all agreed that Hanna's behaviour was unacceptable and they discussed different ways of reacting. Amy's final remark was 'I thought 1–0 to Hanna, that triggers me, I want to win!'

Later that day, I (AR) heard Hanna discuss the ban on sitting down with Emil in the smoking room, asking him to support her aim by also sitting down when the nurses came. Emil agreed and they spent a part of the day sitting down in the room. During the joint meeting for users and professionals, Hanna complained that all the rules at the ward made her feel worse and that she was feeling very ill. Emil lent her support, calling the rules 'inflexible'. After the meeting, a nurse explained to me that she enjoys working with patients who are very ill – unlike Hanna. She said: 'patients who feel very bad don't think about these things' and stated that Hanna does not really belong at the ward. Two days later when I came to the ward, Hanna had been moved to another ward. The professionals called Hanna's displacement 'a punishment' and congratulated the ward psychiatrist on taking such a firm stance. They explained that Emil had attempted to protest Hanna's removal together with some of the other users, and they jokingly imitated Emil saying 'you only want to separate us'.

Time and space in the smoking room at ward D

The trouble in ward D raises questions such as: how may we understand the actions of the professionals and users in the case? Why does the conflict emerge and intensify? What type of a space constitutes the smoking room since it may trigger such strong reactions for both users and staff? A close analysis indicates that the conflict may be understood as a struggle about two fundamental aspects at a mental health ward: time and bodies. We will start by analysing negotiations of time, which is both an explicit and implicit presence in the case.

Time is a pivotal, though often invisible, factor at ward D. Time is constituent for institutional space (McGrath & Reavey, 2013). A mental health ward is not a *permanent place*. The time of discharge and the duration of hospitalisation is subject to negotiations (Ringer & Holen, 2015). While the users often have their own perception of when hospitalisation and discharge is useful, it is up to the professionals to decide the time frame for they stay. The time *inside* a mental health ward is equally regulated. The days are structured generically, as an ideal picture of how a healthy daily rhythm ought to look, for people who are well. This regulation of time is justified as being conducive to recovery and it is couched in biomedical terms: there is time for treatment, medication time, time for ward rounds and waiting time – all part of the vernacular of a hospital. These are all events in time and space that do not belong to a 'normal' everyday life, but that together constitute the space of the mental health ward, and the time spent in it, as 'treatment'. The ideal picture of normal everyday life, as well as the medical regime that governs life on the ward, participate in the disciplining of time at ward D. Understanding the time structure is crucial for understanding the space of a ward – and for being in the space. Service users who understand the time and space of the ward – i.e. who are able to navigate the unwritten rules by performing and 'citing' appropriate patterns of actions (Butler, 1990, 2004) become recognisable subjects who are understood as efficient and responsible individuals (Holen, 2011). For the users, observing the correct time frame is thus both a picture of one's competence in decoding the implicit norms of the institution, of performing 'patient' in intelligible ways (Holen, 2011; Ringer, 2013a), as well as a picture of one's state of health.

Disciplining time in the smoking room

Initially a hidden presence time became visible as an active participant in defining the smoking room, the time used in the smoking room turns out to be subject to regulation. As Hanna expresses in an interview, 'they have all those rules that for example: you're supposed to go into the smoking room, smoke your fag and then you're supposed to go back inside again'. The quote indicates that visits to the smoking room – i.e. the time spent in the room – is something the ward wishes to limit. The users must first and foremost 'go back inside again' as Hanna puts it. With the little word 'again' she indicates that it is the time spent in the other spaces of the ward that counts, while the time in the smoking room is regarded as 'outside'. In other words, the smoking room is out of line with the ward's time frame.

The ward's time frame is linked to space; for each room there are specific activities, which all have a scheduled timetable. The users' bedrooms are for users to stay in at night; here they should sleep and rest. The sitting room is for sitting in during the day, the dining room is for dining. Yet other rooms are for having meetings, and there are rooms for the professionals to discuss the treatment. In addition to having specific functions, these rooms also exist by virtue of time. There are time frames for when to sleep, when to rise, when to have joint meetings, when to eat and when to have activities such as the daily walk. And there is a time frame for when users can relax and have a good time, by watching television in the television room.

This division and classification of time is important in ward D. In contrast, uncontrollable time – time that is wasted, time that is blurry and fluid – becomes unproductive time, which poses a problem. The daily rhythm of many of the service users is understood in this way, as fluid and undisciplined (many users are unemployed), which intensifies the need for creating structured and productive time on the ward. Foucault notes that the invention of the timetable came about based on a 'principle of non-idleness' (Foucault, 1991, p. 135) to shield against the risk of wasting time, which increasingly became a despicable sin with the development of capitalist societies. Maintaining a productive timetable thus also becomes a moral issue. On the ward, the fact that the institution has to put at the users' disposal a space without a productive function, out of line with the ward's timetable, makes the time the users spend in the smoking room inherently problematic. The time spent in the smoking room cannot be scheduled or made subject to a timetable. Since it has no clinical function, the time spent in the smoking room can only become 'a waste of time'. Rather than asking *why* many users apparently wish to occupy such a space for such a long time, it becomes necessary to intensify discipline of the time spent there.

Negotiations of smoking time

For the users, on the other hand, smoking is not useless or a waste of time. Smoking is indeed considered very productive, as it is a way to pass time in ward D. As Emil expresses it:

> You're bored as hell, the others sit as passive mongols and sit, sit and paint all day, and what's there to do? Smoke fags, smoke fags, smoke fags. You're all alone, everyone has their own stuff they're struggling with, don't they? (mm) so they [the professionals] don't have the time or energy to start with you.

Despite attempts to structure the time at the ward, much of the service users' actual time is spent waiting. As Emil says, they are bored, which indicates that the service users do not necessarily share the professionals' experience of the time on the ward being filled up. The professionals, on the other hand, are busy with their timetables and activities, and initiatives that fall outside of their planned and standardised time and which are difficult to reconcile with their work – in the words of Emil, 'they don't have time [. . .] to start with you'.

Meanwhile, because smoking is a need that the users have independently of the professionals' timetable, it gives the professionals a special authority over the time in the smoking room. Emil tells of an episode when he was not allowed to keep his own cigarettes, but was dependent on the staff's goodwill in providing him with them. However, Emil's approaching the professionals and asking for cigarettes was considered a problem and he was often ignored or told they did not have time. Thus, it was construed as a disruption of the professionals' work and time, since smoking is an activity that does not have a timetable. Without a regulation of time, the smoking room is unscheduled, undisciplined, unproductive and the time in it is not guarded by distinct rules.

On the one hand, the smoking room thus has completely different temporal dimensions than the rest of the spaces of the ward. On the other, these temporal dimensions are also subject to similar discipline and regulation found in other spaces on the ward. Thus, the time in the smoking room participates in constituting the room as a space simultaneously separate and part of the ward. In the next section we will see that the users' and professionals' bodies similarly play a part in constituting the special space of the smoking room.

Smoking bodies in the space of ward D

The bodies of both professionals and users participate in producing the smoking room as an 'other' space. The users' bodies remain static for hours at a time in the smoking room, sometimes smoking, sometimes just talking. In no other spaces of the ward do the users gather and interact with each other for such long periods. All other places on the ward are potentially spaces of 'treatment' where the users are 'being treated' and the professionals are treating them (McGrath, 2012).

Because the smoking room has no clinical function it occupies a special position in the experiences of users; it is a space perhaps produced more as 'theirs' than any other part of the ward. The professionals also participate in producing the smoking room as 'other' – specifically by their bodies' tangible absence. In all other spaces of the ward, their access is self-evident; the professionals effortlessly walk into the activity room, enter the TV room, sit down in the dining room and during scheduled rounds they even effortlessly enter the users' bedrooms. Additionally, they carry with them a material artefact – a key – which indicates access to spaces of the ward that are out of bounds for users, such as the medical cabinet and the kitchen. However, while the professionals have keys and bodies that may enter the other spaces of the ward unhindered, the smoking room is the one space of the ward where their access becomes constrained. Since they are not allowed to smoke at work, the professionals have no role to play in the smoking room. Indeed, if they enter at all, it is only very briefly to open the door, stop by the entrance and call on one of the users. The stopping by the door indicates that their body's presence in the smoking room is not self-evident or clear. Quite the contrary, it becomes uncomfortable, out of place. Meanwhile the users' bodies also react when a professionals enters; they tend to become silent and tense, waiting for the person to leave. The smoking room thus constitutes the only room on the ward where the only bodies that have a naturalised presence belong to the users.

The battle over bodies

Apart from the issue of access, bodies play another important role in the case. Disciplining of time in the smoking room is attempted by regulating the position of users' bodies; the professionals demand that users stand up rather than sit down. Foucault notes that the posture of standing upright culturally constitutes part of a 'bodily rhetoric of honor' (Foucault, 1991, p. 135). As the erect position of army recruits, the posture simultaneously signals alertness and obedience. Conversely, sitting down may signal idleness, inactivity and possibly uselessness (Foucault, 1991, p. 154). Here, we may trace how the disciplining of bodies and the disciplining of time in the smoking room intersects. Whereas standing upright indicates a fleeting, momentary state, where one is ready to start moving at any time, there is no predicting how long a person may remain, once sat down.

Perhaps because of its association with idleness, the act of sitting down carries with it political connotations. In political movements, sitting down has been a way of expressing civil disobedience in the face of power – as in the case of Rosa Parks' refusal to leave a white-only bus seat during the Jim Crow era, or sit-in demonstrations, where protestors sit down to promote political or social change. When Hanna chooses to sit down in the smoking room, she invokes a culturally recognisable expression of passive resistance, an insistence that she has the right to occupy the space. This way, her body becomes a means of protest, and she constructs the smoking room as 'hers' – a comfortable place to stay, not a lay-by to depart from, suddenly.

While these practices of resistance surely must have been frustrating for the professionals, this does not account for the decision to move Hanna to another ward. Hanna was hardly the only user who used her body to express disagreement with staff. Other users would even occasionally scream at or hit professionals. These types of violent actions would lead to users being belt-strapped[2] or secluded – but they did not lead to removals from the ward, which in the hierarchy of sanctions is used only for the worst transgressions (Skorpen et al., 2008, p. 735). How, then, may the unusually hard sanction for Hanna be accounted for? With users whose bodies resorted to violence, the professionals usually agreed that they were 'acting out' some inner core of 'illness' and instability (Ringer & Holen, 2015). In this way, a biomedical discourse could provide the resource for making sense of their actions. However, the problem with Hanna seems to be that her nonviolent sitting down did not follow the recognisable pattern of 'patient acting out'. Her actions could not be meaningfully understood within the usual framework of illness and risk. This in itself calls into question the very legitimacy of her position as a patient, and the professionals start questioning whether she is ill enough to stay on the ward.

However, there seems to be another, even more subversive, aspect to Hanna's actions. In his discussion of disciplinary power, Foucault (1991) argues that modern power works not by violence and incarceration, but by individualising, partitioning and dividing among individuals. Close personal ties between users are discouraged on the ward, and the users are assessed, monitored and treated individually. Precautionary measures and unwritten rules serve to regulate users' bodies' proximity to one another; users are not allowed to share details of emotional distress with each other; they may not engage in sexual relationships; and they are not allowed in each other's rooms. This way, close intimacy is discouraged, contributing to an individualising of each user. When Hanna asks Emil to back her in her struggle and encourages him to position his body like hers, this may be seen as a challenge to these very practices of division and individualising. She may be said to summon Emil to act with her as one collective body. Such a call challenges the very premise of the institution: that users must be separated and divided from each other. From this perspective, it is not so much Hanna's resistance to the rules that becomes unacceptable – but rather her refusal to be individualised. As the health care worker, Marie, explains: 'Hanna might be too well to be here. Patients who feel bad don't think about these things'.

Conclusion

Our analysis has indicated how space should not merely be regarded as a container for actions and subjects, but as matter that is constituted by, and participates in the production of interactions, meaning and subject positions. This chapter illuminates how the smoking room's 'in-between status' creates a space for other ways of being and acting which are deemed separate from the other spaces of the ward. If we follow the argument that the material participates in the production of subjectivity, the smoking room becomes a space that provides occasion for other types of positioning than 'patient being treated'. In the smoking room, bodies that are otherwise separated and divided may become collective bodies, which potentially stand together more strongly and defiantly.

However, while the smoking room is produced as 'other' it is not clearly demarcated from the other spaces of the ward. The analysis illustrates that the space of the smoking room is constituted by negotiations of access. Some bodies are allowed access to the smoking room (users who smoke); other bodies are granted the right to monitor from outside (professionals). Yet other bodies are neither allowed to peek in nor enter the room (users who do not smoke). Even the bodies that have access do not have unlimited access (regulation of time). It is by virtue of these patterns that the smoking room is constituted as a disciplinary space.

We may read the struggles surrounding the smoking room as struggles for territories, for the right to define, to possess the room, to produce a framework of time and shape bodily engagement with the space. The fact that the negotiations give rise to an intensified struggle over bodies and time – resulting in the removal of Hanna, indicating that the room is far from that of a 'free' space. Meanwhile its status as 'other' or 'in-between' allows for an aspect of liberation – it is 'free' enough to allow for the possibility of the existence of a struggle for ownership. It is precisely within these negotiations of access, discipline and resistance that the space becomes the smoking room.

Notes

1 To preserve anonymity, the name of the ward as well as all participants are pseudonyms.
2 Belt-strapping as a means of restraint is legal and still applied in the Danish mental health services.

References

Barrett, R. (1996). *The psychiatric team and the social definition of schizophrenia: An anthropological study of person and illness.* New York, NY: Cambridge University Press.
Butler, J. (1990). *Gender trouble: Feminism and the subversion of identity.* New York, NY: Routledge.
Butler, J. (2004). *Undoing gender.* New York, NY and London: Routledge.
Foucault, M. (1986). Of other spaces. *Diacritics, 16*(1), 22–27.
Foucault, M. (1991). *Discipline and punish: The birth of the prison.* London: Penguin.
Holen, M. (2011). *Medinddragelse og lighed – en god idé? En analyse af patienttilblivelser i det moderne hospital.* Roskilde, Denmark: Roskilde University.
Latour, B. (2005). *Reassembling the social: An introduction to actor-network-theory.* Oxford: Oxford University Press.
McGrath, L. (2012). *Heterotopias of mental health care: The role of space in experiences of distress, madness and mental health service use.* London: South Bank University.
McGrath, L., & Reavey, P. (2013). Heterotopias of control: Placing the material in experiences of mental health service use and community living. *Health and Place, 22,* 123–131.
Parr, H. (2008). *Mental health and social space: Towards inclusionary geographies.* Malden, MA: Blackwell.

Ringer, A. (2013a). *Listening to patients: A study of illness discourses, patient identities, and user involvement in contemporary psychiatric practice*. Roskilde, Denmark: Roskilde University.

Ringer, A. (2013b). Researcher-participant positioning and the discursive work of categories: Experiences from fieldwork in the mental health services. *Qualitative Studies, 4*(1), 1–20.

Ringer, A., & Holen, M. (2015). 'Hell no, they'll think you're mad as a hatter': Illness discourses and their implications for patients in mental health practice. *Health, 20*(2), 161–175.

Rose, N. (1998). Governing risky individuals: The role of psychiatry in new regimes of control. *Psychiatry, Psychology and Law, 5*(2), 177–195.

Skorpen, A., Anderssen, N., Oeye, C., & Bjelland, A. K. (2008). The smoking-room as psychiatric patients' sanctuary: A place for resistance. *Journal of Psychiatric and Mental Health Nursing, 15*(9), 728–736.

Terkelsen, T. B. (2009). Transforming subjectivities in psychiatric care. *Subjectivity, 27*(1), 195–216.

Thomas, S. P., Shattell, M., & Martin, T. (2002). What's therapeutic about the therapeutic milieu? *Archives of Psychiatric Nursing, XVI*(3), 99–107.

2

MADLOVE

A designer asylum

Anna Zorwaska

How would patients design the ideal asylum?

> WHAT IS MADLOVE? Is it possible to go mad in a positive way? How would you create a safe place in which to do so? If you designed your own asylum, what would it look like?
>
> Madlove is a project by the vacuum cleaner (in collaboration with Hannah Hull) based on his personal experience of mental health hospitals, and his desire to find a positive space to experience mental distress . . . and enlightenment.
>
> *(www.madlove.org.uk)*

This is how we are introduced to the project that artists 'the vacuum cleaner' (aka James Leadbitter) and Hannah Hull are now developing. A blueprint for a 'designer asylum' was presented at the Wellcome Collection in September 2016, and an interactive beta-version was exhibited at FACT, Liverpool, in Spring 2015 as a part of a larger project called 'Group Therapy: Mental Distress in a Digital Age'.

For artists 'the vacuum cleaner' and Hannah Hull this project is not just an artistic provocation and self-affirmation. 'Madlove' brings together people with and without mental health experiences in an attempt to create a temporary structure that will be a reflective and responsive space for exploring and redesigning our perceptions around 'madness' (Figure 2.1). Positive change is the most important goal of this project, and anyone is encouraged to participate and share their experiences and suggestions on how to make the environment of psychiatric wards more positive, safe and user-friendly.

This is a good moment to tell you who I am and how I know any of this. I am Anna Zagorska – the 'Madlove' trainee from Latvia. Since October 2014 I have been working with 'the vacuum cleaner' and Hannah Hull as a project

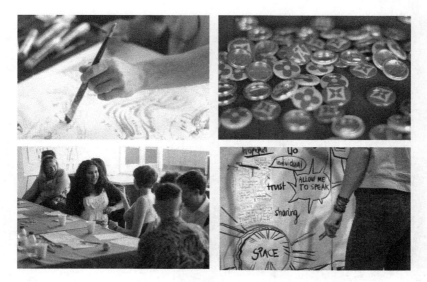

FIGURE 2.1 Madlove workshops: London, Hull, Liverpool.

assistant, taking part in four of seven 'Madlove' workshops, supporting the documentation of the workshops (Figure 2.2). This amazing and extraordinary experience gave me an insight into the creation process of the 'Madlove: A Designer Asylum'.

Since 2014, more than 200 people from diverse backgrounds and with different mental health experiences have contacted the 'Madlove' team with many

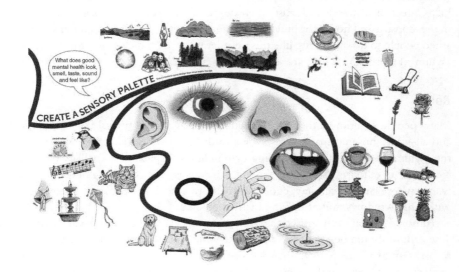

FIGURE 2.2 Illustration of the task 'create a sensory palette'.

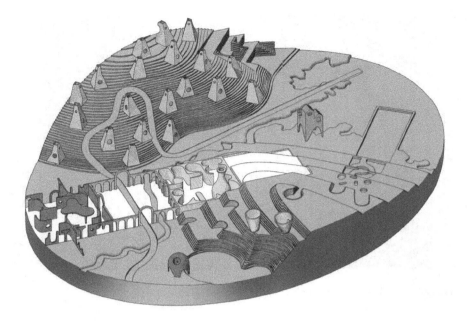

FIGURE 2.3 Illustration of a possible Madlove asylum.

reasonable and practical, imaginative, creative and extraordinary suggestions on how to create the 'designer asylum'.

Some of you probably know the popular simulation video game 'The Sims' where the player creates virtual people called 'Sims', places them in houses and helps direct their moods and satisfy their desires. Players can either place their Sims in pre-constructed homes or build the home themselves. Leadbitter and Hull have asked people to do something like this in order to develop the designs for the 'ideal asylum' (Figure 2.3). These are some of their findings.

Bones

Many people mentioned that they would love to avoid the typical clinical, sterile and all-white hospital space, with its labyrinth of corridors. The general space of the asylum should be a large building or building complex; like a village of giant teepees or tree houses. Someone else suggested an asylum consisting of houses not wards, where families can stay, cook, eat and normalise. It should be an open space, with large windows, full of light and varied colours.

Almost everyone emphasised the importance of access to green areas and nature. The asylum should be located in the countryside with lots of sheep or have access to parks and gardens with fountains, ponds with frogs, bird feeders and butterfly gardens, greenhouses and spaces for growing vegetables, plants and herbs.

The 'designer asylum' should have varied spaces for varied needs: quiet and empty; noisy and chaotic; soft and comfortable; large, light and open; small dark and enclosed. People emphasised how important it is to separate the Private spaces (yes, with capital 'P') and communal spaces, e.g. communal cooking and eating areas.

People should be able to personalise their private rooms, e.g. change the colour of the walls in their rooms, have a room that glows in the dark, have a lighting system connected to the mood of the sounds made, the ability to choose smells and sounds around them, etc. However, some of the suggestions were more modest, e.g. it would be helpful if patients could be allowed to sleep with something of their own – pillow, duvet or stuffed animal, or simply a good quality bed and mattress.

Some people shared their negative experiences of how they were locked out of their room to make them socialise with others (and this 'socialising' consisted of watching overly loud TV or something equally terrifying). The priority of the 'designer asylum' should be respect towards patients' privacy and safety; it should feel safe, supporting, comforting and sustainable.

Flesh

Many imaginative, playful and creative ideas were suggested around the specific spaces in the 'designer asylum'. A common one was a 'soundproof room' for screaming, creating and listening to music. Someone suggested that this soundproof room should function as a recording booth where one can record everything he or she is thinking and use some easy and visual processes to work with those thoughts afterwards.

Another common space suggested for the perfect asylum was a 'washable paint room' where one can explode with colour and easily wash it away when the emotions have been expressed.

For those who need to rid themselves of tension, anger and destructive energy, there should be a stylised 'padded cell', a room where everything is unbreakable, something like an adults' version of a soft playground for children, where you can rant and rave and not damage anything.

In contrast, someone suggested a very simple space – a room where you can hide from everyone else and be alone. This place could be with blocked WiFi and phone signals.

Books, films and music were considered to be a common and important part of the ideal asylum, so there should be a library and the option to watch films and listen to music. In this library there should be a person who can suggest the book you need precisely at that moment and in that state of mind – the 'London black cab driver of books' as someone wittily called it. A step closer to nirvana would be a space where you can listen to music while floating in shallow water.

Blood

Just being in this asylum space is not enough, so people suggested a list of activities that should be a 'must do' for people using the service. Many people emphasised the importance of physical activities – gym, yoga and dance classes, swimming, etc. One person said: 'The arts and education are ways that people can re-establish their identity after going through a system that can really remove all sense of identity.' Different ideas circulated regarding the education and activities, e.g. sharing discussions with other people with mental health experiences, philosophy classes and discussion groups, art and music classes, different kinds of occupational therapy where a sense of achievement could be achieved in a short period of time.

Spirit

'Madlove: A Designer Asylum' is all about kindness, humanity and safety for people who seek asylum. What would be a perfectly designed space with advanced technologies and cool activities without the loving atmosphere? Pets, joyful children, professional huggers and very, very kind helpers are what this space needs the most. People suggested that the general atmosphere should be safe, calm, honest and hopeful. Someone summed it up: 'Asylum should be a place to grow and make new steps. A place to hide from everyone else.' Let's not forget that this is what an 'asylum' means – sanctuary, refuge, a safe place to hide.

3

CHILDREN'S SPACES OF MENTAL HEALTH

Users' experiences of two contrasting child and adolescent mental health outpatients in the UK

Sarah Crafter

Introduction

A series of recent reports examining at the provision of child and adolescent mental health services (CAMHS) in England all point to a service that is under-resourced, over-stretched and in crisis (Children's Commissioner, 2016; Frith, 2016; House of Commons, 2014). Against this backdrop there is some evidence to suggest that there is a significant rise in children's mental health problems (Frith, 2016). The last compelling evidence regarding children and young people's mental health prevalence came from an Office for National Statistics study in 2004. That study, which was discontinued, found 1 in 10 children aged 5–16 years old could be classed as having a mental 'disorder'. Understandably, the aforementioned reports have focused most of their energy on discussing the most pressing issues: the lack of reliable information surrounding children's mental health, the problematic cuts to community prevention schemes, poor waiting times and limited access to outpatient CAMHS services and concerns about the quality and safety within inpatient services. The role of space, or the users' experiences of the 'therapeutic landscape' (Curtis, Gesler, Priebe, & Francis, 2009) do not feature as part of the 'crisis-point' discussions around CAMHS services.

On the one hand, it is understandable that issues of space and design are not one of the key issues concerning a service under strain. However, it is important not to ignore the role of space and materiality in users' experiences of mental health care because space plays a key role in users' subjective involvement in the service (McGrath & Reavey, 2013). A number of commentators have argued, either through descriptions of the 'therapeutic milieu' (Golembiewski, 2010) or through the concept of 'therapeutic landscapes' (Wood et al., 2013), that mental health spaces are a complex interaction between people and the social, material and symbolic environment. In essence, the built environment has an impact on both the physical and the psychological (Evans, 2003). However, much of the work that has looked at mental health spaces has focused on adult settings, while child and adolescent mental health services remain as under-explored as they are under-resourced, particularly outpatient settings. This chapter focuses on users' experiences of the space and built environment of two CAMHS outpatient spaces situated in different towns in the UK. This interrogation will take into account the ways in which conceptualisations of children's mental health, space and constructions of childhood interact with each one.

Children's mental health spaces: an area of neglect

There is little known evidence regarding how outpatient CAMHS services came to occupy particular institutional spaces. Any reference to the historical changes of CAMHS as a service has focused on the impact of changes in policy development (Cottrell & Kraam, 2005). In line with recent approaches to hospital design (Gesler, Bell, Curtis, Hubbard, & Francis, 2004), there appears to have been no coherent agenda associated with the choice of built environment for CAMHS clinic spaces. Outpatient CAMHS services, usually described as Tier 3 provision, exist to provide specialist services for children and young people with moderate to severe mental health needs, and is the key focus of this chapter. Tier 4 provides very specialist services to a small number of children with mental health difficulties, usually in inpatient and residential settings. Tier 1 and Tier 2 focus on a wider group of children who may be vulnerable to mental health difficulties and combine services from education, social care and health. Outpatient CAMHS offers an interesting point of study because people do not stay in the building for prolonged periods of time, as one would in an inpatient setting. Visits are comparatively fleeting, as people come and go for appointment times. The connection, therefore, between the different spaces that users occupy, may have a permeability as they cross the boundaries between other contexts, such as home and the clinic. Although it is a dedicated children's service, it is not a community service per se, as visiting is dependent upon referral. Finally, children may come alone for therapies, or have therapy with the whole family, parent or guardian.

There has been greater attention toward the meanings associated with adult mental health spaces than child-related settings. While adult asylum settings are quite different from children's settings, there remain synergies regarding the highly symbolic and emotional investments in the built environment (Parr, Philo, & Burns, 2003) that are worth exploring. The role of materiality and the implications this has for practices and discourses around risk and danger are particularly salient and have been raised by a number of commentators (McGrath & Reavey, 2013). Emphasis is placed on what McGrath and Reavey (2013) describe as 'risky materiality', where risk is supposedly reduced by including safety observations, locks and barriers and overt staff surveillance, but that can, in fact, enhance a sense of the space as 'risky'. In a review of literature looking across studies on architecture and mental health (Connellan et al., 2013), themes around 'security' and safety were always about keeping staff safe, with little focus on keeping patients safe. Perhaps, this is in part because issues of aggression have been a key concern in adult inpatient settings (Bowers et al., 2005) in ways that might not be relevant for child settings. Yet this chapter will argue that risky materiality features strongly as part of outpatient child and adolescent clinic experiences.

There are other material elements, beyond risk and security measures, which make it hard to deliver therapeutic interventions (Curtis et al., 2013). Interior design features such as light, noise and décor, connect with our emotional experiences or 'place feelings' and enhance health outcomes (Hart, 1997; Ulrich, Zimring, Quan, Joseph, & Choudhary, 2004; Vaaler, Morken, & Linaker, 2005). There has been a growing body of work that has focused on the relationship between health, healing and the built environment and space. These are usually applied to physical health settings but they have found that patients are sensitive to their environment and particularly disliked the lack of control for noise, temperature and light levels (Lawson & Phiri, 2003).

As previously mentioned, much of this work has taken place in adult settings. Children and young people's perspectives on their experiences of internal spaces is relatively rare (James & Curtis, 2012). However, research from hospitals, schools and nurseries provide some sources of information, and the issues raised in those settings do bear some resemblance to problems associated with child mental health contexts. For children of all ages, hospitals can be associated with fear, anxiety and unfamiliarity and should seek to be more child-centred (Lambert, Coad, Hicks, & Glacken, 2013). It may be suggested that mental health settings might amplify such fears because of the stigma associated with social representations of mental health (Ohlsson, 2016). In hospitals, children particularly disliked the lack of control over their space (Birch, Curtis, & James, 2007). They were not able to make changes to noise, temperature or light levels and bedtimes and lights out were a cause for complaint (James & Curtis, 2012).

In studies looking at both hospital and educational settings, colour and comfort are usually key considerations (Ghaziani, 2008; Kraftl & Adey, 2008). Such settings have often attempted to imbue spaces with a sense of 'homeliness', comfort and peace that are strongly associated with affect, and link to feelings of protection. When asked their opinion, children often report wanting bright, colourful spaces (Birch et al., 2007) though in one study, children chose gender-neutral colours alongside artwork (Lambert et al., 2013). Such design features can be contentious in mental health settings because for some therapeutic approaches, colour is said to impact the therapeutic process. In adult mental health settings, particularly inpatient settings, the emotional meanings invested in the building are a great challenge to developing a sense of 'homeliness'. Those features of risky materiality, such as long corridors, heavy doors, locks and cameras, can add to the 'impersonalness' of institutions (Parr et al., 2003). Such features are even more problematic when looking at children's mental health services.

Constructions of childhood: the risky child and the vulnerable child

The discourse of risk in relation to adult mental health has been an area of discussion for some time (Moon, 2000) and in more recent years has become associated with the debate surrounding asylum and community care (Curtis et al., 2009; McGrath & Reavey, 2016). When the focus is on children's mental health spaces, discussions about space are inextricably linked to the often complex and contradictory ways that 'children' and 'childhood' are constructed (Burman, 2008). Commentators working in the sociology of childhood and critical-developmental psychology have been discussing the binaries associated with how society constructs or represents childhood and children across a variety of settings, topics and situations (Burman, 2008; James & Prout, 1997). So, on the one hand, children are seen as vulnerable, innocent and in need of protection and, on the other hand, viewed as dangerous, risky and requiring surveillance. The former maps on to societal ideas of the 'ideal childhood' whereby, under careful adult supervision, children enjoy a life that revolves around school, play and socialisation (Jans, 2004). However, children whose lives transgress these representational boundaries become 'othered' and push the limit of adult concerns (O'Dell, Brownlow, & Bertilsdotter Rosqvist, 2017).

There are a number of examples of 'othered' children within the wider literature that may enact similar meanings for children with mental health needs. A study by Crawley (2011) researching separated migrant children is a good example of how contestations of age boundaries mark them as sitting outside the boundaries of 'childhood'. Experiences of trauma and rape, particularly if that resulted in pregnancy, often led asylum claims being turned down because children were too 'adult-like'. Or, separated migrant children are often talked about as being 'risky' and therefore treated, because of their experience and status, as akin to an adult (Bryan & Denov, 2011; Rosen & Crafter, in submission). Similar phenomenon can be seen in other areas of experience, such as children whose supposed innocence is 'lost' after child sexual abuse, thereby putting them into a grey area between adulthood and childhood (O'Dell, 2008). Child language brokers, children and young people who translate for family following migration, are often positioned as 'parentified' because of their extended knowledge of family 'adult' matters such as banking and finance (Cline, Abreu, O'Dell, & Crafter, 2010; Weisskirch, 2007). Young people are often excluded from outside spaces such as streets and neighbourhoods because they are perceived as a risky presence (Gough & Franch, 2005) inciting 'moral panic' within the neighbourhood (Lucas, 1998). In these examples, social representations of the risky child (as too adult-like) is conflated with spaces that the 'risky' child might occupy (e.g. the streets). It is argued that the same conflations are evident for children who attend mental health services for their mental health needs.

This study was designed to fill the gap in published research by looking at both the users' experiences of a CAMHS outpatient space and the ways in which their experiences are mediated by conceptualisations of 'childhood' when those children occupy 'othered' positions through their mental health diagnosis.

The study

This chapter draws from a wider qualitative study aiming to explore how staff, parents and children and young people experienced their CAMHS built environment (Crafter, Prokopiou, & Stein, 2010).[1] The team collected data from two CAMHS outpatient clinics in different towns within the same NHS primary care trust. Both offered an interesting point of comparison because they were situated in two very different buildings. Clinic A had been occupied by CAMHS for a number of years and was placed in a building with other health services (doctors and dentists). The CAMHS team occupied the second floor and contained a very small waiting room, a reception window with a room behind it, (which housed the office staff), eight therapy rooms and a small kitchen. The clinic was located in the centre of town near a central pedestrian area with shops at the front and parkland at the back.[2]

Clinic B occupied its own building, which was fairly old and had been specially redesigned and decorated for its purpose. It was located a little way out of the centre of the town, requiring roughly a 15-minute walk from central transport. There was a busy dual carriageway on one side and a housing area on the other. There was little in the way of available parking facilities. Clinic B was quite a bit larger than clinic A, with a comfortably large waiting room, reception for office staff and three floors. The first two floors had 12 therapy rooms and the top floor was used as office space for the clinical staff.

The style and design of the therapy rooms was very similar in both clinics, offering a largely sparse but functional space (see Figure 3.1).

The participants

This chapter will focus on the one-to-one interviews with the staff, parents/carers and children/young people, all of whom were attendees of the two outpatient

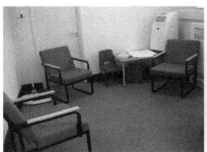 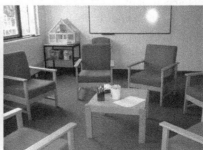

FIGURE 3.1 Clinic A (left) and clinic B (right).

TABLE 3.1 Number of participants by clinic and sample group

Clinic	Child	Parent	Staff
Clinic A	6	16	13
Clinic B	6	13	11

CAMHS clinics. Table 3.1 gives a breakdown of the number of participants who were interviewed.

The youngest child interviewed in the clinics was 11 years of age and the oldest was 18. In clinic A, five of the children were White British or White European, one child was Black Caribbean and one child had a mixed heritage. All the children interviewed in clinic B were either White British or White European. All the interviews undertaken for this project were conducted in the clinics where the therapy took place. Staff were interviewed in the therapy rooms or their offices (if they had one). Parents were interviewed in vacant therapy rooms while their child was having their therapeutic appointment.

Analysis

Data were analysed using a thematic coding technique to look for patterns of similarity and difference across the participants' experiences. In the original report, our analysis focused on different areas or built environment features addressing the 'organisational structure', 'internal space', 'outside space' and 'work space'. The data within this chapter focuses specifically on the 'internal space', inclusive of the waiting room, corridors and therapy rooms.

Analysis: the role of internal spaces for staff, parents and young people

Quite a significant amount of previous work on adult mental health asylum experiences have recognised the underlying uncertainty and trepidation of entering into, or being part of these spaces. Parr (2008) for example, describes the stigma and anxiety she felt attending counselling in an adolescent psychology department located in a hospital asylum. These feelings are not only relevant to inpatient settings, but were felt keenly by some of our interviewees attending the outpatient setting. Moreover, the stigma and anxiety felt by attendees also extended to the parents and guardians who accompany their children. This quote by the father of a 9-year-old boy attending CAMHS, suggests a range of broader symbolic associations between child and adolescent mental health spaces and other institutional spaces:

> You wonder what it's gonna [going to] be like because, I mean, what's its name, 'mental health' so you don't know quite what to expect and it's a bit like, behind glass doors you know, it reminds me of a benefit office or

somewhere where they expect you to be violent people so, I don't know, maybe they are (laughs) . . . yeah um, it's a Government run State thingy that you're . . . um yeah it implies you're, it's almost, it's got that atmosphere of um, you're coming for a service that we need to protect ourselves from you (laughs) yeah?

(Glenn, parent, clinic B)

Spaces and places can have a deeply powerful impact on our sense of identity, and are replete with symbolic meanings (Taylor, 2009). For Glenn, CAMHS signified a range of associations with places of institutional officialdom that represent the State, governance, control and power. The resulting 'atmosphere', he seems to suggest, is a space where the attendees are expected to be dangerous and violent, which the service needs to protect itself from. On the other hand, the clients of this service are children and the principle purpose of the service is to care for vulnerable children. It is this tension between the space, symbolic associations and constructions of childhood that form the analytic focus here.

The analysis is going to first focus on the talk by users of these two CAMHS clinics, noting that their discussions tend to concentrate on their CAMHS clinic as spaces of neglect or spaces of risky materiality. This is not to say that parents and children were not grateful for their treatment, or cognisant of the fact that CAMHS had no money for improving the space and built environment. However, it is argued that their talk about the space is indicative of the broader negative associations with mental health that take on a different type of exacerbation that intersects with representations of the 'child' and 'childhood'.

Space, materiality of neglect and a sense of 'homeliness'

Running through a number of respondents' commentaries was an inferred link between the indicative valued placed on the service and the meanings associated with the material space. Vanessa, a clinical psychologist, was a member of staff from clinic B. When asked about the therapy rooms she replied:

I think they're OK, they're not brilliant, they're, well some of them, the décor could be better, some of them. Well, the room downstairs the wall is all damp which is not, it doesn't give a good impression, it's not good . . . I think some of the clinical rooms need updating, they're a bit you know, the carpets are a bit dirty, the toys are, well, some of the rooms the toys are a bit like a jumble sale, you know, or from a charity shop. Well they need, they need sorting out, there needs to be decent cupboards for toys but I think they're fairly minor things.

(Vanessa, staff, clinic B)

Vanessa ends her list by suggesting that these are 'minor things'. In many ways Vanessa is probably right, that individually the dampness, décor, dirty carpets and jumble-sale toys are a collection of low-level or minor features of the material space. However, collectively, they paint of picture of a space of neglect. As discussed earlier, many material spaces associated with children, such as nurseries, primary schools and children's wards in hospitals, have focused on imbuing the space with associations of comfort and care (Ghaziani, 2008; Kraftl & Adey, 2008). Such landscapes of care are clearly not evident in Vanessa's description of this mental health space. Smith, a young person aged 15, was asked how he felt the building might affect his treatment. He replied:

> Well if it's really messy and disgusting then you wouldn't feel as if you're getting any better but if it's bright and colourful and it's great then you'd feel more as I say you'd feel as if you're feeling much better . . . and you'll recover quicker.
>
> *(Smith, child, Dunstable)*

Smith talked about 'messy' and 'disgusting' as being synonymous with a lack of therapeutic progress. From his perspective, you might be 'getting better', but you 'wouldn't feel' as if you were getting better. His reference to colour was not unusual across the whole sample but was particularly salient for the children and young people's responses to questions about the internal space. This reflects a similar finding in the small amount of research set in children's hospitals (Birch et al., 2007; Lambert et al., 2013). All the children, with one exception, valued colour. As Sarah, who was 15 years old and had been attending the clinic for 5 months said, "The rooms are quite cosy but they're not, they don't have attractive colours so um they could be improved" (Sarah, child, clinic B). Rivva-mae, who was 12 years old, made a more direct connection between colour, affect and mental health:

> I: *How does this building affect how you see your treatment here?*
>
> Um it sort of makes me a bit upset because it's not as nice and colourful as I would like it to be 'cause when you come here, you'd like it to be colourful, a bit more cheery . . . I think the people who come here should, because they're very upset, I think they should have like a bit more colour in the rooms to sort of make you feel a bit more happier.
>
> *(Rivva-Mae, child, clinic B)*

Rivva-Mae had, at the time of interview, only attended two appointments, therefore her experience of the space was relatively fresh and new. For her, the use of colour in the space did not signify that a setting where the aim was to make you feel 'cheery'. When the children were asked to both draw and describe their ideal internal CAMHS space, they too put an emphasis on materiality that enhanced feelings of 'homeliness'. Equally though, they maintained a very functional or practical approach to the therapeutic space. For example, they nearly all included the usual furniture, such as a table (for doing drawings usually) and chairs. Sarah, from clinic B, also mentioned having a dark carpet, which wouldn't show stains so easily. To this they added, couches/sofas, plants or flowers, large windows offering nice views, a 'playing table' for young children, posters and paintings (similar to what you might see in school) and in one case, a welcome mat. The wall colours were invariably chosen for their relaxing qualities: blues, greens or purples because they are relaxing, orange for Dillen (aged 15) because it is both bright but gender neutral. Overall, the prevailing desire was for an atmosphere of 'homeliness' signifying a permeability in the boundaries between the outpatient clinic and other significant contexts like 'home'.

The desire from the children for a more 'homely' or comforting space sat in direct conflict with the therapeutic needs of some of the staff and may explain the very functional and 'adult-like' approach within the clinics. Some therapeutic approaches would hold that room colour, pictures and other symbols of materiality could impact on the therapy. This was the case for Vanessa, the clinical psychologist: "I would want rooms to be plain, I wouldn't want pictures on the walls 'cause I think that could interfere with the therapy as well so . . ." (Vanessa, staff, Luton). In Vanessa's descriptions of her ideal space, the therapy is foreground above a space orientated to the material needs of children, so often sought in other children's spaces. Alexis, a systemic family therapist with a background in social work, held a different perspective and would have been pleased to personalise a room. When asked what she liked least about the building she replied:

> [N]ot having a space which is mine, err, I mean when I would have my own room, I didn't – I'd be glad [to have] my own clinical room, I can then, I could put up my pictures full of [Nelson] Mandela, you know, I had, I made it as multi-cultural as I could because the County's bloody awful at that. But now I can't create my own personal space.
>
> *(Alexis, staff, clinic A)*

Alexis oscillates between describing a time when she had her own designated room and the current situation where staff constantly had to move to different rooms throughout the day. Her own interest in issues of cultural diversity meant that when she had her own room, she could tailor the wall decorations to reflect this. Additionally, she found it helped the therapy because the children would ask about her posters and it would help to initiate a conversation. In the end, the therapeutic divergences, coupled with a policy that avoided providing dedicated therapy rooms to individual therapists, meant that the clinic maintained the 'beigeness' associated with many other, arguably adult-orientated, institutional spaces.

There were other spaces within the clinics that were clearly not developed as spaces with the care of children in mind. The waiting room in clinic A was universally disliked. In many ways, it may seem like the waiting room is of little importance. It is not where the therapy takes place and it is a temporary 'holding-place', usually for the parent or guardian waiting for their child to finish their appointment. As one parent said it "felt like any other medical reception that I've been to really" (Kate, parent, clinic B). While this is true, it is also worth bearing in mind that, after the first impressions provided by the building façade, the waiting room sets the tone for all subsequent therapeutic experiences and is therefore representationally very important. In clinic A, the waiting room was exceedingly small. It was only able to seat five or six people and there was no window or fresh air. Even with a glass window to the reception staff, conversations could be overheard. As one parent said "it's horrible in there" (Kate, parent, clinic B).

Staff were very aware that the waiting room, and other areas like corridors, contributed to a negative emotional ecology (Reavey et al., 2017) that was problematic for clients who attended CAMHS:

> I think the waiting room is appalling, it is claustrophobic and I have a foster carer who can't wait there because there is claustrophobia, I think, er, it doesn't have wheelchair access, it's, er, and it's a long corridor that's seems very institutional. I think the individual rooms are not bad but the actual environment itself, I don't think it's very good.
>
> *(Alexis, staff, clinic A)*

Alexis' quote highlights an important point about who is impacted by the mental health space. Our focus is often on those receiving treatment, yet staff and parents/guardians are also integral users of mental health spaces. For the children, and indeed the parent in the next quote, it was clear after asking them to describe their ideal internal space, that they would marry together functionality with a sense of 'homeliness'. This parent was asked what they would like the waiting room to look like:

> *What would you like it to be?*
> I don't know um, a bit more homely I suppose, bit like well, not just sitting on these [functional chairs] but a big nice sofa and . . .
>
> *So, a sofa in the waiting area?*
> Um yeah or maybe when you go and talk to them, well something just to put your mind at ease really um, put yourself at ease, a bit more homely.
>
> *(Katie, parent, clinic B)*

This section has focused on the CAMHS clinics as representing spaces of material neglect alongside a material functionalism. Whilst staff in the clinic were clearly highly dedicated to the therapeutic care of children, it is argued here that the material space neither matched that commitment, nor did it justice. If we treat mental health settings as a transactional relationship between the space and the person using that space (Golembiewski, 2010) or a place of refuge (Curtis et al., 2009) then what value is placed on therapy when there are damp walls, dirty carpets and jumble-sale toys? The call to 'homeliness' (through brighter colours and environmental neglect) suggests that CAMHS should be a service that cares for children therapeutically, while also demonstrating a commitment to care through its material and symbolic space.

Conceptualising 'childhood' in spaces of mental health

Many of the issues discussed above, relating to clinic space as an area of material neglect or material 'homeliness', have strong intersections with conceptualisations of the 'child' and 'childhood'. Critical-developmental psychological theorising posits that the way we think about the ideal childhood, as a time of innocence, play and protection from the negative concerns of the adult world, sit at odds with the actual lived experiences of many children (Burman, 2008). Traditional developmental psychology proposes a set of 'normative' age-related trajectories, which see children steadily reaching an end point of physical and emotional maturity. Many children though, find themselves in challenging situations and settings that sit at odds with these 'normative' ideas and a mental health setting like CAMHS is one example.

As a service that catered for children between 5 and 18 years old, there was a tension surrounding how to arrange the space so that it catered for this age range. Both clinics tended to centre on the needs of younger children, which manifested itself in the open display of toys. However, as the following quotes suggest, even this is complex as some adolescents liked to use the toys while others would find them babyish. The first quote is from Alexis and the second from Henry, both are members of staff from clinic A. They talked about the dangers of having an adolescent room full of childish toys. At the same time, they were cautious about generalised assumptions on behalf of adolescents:

> Yeah, I think, I think it's naff coming to a place that has got toys for little ones, for me, you know, I think it's [an] insult to them. Don't think it should be divided by age but by the appropriate fit of the kid, so that would be a clinical decision really. Because I've got 15-year-olds who use the playroom, they use sand and toys and they're 15, so it's not the age it's the appropriateness of developmental stage.
>
> *(Alexis, staff, clinic A)*

> I think it's a mistake to generalise, I'd think most adolescents would prefer a room without toys although, I don't have it now but there used to be a cupboard in the room that I always used next door and it had toys in it and I had some, well some teenagers' boundaries are difficult so they'd open the cupboard and they'd take the toys out and get down on the floor and play with them but it was there, you know, but then, so it's hard to say but in general if I have a family session say in here or across the corridor I would get rid of dolls' houses personally.
>
> *(Henry, staff, clinic A)*

Both Alexis and Henry were wrestling here with the therapeutic needs of the children alongside or against the 'normative' age-graded conceptualisation of childhood. The prevailing view of a normative pattern of development prevalent within developmental psychology, would suggest that the move towards adolescence would involve dispensing with toys meant for younger children. The traditional and quite pervasive characterisation of adolescence laid out by Erikson (1950), which has been criticised by some scholars, would suggest that during adolescence, young people become focused on future adult responsibilities in relation to their vocational future. Arguably, it is this generalised view of adolescence that Alexis and Henry draw on to describe the most ideal or appropriate therapeutic space for this age group. Equally though, their adolescent clients transgress these normative expectations by playing with the toys. The difficult dichotomies raised by Alexis and Henry speak to the role mental health spaces might play in 'othering' this group of children and young people (Philo, 1992), those whose lives are rendered less 'visible' because they fall uncomfortably outside the boundaries of the 'ideal childhood'.

Other settings, where the care of children is a central tenet of the practice, demonstrate a very different approach to the material space. The hospital literature, for example, has shown some inroads into creating spaces that have children's own preferences as a driving force for how spaces are developed (James & Curtis, 2012). Educational spaces, particularly primary schools, have a long history in linking the materiality of the space with benefits in say, teaching and learning. This next quote is interesting because this parent worked as a teacher in a school, thereby offering an interesting contrast to how children's spaces are conceptualised:

> They're a bit drab you know, considering it's for children and I, I think they could maybe make a bit more effort with um decoration, posters and other things of distraction . . . it's lovely that somebody has taken posters out of the newspaper and stuff and put them on the wall um, but as a teacher I know the importance of display and how it appeals to children and it would be nice, somebody, somebody's kindly done that and it hasn't cost anything but a bit of effort but it would be nice if money had been invested to make more child-friendly displays.
>
> *(Kate, parent, clinic B)*

Kate's assumption, coming from a formal school setting, is that the building would be designed to appeal to children. In fact, throughout this analysis, 'the therapy' has been foregrounded over and above 'the child'. For example, the lack of colour and display is not just about the lack of money, it is also related to therapeutic preference.

In an interesting contrast to the perspective of the two staff members, Alexis and Henry, Emily (12 years old) perceives CAMHS to be a space that is more for older children. The plainness of the clinic is partly why she suggests this:

Um, I think it's like more, it's like more for like older people rather than younger people um, but I think if they just made, even little changes like painting something on the wall, maybe that would make a big difference and I like, there's like colouring pencils and play houses for like the younger children.

(*Emily, child, clinic B*)

Until this point, discussions about age and how it links with conceptualisations of childhood have pointed to fairly benign aspects of the material space. Other material features of the clinic space speak to the troubling of the 'risky' child and 'at-risk' child. This manifested itself most strongly during discussions about the glass reception window or 'hatch', which is where the children and their parents check in for their appointment. Figure 3.2 shows the hatch from both clinic A and clinic B.

It was the parents attending clinic appointments with their children who were particularly concerned with the reception window. Amy begins her quote by discussing the cramped waiting room, an issue already addressed earlier in the chapter. However, the glass window is an extension of this space, as children and carers must walk through this space to check in for their appointment:

I didn't like the waiting room, it's too small um, it's very cramped. People walking through all the time and if you've got a nervous child like P, he becomes very sort of like insecure and he can't deal with that sort of situation at all and obviously realising that, obviously the glass needs to be there between reception and the public patient area [but] it doesn't, it looks like you're completely cut off, it's just a sliding glass, it's not patient-friendly I don't think.

(*Amy, parent, clinic A*)

The glass window then, becomes an integrated part of the general anxiety discussed by many who need to attend CAMHS outpatients. The glass window symbolically

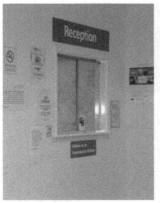
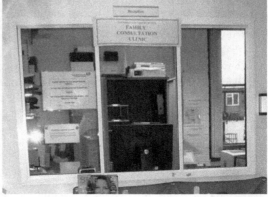

FIGURE 3.2 The reception window for both clinics: clinic A (left) and clinic B (right).

represents a 'risky' materiality in much the same way that risky materiality in adult settings are used to manage aggressive behaviour (Bowers et al., 2005). Amy talked about the glass 'obviously' needing to be there, however, it is not clear why a glass petition is needed. It did not act as a soundproof barrier, so this level of functionality was redundant. One obvious assumption is that it is there as a form of protection for the reception staff. If it is the staff, then, who are in need of protection by extension, it is the children they need protecting from. One office manager, who had been working in clinic A for eight years, was asked whether there had ever been any violent or aggressive incidences that would require a glass partition; she had never experienced anything that would suggest it was needed.

From the children's perspective, the glass window is indicative of the way they are excluded as active participants in the process of their care. Spaces of care often involve power inequalities, in part because the labour of care suggests some sense of vulnerability in those being 'cared for' (Bowlby, 2012). The barriers created by inequalities can certainly be evident when they involve children. The glass window was built so high up on the wall that younger children were unable to check themselves into the clinic. Glenn, one of the fathers who visited CAMHS with his son, was asked what he would do to improve the space. He said, "So I'd lower the walls so for J, well J, he's 9 and he loves to go and do himself and take responsibility, so has to sort of peek over the sliding window" (Glenn, parent, clinic B).

It was argued earlier that children in 'othered' positions can be treated as simultaneously 'at risk' and as 'risky' by the adult world. Equally, commentators working in adult asylums have discussed how the materiality around mental health spaces is suggestive of the containment of risky people. Such risky materiality, like locked doors, dark corridors and cameras can have a deeply distressing impact on those with mental health issues (McGrath & Reavey, 2013). The two outpatient CAMHS clinics in this study also contained many signifiers of risky materiality. Interestingly though, this materiality was interpreted in quite different ways by two boys in our sample. The first quote is from Smith, who was 18 years old at the time of interview. In this quote Smith talks about a range of material objects that signified to him that the space was a dangerous place to be:

> I was in a bit of a mood when I first came but it didn't really make me happy and when I came in here and the doors were opened and the mirror up and I could see people behind the mirror and the camera was on and they were watching us and I didn't, I was worried about that and it made me angry, so it made me think that the clinic; it isn't all as they say it is because of the danger.
>
> *(Smith, child, clinic A)*

On the one hand, leaving doors open could give the impression that the space is open and safe. Interestingly, Smith's interpretation is the opposite and makes him feel unsafe. The mirror he refers to is the one-way mirror that is supposedly used for training purposes although clearly, it was possible to still see people moving around behind the mirrors. All the therapy rooms still had cameras in the corners, though we were informed by one of the leading psychiatrists that it had been a long time since they had been used but had never been removed. Overall though, Smith presents these aspects of materiality as symbols of deceptiveness. A clinic that promises it is safe while signalling the opposite.

Dillen, aged 15, took a different viewpoint. For him, symbols that might be perceived as risky materiality signified to him features of safety: "When I come in um like the secure locks, like you have to touch to open which I thought was really clever so like no-one can come in like and do anything, do any damage" (Dillen, child, clinic B). It is not clear who the dangerous 'someone' is who could come in and do damage. It could be that Dillen is worried about an outside force that could come in and 'do any damage' or equally, the risk is perceived to be from within its own walls, from those who attend the clinic.

The users of these CAMHS outpatient settings wrestled with their own conceptualisations of childhood, the needs and requirements of a mental health setting and the demands of security versus risky environment. Overall, discussions about space within CAMHS are often integrally tied to age-related understandings of childhood. Yet there is a constant tussle between providing a service that fits a range of children and adolescence, while the materiality of the space, such as the cameras, mirrors, glass windows and locked doors, all speak to a service that contain risky and dangerous individuals.

Concluding thoughts

It is the institutional ordinariness that I propose is the biggest challenge to the space and built environment of outpatient CAMHS clinics. That they represent themselves like any other institutional services such as a medical reception, a government office or a borough council suggests that these spaces struggle with a dual identity. On the one hand CAMHS have care at the heart of their practice – this is the aim of therapy, and the staff we interviewed were very committed to their therapeutic practice. The space, however, has all the hallmarks of a service that caters for the needs of adults, rather than children. The clinics 'beigeness', its lack of wall displays or artwork, child-orientated furniture and overall sense of 'homeliness', speak to spaces that are dictated by adult needs. There is the argument that some therapeutic approaches require a plain room. Perhaps then, it would make sense to design fit-for-purpose rooms that cater for different approaches and indeed, different ages groups. Equally, why does this plainness slip into other areas of the clinic like the waiting room and corridors?

Perhaps, like other mental health services, CAMHS suffers from a long history of negative social representations surrounding mental health (Foster, 2006). However, CAMHS, as a service for children, adds another dimension, or perhaps an explanation, for why it is a service under-resourced in both monetary terms, and with respect to space and materiality. CAMHS clinics foreground the presence of those 'othered' children that confound the ideal childhood of innocence and joyfulness. More than that, children with mental health difficulties fit into the mould of the 'risky' child, who others may need protecting from, and the mental health setting as the 'risky' space they occupy. In this study, there were a number of material signifiers that represented the space as symbolically risky. The locked doors, the cameras in the corners of the therapy rooms, the one-way mirror and the glass window at the reception desk, are all pertinent examples. The two examples from the young people, Smith and Dillen, are interesting in this regard, however. Smith finds this 'risky' materiality disconcerting because it signifies to him that CAMHS cannot promise he is safe. Dillen though, sees the locks on the doors as a reassurance of this safety. The big question is, who needs protecting from whom? Who or where are the dangerous people?

It is interesting that some of the staff and parents are very cognisant of the lack of resources within CAMHS. They were torn between feeling negatively towards the material neglect within the space, such as the damp walls, dirty carpets and 'jumble-sale' looking toys. At the same time, they qualify that these are perhaps 'minor' issues when set against the many other challenges facing mental health provision. I return though to the point about people being in a transactional relationship with their therapeutic space (Golembiewski, 2010). Golembiewski (2010) proposes that objects occupying our spaces are not just a matter for our senses (e.g. sight, smell) but 'experienced' in a variety of ways. The notion that space is experienced subjectively also features strongly in the work of McGrath and Reavey (2013, 2016). If this is the case, then the value of material neglect and the impact on the therapeutic process should not be underestimated. Clearly, a key limitation of this study is that only two outpatient clinics were accessed for this research. Given that CAMHS outpatients appear to occupy such a variety of built environments, it would be fruitful to extend this study to clinics across the country, covering a broader socio-economic terrain. However, this does not take away from the importance of these findings. For example, mentioned by both the children and the parents was a need for a sense of 'homeliness' within the clinic. The call for a greater feeling of 'homeliness' to improve the experience of institutionalisation has been evident in debates about adult asylums (Foster, 2014) but could be the focus for child and adolescent settings, across both inpatient and outpatient services.

Notes

1 Detailed information about the full study can be found in this report.
2 Since this study clinic A has moved to a different location.

References

Birch, J., Curtis, P., & James, A. (2007). Sense and sensibilities: In search of the child-friendly hospital. *Built Environment*, *33*, 405–416.

Bowers, L., Simpson, A., Alexander, J., Hackney, D., Nijman, H., Grange, A., & Warren, J. (2005). The nature and purpose of acute psychiatric wards: The Tompkins Acute Ward Study. *Journal of Mental Health, 14*, 625–635.

Bowlby, S. (2012). Recognising the time–space dimensions of care: Caringscapes and carescapes. *Environment and Planning A, 44*(9), 2101–2118. doi: 10.1068/a44492.

Bryan, C., & Denov, M. (2011). Separated refugee children in Canada: The construction of risk identity. *Journal of Immigrant & Refugee Studies, 9*(3), 242–266.

Burman, E. (2008). *Deconstructing developmental psychology*. Hove: Routledge.

Children's Commissioner. (2016). *Lightning review: Access to children and adolescent mental health services*. Retrieved from www.childrenscommissioner.gov.uk.

Cline, T., Abreu, D. G., O'Dell, L., & Crafter, S. (2010). Recent research on child language brokering in the United Kingdom. *MediAziono: Journal of Interdisciplinary Studies on Language and Cultures, 10*, 105–124.

Connellan, K., Gaardboe, M., Riggs, D., Due, C., Reinschmidt, A., & Mustillo, L. (2013). Stressed spaces: Mental health and architecture. *Mental Health and Architecture, 6*, 127–168.

Cottrell, D., & Kraam, A. (2005). Growing up? A history of CAMHS (1987–2005). *Child and Adolescent Mental Health, 10*, 111–117.

Crafter, S., Prokopiou, E., & Stein, S. (2010). *Exploring the build and space environment for users of the Child and Adolescent Mental Health Service*. Retrieved from https://centreforum.org/.../children-young-peoples-mental-health-state-nation.

Crawley, H. (2011). 'Asexual, apolitical beings': The interpretation of children's identities and experiences in the UK asylum system. *Journal of Ethnic and Migration Studies, 37*(8), 1171–1184. doi: 10.1080/1369183x.2011.590645.

Curtis, S., Gesler, W., Priebe, S., & Francis, S. (2009). New spaces of inpatient care for people with mental illness: A complex 'rebirth' of the clinic? *Health & Place, 15*, 340–348.

Curtis, S., Gesler, W., Wood, V., Spencer, I., Mason, J., Close, H., & Reilly, J. (2013). Compassionate containment? Balancing technical safety and therapy in the design of psychiatric wards. *Social Science & Medicine, 97*, 201–209.

Erikson, E. (1950). *Childhood and society*. London: Imago.

Evans, G. W. (2003). The built environment and mental health. *Journal of Urban Health, 80*, 536–555.

Foster, J. L. H. (2006). Media presentation of the mental health bill and representations of mental health problems. *Journal of Community & Applied Social Psychology, 16*(4), 285–300. doi: 10.1002/casp.863.

Foster, J. L. H. (2014). What can social psychologists learn from architecture? The asylum as example. *Journal for the Theory of Social Behaviour, 44*(2), 131–147.

Frith, E. (2016). *Centre Forum Commission on children and young people's mental health: State of the nation*. Retrieved from https://centreforum.org/.../children-young-peoples-mental-health-state-nation.

Gesler, W., Bell, M., Curtis, S., Hubbard, P., & Francis, S. (2004). Therapy by design: evaluating the UK hospital building program. *Health & Place, 10*, 117–128.

Ghaziani, R. (2008). Children's voices: Raised issues for school design. *CoDesign, 4*(4), 225–236. doi: 10.1080/15710880802536403.

Golembiewski, J. A. (2010). Start making sense: Applying a salutogenic model to architectural design for psychiatric care. *Facilities, 28*(3/4), 100–117. doi: 10.1108/02632771011023096.

Gough, K. V., & Franch, M. (2005). Spaces of the street: socio-spatial mobility and exclusion of youth in Recife. *Children's Geographies, 3*(2), 149–166.

Hart, R. (1997). *Children's experience of place*. New York, NY: Irvington.

House of Commons. (2014). *Children's and adolescents' mental health and CAMHS: Third Report of Session*. Retrieved from https://publications.parliament.uk/pa/cm201415/cmselect/cmhealth/342/342.pdf.

James, A., & Curtis, P. (2012). Constructing the sick child: The cultural politics of children's hospitals. *Sociological Review*, *60*, 754–772.

James, A., & Prout, A. (1997). *Constructing and reconstructing childhood: Contemporary issues in the sociological study of childhood*. London: Falmer.

Jans, M. (2004). Children as citizens: Towards a contemporary notion of child participation. *Childhood*, *11*, 27–44.

Kraftl, P., & Adey, P. (2008). Architecture/affect/inhabitation: Geographies of being-in buildings. *Annals of the Association of American Geographers*, *98*(1), 213–231. doi: 10.1080/00045600701734687.

Lambert, V., Coad, J., Hicks, P., & Glacken, M. (2013). Young children's perspectives of ideal physical design features for hospital-built environments. *Journal of Child Health Care*, *18*, 57–71.

Lawson, B., & Phiri, M. (2003). *The architectural healthcare environment of its effects of patient health outcomes: A report on an NHS Estates funded research project*. Retrieved from www.artshealthresources.org.uk.

Lucas, T. (1998). Youth gangs and moral panics in Santa Cruz, California. In T. Skelton & G. Valentine (Eds.), *Cool places: Geographies of youth cultures* (pp. 145–160). London: Routledge.

McGrath, L., & Reavey, P. (2013). Heterotopias of control: placing the material in experiences of mental health service use and community living. *Health Place*, *22*, 123–131. doi: 10.1016/j.healthplace.2013.03.010.

McGrath, L., & Reavey, P. (2016). 'Zip me up, and cool me down': Molar narratives and molecular intensities in 'helicopter' mental health services. *Health Place*, *38*, 61–69. doi: 10.1016/j.healthplace.2015.12.005.

Moon, G. (2000). Risk and protection: The discourse of confinement in contemporary mental health policy. *Health & Place*, *6*, 239–250.

O'Dell, L. (2008). Representations of the 'damaged' child: 'Child saving' in a British children's charity ad campaign. *Children & Society*, *22*(5), 383–392.

O'Dell, L., Brownlow, C., & Bertilsdotter Rosqvist, H. (2017). *Different childhoods: Non/normative development and transgressive trajectories*. London: Routledge.

Ohlsson, R. (2016). Diagnosis as a resource in the social representation of mental illness. *Papers on Social Representations*, *25*(1), 12.11–12.24.

Parr, H. (2008). *Mental health and social space: Towards inclusionary geographies?* Malden, MA: Blackwell.

Parr, H., Philo, C., & Burns, N. (2003). 'That awful place was home': Reflections on the contested meanings of Craig Dunain Asylum. *Scottish Geographical Journal*, *119*(4), 341–360.

Philo, C. (1992). Neglected rural geographies: A review. *Journal of Rural Studies*, *8*(2), 193–207.

Reavey, P., Poole, J., Corrigall, R., Zundel, T., Byford, D., Sarhane, S., . . . Ougrin, D. (2017). The ward as emotional ecology: Adolescent experiences of managing mental health and distress in psychiatric inpatient settings. *Health & Place*, *46*, 210–218. doi: https://doi.org/10.1016/j.healthplace.2017.05.008.

Rosen, R., & Crafter, S. (in submission). Media representations of separated child migrants: From Dubs to doubt. *Sociology*.

Taylor, S. (2009). *Narratives of identity and place*. London: Routledge.

Ulrich, R. S., Zimring, C., Quan, X., Joseph, A., & Choudhary, R. (2004). *The role of the physical environment in the hospital of the 21st century*. Retrieved from www.healthdesign.org.

Vaaler, A. E., Morken, G., & Linaker, O. M. (2005). Effects of different interior decorations in the seclusion area of a psychiatric acute ward. *Nordic Journal of Psychiatry, 59*, 9–24.

Weisskirch, R. S. (2007). Feelings about language brokering and family relations among Mexican American early adolescents. *Journal of Early Adolescence, 27*(4), 545–561.

Wood, V. J., Curtis, S. E., Gesler, W., Spencer, I. H., Close, H. J., Mason, J., & Reilly, J. G. (2013). Creating 'therapeutic landscapes' for mental health carers in inpatient settings: A dynamic perspective on permeability and inclusivity. *Social Science & Medicine, 91*, 122–129.

4

NEGOTIATING ADULT AUTHORITY

Young people's experience of adolescent mental health wards

Jason Poole and Paula Reavey

Introduction

This chapter explores the ways in which child and adolescent mental health services (CAMHS) inpatients interpret expressions of adult institutional power within the ward-place where they enact strategies of negotiation and resistance. This account understands age and mental distress as intersecting, mutually constituted axes of social inequality (Cromby, Harper, & Reavey, 2013; Gordon, 2007; Haslam & Ernst, 2002). The adolescent inpatient unit itself is examined here as a unique therapeutic landscape within which these inequalities become crystallised as expressions of panoptic power (Foucault, 1975).

Literature review

Adolescence

Within dominant Western discourses, adolescence and other life-cycle stages are treated as though they are absolute, natural categories that occur across the span of human development (Elder, 1994). This perspective, though prevalent, omits the identifiable processes by which societal perceptions of youth transitioned through the late eighteenth and early nineteenth centuries. During this time the average age of first employment in Britain was 10 years and half of the total workforce was under the age of 20. Following industrialisation, a new understanding of youth emerged, which perceived children and adolescents as requiring education, guidance, and protection, preferably provided by adults (Cunningham, 2003; Griffin, 1993; Humphries, 2013). In this context, adolescence was constructed for the first time as a transitional phase concerned with the cessation of *being* a child and instead engaging in the work of *becoming* an adult. The direction of this metamorphosis implicitly enforces a hierarchical adult/child dualism, by defining the importance of adolescence as establishing the identity of the person who will one day *be* rather than acknowledging value in, or even the stable existence of, the person who presently *is* (Griffin, 1993; Uprichard, 2008). The responsibility for negotiating this discursive tension between *being* and *becoming* was assumed by adult actors within the machinery of state, for whom the guiding of youth into adulthood represented an ethical obligation; a necessity if society were to avoid descent into moral anarchy (Lesko, 2001).

Presently, Western discourses surrounding youth frequently describe adolescents as essentially immoral beings of 'unreason', framing their bodies with narratives of sexuality, criminality, unreliability and naivety; defining the 'reasonable' domain of adulthood with this juxtaposition (Gordon, 2007; Lesko, 2001). Youth voices are commonly suppressed or ignored by systemic/institutional power, and young people themselves popularly conceived as passive objects broadly removed from societal problems rather than as active subjects (Gordon, 2007). Meaningful avenues for understanding youth, including the research, media and technology that frame their lives, are limited by their almost exclusively having been constituted by adults (Herring, 2008). Increasingly, adult influence is exerted over the public spaces in which adolescents traditionally express themselves, and risk-based narratives are used to justify a growing prevalence of surveillance, detentions and exclusionary practices which specifically target youth (McCahill, 2007; Malone, 2002; Valentine, 1996). Moreover, economic systems committed to providing free education and full employment are now replaced by policies encouraging competition in the global market in lieu of supporting the young (Mizen, 2004). It is therefore unsurprising that adolescents regularly perceive themselves as irrelevant to the institutions that exercise control over their daily lives. Research indicates that the significant majority of UK youth experience feelings of societal disenfranchisement and an inability to affect political decision-making processes (Henn & Foard, 2012; Rayle, 2005). This uneven distribution of social power between adults and adolescents colours present day British political discourses relating to the rights of institutions to detain youth, with these broadly featuring strong currents of authoritarianism and remoralisation: The state not only possesses the *right* to incarcerate adolescents for breaking with the (adult) social contract; it is bound by *duty* to do so, in order to promote young people's moral improvement (Fergusson, 2007; Muncie & Hughes, 2002).

Young 'mental patients'

Conceptualising adolescents as a socially marginalised group contributes to our understanding of young people as mental health service users. Just as British society's notions of youth shifted dramatically in response to industrialisation, so too did its understanding of those individuals exhibiting markers of what would come to be known as mental illness. During this period, owing to the increasing credence afforded to new, capitalistic thought, individuals' value to society was reconstituted around their ability to produce and the presence of those who could not do so was problematised (Foucault, 1967). Whereas many wealthy sufferers of mental illness could quietly retreat to relatively comfortable, for-profit private asylums, those working-class individuals experiencing debilitating madness rapidly came to be understood not only as troublesome to society but also as inherently immoral and unfit to continue in their sharing of public spaces (Parr & Davidson, 2009). Mirroring the government-sanctioned movement and detention of youth in postmodernity (Valentine, 1996), the removal of the 'lunatic poor' from visible British society became a role of the state, and was conducted en masse. With time, attempts to categorise and manage the overwhelming numbers of confined individuals contributed toward the emergence of psychiatry as a new field of scientific inquiry and medicine, and the low-class inhabitants of state-run asylums were gradually reconceptualised as 'mental patients' whose problematised behaviours could now be categorised as particular symptoms and illnesses (Foucault, 1967; Rogers & Pilgrim, 2010).

In current clinical research and practice, social inequalities are increasingly understood as major correlational risk factors for the development of mental illness (see Fryers, Melzer, & Jenkins, 2003 for a review). Furthermore, the research literature suggests that the onset of debilitating distress typically has roots in adolescence (Jones, 2013), and the relationship between socioeconomic disparity and distress would appear to be strongest during this period (Dorling, 2011; Wilkinson & Pickett, 2010; Wright & Ord, 2015). However, most accounts continue to treat adolescence as a period of increased vulnerability to traumatogenic factors rather than acknowledging youth as being an axis of inequality that may itself provoke the onset of mental illness: Major social domains determining mental well-being, such as access to material resources, control over one's own life, and ability to participate in political decision-making (CSDH, 2008) require negotiation of markedly more stubborn and numerous barriers for young people than their adult counterparts (Doyle, 2009; Henn & Foard, 2012; The Prince's Trust, 2017), and thus these may be discussed as issues of *youth specifically*. These enhanced vulnerabilities notwithstanding, and perhaps holding as an example of institutional inequality, statutory mental health services are "arguably at their weakest" in their provision of care to young people (Purcell et al., 2011, p. 16), who find it especially difficult to access services and often experience those clinicians they do encounter as unsympathetic or insensitive (Wright & Ord, 2015). Young service users are routinely described by professionals and researchers as being particularly difficult to engage in treatment (Green, Wisdom, Wolfe, & Firemark, 2012; Rickwood, Deane, & Wilson, 2007), whereas young people themselves report experiencing mental health professionals and institutions as key sources of stigmatisation and coercion. It is of note that research addressing the experiences of adolescents in this area is sparse and usually based on previous work with adults (Heflinger & Hinshaw, 2010; Reavey et al., 2017). Throughout the adult literature service users explain stigmatising and coercive practices by professionals in terms of *infantilisation*; they know that they are being mistreated because they are made to feel like youth (e.g. Angell, Cooke, & Kovac, 2005; Chamberlin, 1995; Mancini & Rogers, 2007; Sweeney, Gillard, Wykes, & Rose, 2015).

Inpatient spaces

The historical ideals underpinning the asylum are evidenced by its nomenclature: These were to be devolved sanctuaries in which people could pursue a period of respite from the traumatic events of their lives. In much the same way that postmodern popular discourses surrounding the act of 'asylum seeking' emphasise the geographical movement of a body from a place of fear, persecution and violence to one that is less threatening, the spatial identity of the asylum was initially tied to its physical removedness from the centres of urban living that were implicitly understood to generate distress (Foucault, 1967; Philo, 1987). The modern inpatient unit may now often be found within the very cities from which they would once have provided refuge, yet their structures and inhabitants remain subject to a persistent and stigmatising discursive demarcation from broader society that colours both with a sense of uneasy Otherness (Angermeyer, van der Auwera, Carta, & Schomerus, 2017; Parr & Davidson, 2009). This distance is made manifest in its most extreme form as an association between psychiatric inpatient spaces and the darkly paranormal, as perpetuated by entertainment media (Goodwin, 2014). The inpatient unit could therefore be understood by those situated externally to it as a fundamentally frightening holding place for mysterious and perhaps malevolent beings whose essential immorality, unpredictability and potential for frenzy render them unfit to continue as active participants in public arenas (Clark & Dear, 1984; Foucault, 1967).

Viewed from within, however, the ward space can be conceptualised much like any other; as inherently social and political, featuring complex collective systems, trajectories and practices and saturated by inequalities, power and resistance. Differing understandings of what the space is *for* and *should be* shape ongoing negotiations and conflicts between the individuals and groups who govern and/ or inhabit the adolescent unit, establishing the space as an 'ongoing construction' that, much like its inhabitants, is engaged in the perpetual work of *becoming* (Massey, 1992, 2005; Renedo & Marston, 2015). Crucially, it is within the bounds of the ward space that socio-cultural constructions of youth and madness intersect and a form of inversion occurs: The young and the mad, increasingly relegated to the spatial margins in wider society, inhabit the central position within the inpatient unit and come to present a potential threat to the established structures of adult/medical power (Foucault, 2006; Malone, 2002). As is the norm, intensive regulatory practices are enacted to contain this centring of an 'alternative' group, in this instance constituted by highly authoritarian staff policies and procedures that are often experienced by young inpatients as detrimental to their pursuit of wellness (Marriage, Petrie, & Worling, 2001; Moses, 2011; Reavey et al., 2017; Tulloch et al., 2008). Access to responsive, individualised care in these spaces requires negotiation of the biases of adult actors, with young people's views of their treatment only given sufficient validation to affect change when deemed 'age-appropriate' by staff. Voices that do not meet this expectation are problematised or silenced (LeFrançois, 2007).

Research methodology

A total of 20 participants (8 male, 12 female) were interviewed regarding their experiences of inpatient treatment. Participants were aged between 14 and 19 years, with a mean age of 16.8 years. All participants had experienced a UK CAMHS inpatient stay within six months prior to interview. The average length of inpatient stay was 91 days. All participants had received diagnoses of mental disorder using ICD-10. The participants' ethnic backgrounds included: 13 White British; 3 Black British (2 British Caribbean); 1 Black Jamaican; 1 Lithuanian; 1 Polish; and 1 Bengali. Participants' self-reported social class (based on primary household earners' occupations): 2 upper middle class; 1 middle class; 6 lower middle class; 6 working class; 5 unemployed.

These interviews utilised a combination of photo-elicitation and photo-production methodologies, in which participants compared and discussed ready-produced photographs of the inpatient spaces they had inhabited, alongside photographs they had taken of their everyday lives prior to first contact with CAMHS (see Reavey, 2011). Participants were asked to choose inpatient photographs based on their having "strong memories" attached to them, but were otherwise given no guidance. Once participants were satisfied with their chosen photos, their reasons for selection were discussed and significant memories and emotions connecting participants to each space were explored. This multi-modal combination of visual and verbal methodologies assists participants in accessing and articulating their situated, embodied knowledges of their experiences by enabling them to transcend the here and now and anchor themselves on to the landscapes to which they were once attached (Frith, Riley, Archer, & Gleeson, 2004; Stedman, Beckley, Wallace, & Ambard, 2004). The interview schedule explored participants' perceptions of diagnosis, inpatient treatment, the role of CAMHS staff, and the broader impact of inpatient admission on their wider social contexts. Semi-structured interviews were transcribed verbatim and analysed using an extended version of Colaizzi's (1978) method of phenomenological enquiry, in which an additional step specifically attending to participants' articulation of symbolic representations is included (Edward & Welch, 2011).

Analysis

Two over-arching domains of control and resistance were identified and are presented here, entitled (a) situated resistances; and b) allies and performances. These do not represent the total number of themes that emerged from the analysis, but do answer the research question 'How is institutional power experienced and negotiated by adolescent inpatients?' Extracts from the transcripts are presented here to demonstrate the major themes that emerged throughout the interviews.

Situated resistances

Most participants understood the wards they had inhabited as being spaces of detention whose principal concern was situating their residents' bodies, both in relation to the confines of the hospital buildings themselves and the surrounding communities. Two primary strategies were relied upon by staff when enforcing these controls: reliance upon the physical structures of the ward itself and an intense degree of behavioural surveillance (Foucault, 1975). Young people experienced wards as being highly ordered environments, movement through which often entailed complex negotiations of obstacles presented by staff members and the ever-present locked doors. Many participants described being an inpatient as similar to inhabiting a 'prison' or 'zoo' (Moses, 2011; Reavey et al., 2017). Nursing stations held particular significance for the young people interviewed, who found that they acted as central spatial focuses in which expressions of institutional power would be performed. The stations' large windows, which enabled patients to see the staff inside but otherwise blocked any attempts at meaningful communication, reinforced the felt presence of barriers on the ward and served as a reminder to some of the unequal balance of power:

> The door's like meant to be open and that, but then sometimes you're knocking on the door and they're like, "Oh, you're going to have to wait a minute," but like it could be an emergency and they're not even answering the door. They don't even know if it could be like an emergency or just a normal conversation.

Many participants disclosed experiencing periods of escalating confinement and seclusion during their inpatient stays. These instances were overwhelmingly perceived as a form of punishment for engaging in problematised behaviours, despite staff members' framing of them exclusively in terms of risk and safety. Young people described being detained in particular rooms for uncertain periods of time, often in response to noncompliance with ward rules but also when staff anticipated that their distress would interfere with the efficient completion of a given task, such as dispensing medication. Where the extant spaces of seclusion within the boundaries of the ward would fail to produce desired behaviours, staff would sometimes fall back upon a secondary strategy of openly discussing alternative, more authoritarian spaces for the resistant young person to potentially inhabit, be they within increasingly restrictive legal frameworks or different geographical locations altogether. In the following extract a participant describes the institutional response to an incident in which he shouted at several members of staff, pressed a fire alarm, absconded from the ward and set a small fire in a car park that caused no damage; a sequence of events that he understood as his reaction to having been unfairly told off by a nurse when intensely distressed:

> Sixty hours in the isolation room. The room was tiny. There was a toilet and a sofa in there though, but yeah, I was there for days. They first said I might not get transferred. Met two doctors, both put me on section for a month, 28 days. Then they were discussing about moving me to a PICU (Psychiatric Intensive Care Unit). Then they discussed with my parents about pressing charges and moving me to a forensic unit.

The primacy given to the physical structure of the ward space in planning and enacting strategies of control resulted in it being a central feature in many young people's acts of resistance. A number of participants described absconsion from wards in urban locales as a common means for some to express their dissatisfaction, with particular individuals or small groups repeatedly utilising this approach to avoid observation for short periods of time. Young people who found themselves inhabiting rural areas were more inventive, finding ways to go missing that did not require leaving the ward:

> You just feel like everyone's watching you, you can't do anything. A few of us would just like try to sneak, and we were quite sneaky, so when they weren't looking we used to open the door, we used to go in the lift and I used to nick the keys and put them in the lift, and so we'd sit in the lift 'cause they couldn't find us then unless they did the lift, and then we'd come down and we'd go "Hello!" (laughs) . . . You don't want to be watched all the time, so that's why we used to go up there, 'cause no one could actually see us. It's not allowed, I know, but it's still fun and we enjoyed ourselves playing cards.

The previous extract details the unsanctioned occupation of a restricted space, an action that features frequently in the disruptive strategies of youth political movements across the world (e.g. Castañeda, 2012; Ruiz, 2016). However, of note here is the unusual purpose that this occupation serves: Whereas youth activists in wider society are often engaged in battles for *visibility* in which they seek to overcome systems that silence their voices (Gordon, 2007; Ruiz, 2016), the panoptic nature of institutional power within the adolescent unit, in tandem with the aforementioned spatial inversion that it enforces, transforms *becoming hidden* into a revolutionary act that provokes a marked response from adult actors. In this example it is clear that the elevator did not present any exciting opportunities for the young people involved beyond a chance to subvert the power of constant surveillance, as evidenced by their simply remaining and playing cards upon having successfully disappeared.

Many participants expressed confusion and dismay at ward policies surrounding their 'personal space', in particular a complete moratorium on physical contact. This was reportedly due to concerns around risk and appropriateness, reflecting wider societal discourses framing young bodies as objects of suspicion

(Lesko, 2001). Moreover, young people were not allowed to set foot in one another's bedrooms, though these rules were experienced by our sample as the most routinely broken and most often ignored by staff. Participants found that where these 'personal space' policies were not enforced, it often appeared to be due to an assumption by staff that pairs of adolescent women would not wish to form sexual relationships with one another, which a number of our sample considered to be an amusing and occasionally offensive oversight. This uneven application of the rules would sometimes culminate in more visible protests being staged within young people's bedrooms, with participants describing the erection of new structures such as tents, pillow forts and barricades to obfuscate the presence of guests and stymie staff attempts to enforce ward policies:

P: Yeah, we got dragged out . . . no one's allowed to go into each other's rooms, which is understandable, but me and K were like best friends and she only lives around the corner from me so we decided one night that we were both a bit bored and I went into her room without anyone knowing and we slept under her desk, and we got all the pillows and we made it into a camping kind of tent, and then people came in and said I'm not allowed to be in there and stuff but she was kind of blocking the entry so they couldn't get me out, which was quite fun. Not fun for them, but it was quite fun.
I: Was that physically dragging you?
P: Oh, physically. I had five people on me. It was a restraint and it lasted four hours on the floor. Yeah. They injected me (laughs).

Over half of our sample reported having been pushed, pulled or pinned by staff members at some point during their admission, with three disclosing experiences of threatened or inflicted (unsanctioned) physical violence by members of ward staff. The participants broadly lacked effective strategies to counter instances of restraint and/or violence. A number reported intentionally instigating situations in which they knew they would be restrained as a form of protest in itself, placing significant demands on the ward's resources and perhaps utilising an understanding of how intensely distressing such occurrences can be for the majority of staff (Bonner, Lowe, Rawcliffe, & Wellman, 2002). On occasions when participants felt themselves to be at risk of violence at the hands of staff they would often find the systems of adult institutional power to be at their most inflexible, with complaints procedures promising no certain results and external agencies such as, in one instance, the police refusing to help when contacted by youth. It was in such instances that young people would rely on alliances with peers and particular staff members for support, and focus on performing docility in pursuit of discharge.

Allies and performance

Many participants described the formation of supportive relationships as being crucial to maintaining well-being on the ward, particularly when these alliances were built on feelings of openness and equality (Freake, Barley, & Kent, 2007; Gilburt, Rose, & Slade, 2008; Reavey et al., 2017). Such relationships with peers were valued above all others for their facilitation of enhanced resilience and recovery, due to a sense of communal empathy and understanding among service users (Moos, 1997; Moses, 2011), which for a number of our participants was interwoven with a distrust of adults' motivations:

I: Do you think other people your age have a better view of mental health?
P: Yeah, than adults. Yeah.
I: Why do you think that might be?
P: Just because they understand us. Adults like judging.

This need to be understood rather than judged ran central to many participants' sense-making around interactions with adults on the ward, and was often the yardstick against which individual staff members' potential worth as an ally would be measured. Young people often experienced overly medical or scientific framings of their distress as disingenuous or, at worst, an unwanted practice by which their most meaningful and often traumatic experiences would be reformatted to meet adult expectations and understandings. As such, many participants described their most important and helpful exchanges with trusted members of ward staff as being overtly *non-therapeutic*, a term that in this instance refers to interactions that were felt to fall outside of the strict boundaries of the 'therapeutic relationship'. Rather than offering formal guidance or support in combating aspects of the ward space that young people found to be oppressive, these adults' value lay in their ability to disrupt the highly ordered ward environments through initiating or engaging in unstructured, non-therapeutic activities, or by quietly ignoring policies that they did not feel were useful at a given moment in time:

> He didn't know I was going for a fag and obviously I'm not allowed to and I went, "Do you smoke?" He was like, "No." I was like, "Did you used to smoke at all?" He was like, "Yeah." I was like, "Oh, you understand then. Can I have a fag?" He went, "Yeah, alright then." (Laughs) He was like, he had a lighter in his pocket.

Where participants were unable to have their needs met through the formation of genuine alliances with adult actors, some would learn to disguise themselves as having bought in to the dominant institutional discourses, superficially performing 'wellness' in a manner they felt would please their observers. Many young people described actively monitoring staff members' behaviours as a matter of course. Most would do this to assuage the anxieties provoked by inhabiting such an unfamiliar space, or simply to pass the time, but for some this counter-observation facilitated the development of resistances through mimicry, which, when engaged in by youth movements, typically rely upon imitating those aspects of adulthood conceptualised as being particularly moral (Avdela, 2008). Within the ward space, such performances of morality rely upon an acknowledgement of the value of reason and docility despite one's inner turmoil. These acts must deviate from clinicians' preconceptions of both youth and madness:

> I knew that kind of being relaxed and controlled and back straight and I have a shirt on, my hair's done and I don't have weird stubble growing or anything. Like, I looked the part. I looked like a person who could be integrated into society and I kind of painted that picture and I made them laugh with something. Yeah, they were saying, "When you came in, you said that you wanted to give up smoking. Was that something you want us to help you with?" and I probably said something like, "No, that was part of the psychosis." They giggled, and I felt like I had all of them in my pocket. They kind of ticked the box and I was, yeah, I got let out. That felt like a real victory for me.

This excerpt describes one participant's successful attempt to be discharged from hospital, despite their still being "quite heavily in psychosis at the time". Here the ability to anticipate and perform to the expectations of adult actors on the ward reveals itself as perhaps the most effective means of resistance available to young people, granting freedom where other strategies serve as statements of discontent. Of note here is that the only participants who reported successfully utilising these approaches were White British, a group that is underrepresented in UK CAMHS inpatient services (Faulconbridge, Law, & Laffan, 2015), and of upper middle-class backgrounds. These factors doubtlessly provided those participants with the resources to more effectively engage with Western medical discourses and forms of legitimised self-presentation, which perhaps rendered staff more likely to take their claims seriously (Fiske, 2012).

Discussion

In this chapter we have sought to explore how young inpatients negotiate and resist adult authority within the confines of the ward space. Our findings have identified several core strategies utilised by young people to challenge those expressions of institutional power that they find to be most problematic, broadly taking the form of acts that are disruptive (occupation, absconscion, direct confrontation) or surreptitious (counter-observation, rule-breaking with adult support, mimicry). Of particular interest to us is the extent to which these resistances reflect those engaged in by youth political movements in wider society, where young people must increasingly fight for their right to spatial agency (Gordon, 2007; Malone, 2002). The adolescent inpatient unit presents a unique arena in which to examine these negotiations, as those factors relied upon by the state to restrict the movements and actions of youth, in particular surveillance and the risk of (further) detention, are made overt and openly discussed on the ward, though often exclusively in the context of risk and safety (Gilburt et al., 2008). In these spaces behavioural surveillance shifts from an obliquely presented societal force serving to marginalise youth to an explicit expression of panopticism designed to centre and contain them (Foucault, 2006; Malone, 2002). The resistances enacted by young people within the ward are then themselves inverted: Where youth movements typically struggle to be heard, young inpatients may learn that the most effective means of resistance is to go unseen, potentially negatively impacting their willingness to engage in future help-seeking.

Though they are ostensibly spaces developed to facilitate wellness and recovery, we must acknowledge that inpatient units are primarily experienced by some residents as places of involuntary detention, coercion or punishment, whether held under section or otherwise (Gilburt et al., 2008; Reavey et al., 2017). Given the traumatogenic social power imbalances that lead so many young people to mental health service involvement (Fryers et al., 2003), it is crucial that we address and challenge factors that may cause these inequalities to become crystallised within the ward space, be they issues of ethnicity, gender, sexuality, class or youth specifically.

References

Angell, B., Cooke, A., & Kovac, K. (2005). First-person accounts of stigma. In P. W. Corrigan (Ed.), *On the stigma of mental illness: Practical strategies for research and social change* (pp. 69–98). Washington, DC: American Psychological Association.

Angermeyer, M. C., van der Auwera, S., Carta, M. G., & Schomerus, G. (2017). Public attitudes towards psychiatry and psychiatric treatment at the beginning of the 21st century: A systematic review and meta-analysis of population surveys. *World Psychiatry, 16*, 50–61.

Avdela, E. (2008). 'Corrupting and uncontrollable activities': Moral panic about youth in post-civil-war Greece. *Journal of Contemporary History, 43*(1), 25–44.

Bonner, G., Lowe, T., Rawcliffe, D., & Wellman, N. (2002). Trauma for all: A pilot study of the subjective experience of physical restraint for mental health inpatients and staff in the UK. *Journal of Psychiatric and Mental Health Nursing, 9*(4), 465–473.

Castañeda, E. (2012). The Indignados of Spain: A precedent to Occupy Wall Street. *Social Movement Studies, 11*(3–4), 309–319.

Chamberlin, J. (1995). Rehabilitating ourselves: The psychiatric survivor movement. *International Journal of Mental Health, 24*(1), 39–46.

Clark, G. L., & Dear, M. (1984). State apparatus and everyday life. In G. L. Clark & M. Dear (Eds.), *State apparatus: Structures of language and legitimacy* (pp. 15–34). London: Routledge.

Colaizzi, P. (1978). Psychological research as the phenomenologists view it. In R. Vale & M. King (Eds.), *Existential-phenomenological alternatives for psychology* (pp. 48–71). New York, NY: Oxford University Press.

Commission on Social Determinants of Health. (2008). *Closing the gap in a generation: Health equity through action on the social determinants of health. Final report of the Commission on Social Determinants of Health.* Geneva: World Health Organisation.

Cromby, J., Harper, D., & Reavey, P. (2013). *Psychology, mental health and distress.* Basingstoke: Palgrave Macmillan.

Cunningham, H. (2003). *The invention of childhood.* London: BBC Books.

Dorling, D. (2011). *Injustice: Why social inequality persists.* Bristol: Policy Press.

Doyle, R. (2009). Youth, development, and sustainability. In R. C. Elliot (Ed.), *Institutional issues involving ethics and justice* (vol. 2, pp. 176–201). Oxford: Eolss.

Edward, K. L., & Welch, T. (2011). The extension of Colaizzi's method of phenomenological enquiry. *Contemporary Nurse, 39*(2), 163–171.

Elder, G. H. (1994). Time, human agency, and social change: Perspectives on the life course. *Social Psychology Quarterly*, *57*(1), 4–15.

Faulconbridge, J., Law, D., & Laffan, A. (2015). What good looks like in psychological services for children, young people and their families. *The Child & Family Clinical Psychology Review*, *3*(Summer). Leicester: British Psychological Society.

Fergusson, R. (2007). Making sense of the melting pot: Multiple discourses in youth justice policy. *Youth Justice*, *73*(3), 179–194.

Fiske, S. T. (2012). Warmth and competence: Stereotype content issues for clinicians and researchers. *Canadian Psychology*, *53*(1), 14–20.

Foucault, M. (1967). *Madness and civilisation: The history of madness in an age of reason*. London: Vintage Books.

Foucault, M. (1975). *Disciple and punish: The birth of the prison*. New York, NY: Random House.

Foucault, M. (2006). 23 January 1974. In J. Lagrange, F. Ewald, & A. Fontana (Eds.), *Psychiatric power: Michel Foucault lectures at the Collège de France* (pp. 90–100). London: Palgrave Macmillan.

Freake, H., Barley, V., & Kent, G. (2007). Adolescents' views of helping professionals: A review of the literature. *Journal of Adolescence*, *30*, 639–653.

Frith, H., Riley, S., Archer, L., & Gleeson, K. (2005). Imag(in)ing visual methodologies. *Qualitative Research in Psychology*, *2*(3), 187–198.

Fryers, T., Melzer, D., & Jenkins, R. (2003). Social inequalities and the common mental disorders: A systematic review of the evidence. *Social Psychiatry and Psychiatric Epidemiology*, *38*(5), 229–237.

Gilburt, H., Rose, D., & Slade, M. (2008). The importance of relationships in mental health care: A qualitative study of service users' experiences of psychiatric hospital admission in the UK. *BMC Health Services Research*, *8*(1), 92.

Goodwin, J. (2014). The horror of stigma: Psychosis and mental health care environments in twenty-first-century horror film (part I). *Perspectives in Psychiatric Care*, *50*(3), 201–209.

Gordon, H. R. (2007). Allies within and without: How adolescent activists conceptualize ageism and navigate adult power in youth social movements. *Journal of Contemporary Ethnography*, *36*(6), 631–668.

Green, C. A., Wisdom, J. P., Wolfe, L., & Firemark, A. (2012). Engaging youths with serious mental illness in treatment: STARS study consumer recommendations. *Psychiatric Rehabilitation Journal*, *35*(5), 360–368.

Griffin, C. (1993). *Representations of youth: The study of youth and adolescence in Britain and America (feminist perspectives)*. Cambridge: Polity Press.

Haslam, N., & Ernst, D. (2002). Essentialist beliefs about mental disorders. *Journal of Social & Clinical Psychology*, *21*(6), 628–644.

Heflinger, C. A., & Hinshaw, S. P. (2010). Stigma in child and adolescent mental health services research: Understanding professional and institutional stigmatization of youth with mental health problems and their families. *Policy Mental Health*, *37*(1–2), 61–70.

Henn, M., & Foard, N. (2012). Young people, political participation and trust in Britain. *Parliamentary Affairs*, *65*(1), 47–67.

Herring, S. C. (2008). Questioning the generational divide: Technological exoticism and adult constructions of online youth identity. In D. Buckingham (Ed.), *Youth, identity, and digital media* (pp. 71–94). Cambridge, MA: MIT Press.

Humphries, J. (2013). Childhood and child labour in the British industrial revolution. *Economic History Review*, *66*(2), 395–418.

Jones, P. B. (2013). Adult mental health disorders and their age at onset. *British Journal of Psychiatry*, *202*(suppl. 54), 5–10.

LeFrançois, B. (2007). Children's participation rights: Voicing opinions in inpatient care. *Child & Adolescent Mental Health, 12*(2), 94–97.
Lesko, N. (2001). *Act your age! The cultural construction of adolescence*. London: Routledge.
McCahill, M. (2007). Us and them: The social impact of 'new surveillance' technologies. *Criminal Justice Matters, 68*(1), 14–15.
Malone, K. (2002). Street life: Youth, culture and competing uses of public space. *Environment & Urbanization, 14*(2), 157–168.
Mancini, M. A., & Rogers, R. (2007). Narratives of recovery from serious psychiatric disabilities: A critical discourse analysis. *Critical Approaches to Discourse Analysis across Disciplines, 1*(2), 35–50.
Marriage, K., Petrie, J., & Worling, D. (2001). Consumer satisfaction with an adolescent inpatient psychiatric unit. *Canadian Journal of Psychiatry, 46*(10), 969–975.
Massey, D. (1992). Politics and space/time. *New Left Review, 196*, 65–84.
Massey, D. (2005). *For space*. London: Sage.
Mizen, P. (2004). *The changing state of youth*. Basingstoke: Palgrave Macmillan.
Moos, R. H. (1997). The social climate of hospital programs. In R. H. Moos (Ed.), *Evaluating treatment environments: The quality of psychiatric and substance abuse programs* (2nd ed., pp. 23–44). New Brunswick, NJ: Transaction Publishers.
Moses, T. (2011). Adolescents' perspectives about brief psychiatric hospitalization: What is helpful and what is not? *Psychiatric Quarterly, 82*(2), 121–37.
Muncie, J., & Hughes, G. (2002). Modes of youth governance: Political rationalities, criminalisation and resistance. In J. Muncie, G. Hughes, & E. Mclaughlin (Eds.), *Youth justice: Critical readings* (pp. 1–18). London: Sage.
Parr, H., & Davidson, J. (2009). Mental and emotional health. In T. Brown, S. McLafferty, & G. Moon (Eds.), *A companion to health and medical geography* (pp. 258–277). London: Wiley-Blackwell.
Philo, C. (1987). 'Fit localities for an asylum': The historical geography of the nineteenth-century 'mad-business' in England as viewed through the pages of the asylum journal. *Journal of Historical Geography, 13*(4), 398–415.
The Prince's Trust (2017). *The Prince's Trust Macquarie Youth Index 2017*. London: The Prince's Trust.
Purcell, R., Goldstone, S., Moran, J., Albiston, D., Edwards, J., Pennell, K., & McGorry, P. (2011). Toward a twenty-first century approach to youth mental health care. *International Journal of Mental Health, 40*(2), 72–87.
Rayle, A. D. (2005). Adolescent gender differences in mattering and wellness. *Journal of Adolescence, 28*, 753–763.
Reavey, P. (Ed.) (2011). *Visual methods in psychology: using and interpreting images in qualiative research*. London: Routledge.
Reavey, P., Poole, J., Corrigall, R., Zundel, T., Byford, S., Sarhane, M., . . . Ougrin, D. (2017). The ward as emotional ecology: Adolescent experiences of managing mental health and distress in psychiatric inpatient settings. *Health & Place, 46*, 210–218.
Renedo, A., & Marston, C. (2015). Spaces for citizen involvement in healthcare: An ethnographic study. *Sociology, 49*(3), 488–504.
Rickwood, D. J., Deane, F. P., & Wilson, C. J. (2007). When and how do young people seek professional help for mental health problems? *Medical Journal of Australia, 187*, S35–S39.
Rogers, A., & Pilgrim, D. (2010). *A sociology of mental health and illness*. Buckingham, UK: Open University Press.

Ruiz, Ó. A. (2016). Youth movements, politics of identity and battles for visibility in neo-liberal Chile: Penguin generations. In C. Feixa, C. Leccardi, & P. Nilan (Eds.), *Youth, space, and time: Agoras and chronotopes in the global city* (pp. 342–365). Leiden: Brill.

Stedman, R., Beckley, T., Wallace, S., & Ambard, M. (2004). A picture and 1000 words: Using resident-employed photography to understand attachment to high amenity places. *Journal of Leisure Research, 36*(4), 580–606.

Sweeney, A., Gillard, S., Wykes, T., & Rose, D. (2015). The role of fear in mental health service users' experiences: A qualitative exploration. *Social Psychiatry and Psychiatric Epidemiology, 50*(7), 1079–1087.

Tulloch, S., Lelliott, P., Bannister, D., Andiappan, M., O'Herlihy, A., Beecham, J., & Ayton, A. (2008). *The costs, outcomes and satisfaction for inpatient child and adolescent psychiatric services (COSI-CAPS) study: Report for the National Co-Ordinating Centre for NHS Service Delivery and Organisation R&D*. Retrieved from http://rcpsych.ac.uk/pdf/COSI%20 CAPS.pdf.

Uprichard, E. (2008). Children as 'being and becomings': Children, childhood and temporality. *Children & Society, 22*(4), 303–313.

Valentine, G. (1996). Children should be seen and not heard: The production and transgression of adults' public space. *Urban Geography, 17*(3), 205–220.

Wilkinson, R., & Pickett, K. (2010). *The spirit level: Why equality is better for everyone*. London: Penguin.

Wright, E., & Ord, J. (2015). Youth work and the power of 'giving voice': A reframing of mental health services for young people. *Youth & Policy, 115*, 63–84.

5
USING EXPERIENCE-BASED CO-DESIGN TO IMPROVE INPATIENT MENTAL HEALTH SPACES

Zoë Boden, Michael Larkin and Neil Springham

Inpatient spaces: challenges in acute mental health services

While some inpatient mental health services provide pockets of excellence (NICE, 2012), a major UK government report (Crisp, Smith, & Nicholson, 2016) has recently found many under great pressure. Staff are often demoralised and locked into cycles of crisis management and service users and families may feel disenfranchised and excluded. Dangerous and chaotic wards, diverse case-mixes, the lack of therapeutic input and the excessive focus on community services at the expense of inpatient settings, all threaten the quality of acute care (Lelliot, Bennett, McGeorge, & Turner, 2006). Service users (Mind, 2011), families, (Hickman et al., 2015) and staff (Garcia, Kennet, Quarishi, & Durcan, 2005) all agree that acute mental health care is unsatisfactory, frightening and stigmatising. There is even evidence that being hospitalised for a mental health problem can be, in itself, traumatic (Morrison, Bowe, Larkin, & Nothard, 1999). This may be unsurprising given the coercive and controlling practices that take place there, including detention, seclusion, restraint and being forcibly compelled to undergo pharmacological treatments or electro-convulsive therapy.

It is worth questioning how a health care environment ever came to be associated with these types of coercive practices. In contemporary society, problems of psychological distress are generally conceptualised as problems of 'mental health'. At times of acute distress, such experiences are subject to psychiatric care, and if the distress involves risk of harm to self or others, then such care is usually provided in an inpatient environment, and the Mental Health Act can be invoked. Currently the majority of service users on an NHS inpatient ward are there involuntarily (Keown et al., 2016). This view – of what is problematic, who it affects and how it should be dealt with – is the consequence of a series of historical developments as much as it is a consequence of any experiential reality of 'feeling distressed'. In Foucault's (1964/2006) reading, mental health problems first emerged as a category of 'otherness', which needed to be managed alongside a number of other marginal or problematic forms of identity. In his account, people experiencing psychological distress are among several categories of people who may threaten the smooth running of the state. The state therefore, steps in to provide institutional control, meaning the early asylums emerge primarily to control the external environment, rather than for the benefit of those people who found themselves inside. However, it is also notable that distress is medicalised early on in these developments: medical assessment and intervention was developed in tandem with the control and surveillance. As a consequence, inpatient wards have retained some features of both cultures, in an "an uneasy compromise between a general hospital and a prison" (WHO, 1953). This remains the case for modern wards (Haigh, 2002).

In 1945, there was uncertainty about whether 'mental health' should be situated within the NHS (Kinderman, 2014). If it had not been given to health professionals to meet this need, then acute mental health treatment might have been quite different. It can be helpful to consider how the needs of people in psychological distress might be met from a design perspective. When designing a service or product, three domains are considered: performance, engineering and aesthetics (Berkun, 2004). Performance concerns whether the product or service works, so designers would likely introduce evidence-based interventions. Engineering involves ensuring those interventions are safe and reliable. Lastly, aesthetics focuses both on the physical environment, such as decoration and furnishing, and on the human and social world, that is how a service or product *feels*. Performance, engineering and aesthetics must work together. The design process involves testing this, experientially. Designers want to understand the emotional touchpoints; how a service user feels when interacting with the service. Problems occur if performance, engineering and aesthetics do not work together or if testing has been insufficient. At first glance, the NHS quality streams map reasonably well on to this design process. Performance is currently covered by clinical effectiveness, engineering by patient safety and aesthetics by patient experience. However, despite a number of more recent initiatives, such as Enhancing the Healing Environment (DoH, 2008), which have attempted to focus on the aesthetics of mental health services, it has taken the scandal highlighted by the Francis report (Mid Staffordshire NHS Foundation Trust, 2013), to instigate a duty to engage with the patient's human experience of their health care. The NHS has yet to develop consistent and effective practices that use patient experience data to initiate change (Coulter, Locock, Ziebland, & Calabrese, 2014).

When people are taken to mental health wards, typically in crisis, the aesthetic experience will be substantially different from when a person visits hospital with a physical health problem. Societal views of mental distress, the disruption to the individual's social context and the subjective experience itself, make the mental health crisis unique. The projects and the experience-based co-design (EBCD) approach we are going to discuss in this chapter, suggest that key elements of service users', staff members' and carers' experience in inpatient services (the emotional *touchpoints*), evoke strong and universal feelings, including terror, shame and alienation. These experiences are not routinely captured by the NHS quality measures, and those admitted to mental health wards do not have the consumer power to vote with their feet – services are commissioned on their behalf and they have little or no opportunity to choose where they are treated.

Conceptualising spaces as relational, meaningful and psychological

In her article on therapeutic spaces, Fenner (2011) argues that our understanding of the therapeutic relationship should be extended to take into account the material and spatial aspects of the environment in which the relationship occurs. In considering inpatient spaces, the reverse needs to happen; consideration of the environment needs to extend to thinking about the people who occupy these spaces, and how they interact. Spaces are given shape by the practices that are conducted within them; they have functions, atmospheres and cultures. The inpatient ward might be best understood as a 'therapeutic landscape' (Gesler, 1993); a place, expected to be beneficial to well-being, where the physical, social and symbolic aspects of the environment, and their cultural and historical context, will elicit particular experiences and meanings for the people who use it. These subjective experiences and meanings will be contingent upon individuals' and groups' personal attitudes (Corandson, 2005), their emotional experiences and their memories of other therapeutic landscapes, for example those encountered in previous admissions.

The literature on psychologically informed environments suggests that spaces can be changed by careful consideration of who resides there, and particular consideration of their psychological and emotional needs (Johnson & Haigh, 2010). At the most basic level, an inpatient ward needs to be "a good place to be"[1] (Haigh, Harrison, Johnson, Paget, & Williams, 2012, p. 36). In thinking about improving inpatient spaces, it is necessary to include all aspects of the psychosocial environment alongside the physical features. While some mental health hospitals may visually resemble other kinds of hospital, or even office spaces, they are very clearly distinct in terms of their social rules, expectations, practices, affectivity and culture. Some of these distinctive features are best understood as properties of the spaces themselves (rather than say, as norms or ideas held by any specific person or group). The EBCD approach we now turn to is promising because, while it explicitly focuses on changing fairly 'concrete' aspects of the environment, it does so via a relational, collaborative mechanism that seems to work – implicitly – to improve psychosocial aspects of the environment as well.

Experience-based co-design

Services can be developed from a range of rationales, and the role and source of evidence may vary. In conventional evidence-based practice, a line is presumed to run from acceptability, to efficacy under controlled conditions and then to effectiveness in naturalistic settings. Yet many interventions supported by high-quality RCT evidence, such as family therapy interventions for psychosis, have been difficult to implement in front line practice (Berry & Haddock, 2008). NICE often overlooks experiential data as suitable evidence, yet understanding the context in which services or interventions happen (as a staff member, service user or carer) is vital to understanding the local variables that can act as tangential barriers and that may not be apparent in other contexts. To design an effective service or environment, we need to integrate context-bound experiential insights and more traditional sources of (generalised) evidence.

Crisp et al. (2016) recommend that the service design, provision and governance of acute care can be improved by greater collaboration between providers, users and commissioners of inpatient mental health services. EBCD is one such way of working collaboratively to improve health care services. EBCD enables service users, carers and staff (both ground-level and management) to work together to improve services and health care environments. EBCD has roots in participatory action research, user-centred design, learning theory and narrative-based approaches to change (Robert, 2013). It was developed for physical health care and was first piloted in a head and neck cancer service (Bate & Robert, 2007). Subsequently a toolkit was developed (The King's Fund, 2012) to assist local teams in using EBCD in their services.

The EBCD process

EBCD follows a basic six-step process, and although this has evolved with the literature, most projects in physical health care follow this standard sequence (see Figure 5.1). First, experiences are gathered from staff, service users and sometimes carers, via observation and interviews, which are typically filmed. Second, 'touchpoints' are identified by the project team. These are critical moments experienced in relation to the service. Third, these are fed back to the participants, who then prioritise the touchpoints. The penultimate phase is the co-design event, which is the opportunity for different stakeholders to come together and work in small groups to co-design improvements to the service, according to those priorities that have been identified. The final stage is to hold a celebration event to review what has been achieved.

Using EBCD to change inpatient mental health spaces

Mental health contexts are different to physical health ones. Asking service users to share personal stories of hospitalisation for psychosis, for example, requires different considerations than asking people to talk about the treatment they received for broken bones. In the last few years, a few researchers and clinicians have begun to adapt EBCD for use in mental health contexts. EBCD offers a practical and powerful way of improving mental health services, but it requires a great deal of

- **Gathering experiences** from staff, then service uses and carers, via observation and interviews (which are often filmed)

- **Identifying 'touchpoints'**; critical moments experiences in relation to the service

- **Feeding back** these touchpoints to project participants

- The **prioritising of the touchpoints** by the project participants

- Bringing everyone together in a **co-design event**, which they work in small groups to co-design improvements to the service according to the priorities identified

- Holding a **celebration event** to all involved to review what has been achieved

(Donetto, Tsianakas, & Robert, 2014; Robert, 2013)

FIGURE 5.1 The standard EBCD process.

care to ensure the process does not echo the problems of the services it seeks to improve. We have undertaken EBCD projects in two NHS mental health Trusts in the UK. In Coventry and Warwickshire Mental Health Trust (CWMHT; led by Michael Larkin and Lizzie Newton) the project worked to improve inpatient provision, particularly for young people experiencing early psychosis. At Oxleas Mental Health Trust (led by Neil Springham) the project worked to improve the ward environments in acute adult mental health, with the aim of reducing service user complaints (Springham & Robert, 2015) (Figure 5.2). Both projects sought to make positive changes to the inpatient experience, but adapted EBCD in slightly different ways.

Developing trust and cooperation: overcoming the challenges

EBCD is a collaborative approach, and mental health inpatient wards are difficult environments for the development of trust between staff, service users and carers.

Experience-based co-design   93

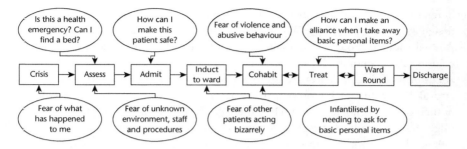

FIGURE 5.2   Generating touchpoints in the Oxleas project. The sequence of clinical procedures is shown as squares. Emotional touchpoints are shown as circles, with staff experience shown above and service user experience below.

The service user perspective has traditionally been denigrated as lacking in insight, and has often been ignored in service planning (Repper & Perkins, 2003). At Oxleas, service users were concerned that what they share in the project could have implications if they needed to return to hospital. The imbalance of power between providers and users of acute inpatient services is heightened in comparison to physical health care. Service users may be frightened of service providers: they have the power to act coercively, and to interpret information provided to them in the light of a 'risk' discourse, which can threaten service users' liberty and autonomy. Service providers may also sometimes be frightened of service users: in acute settings, emotions are intensified and behaviour may seem unpredictable or extreme. There are also very real consequences for staff speaking out in terms of livelihood and career progression. At Oxleas, many staff feared talking freely, in case their feelings were seen as 'un-PC'. They were worried that any negative feelings that they shared would be deemed indicative of personal incompetence, rather than as systemic, service-level issues. Staff may need reassurance that EBCD is a design project about an improved future, and not an investigation raking over the past or allocating blame – perhaps a far more common experience of NHS management processes.

Co-operation between groups with different interests and statuses is improved when there is trust between them. Trust in this context might relate particularly to the transparency of each group's motives, to the reliability of the groups (in terms of honouring its commitments) and to the respect that each group is able to show for other groups' motives and concerns. In mental health services, and particularly in inpatient care, trust can be threatened by the dual role of the service provider, as both coercive and caring. EBCD contains a number of features that are very helpful for developing trust, and producing effective collaborations.

EBCD invites people to identify their individual concerns, but is predicated on high levels of perspective taking. Its structured nature means that participants are encouraged to anticipate sharing their experiences with people who have quite different experiences from them, before they are brought face-to-face at the co-design event. Importantly, EBCD treats everyone's experience as equally relevant. All 'stakeholder' groups are consulted and all contribute data that lead to the generation of touchpoints. It ensures that each group has a say in how touchpoints are prioritised. It also invites groups to consider the perspective of others, which is critical. In the 'feedback groups', participants are consulted in the relatively 'safety' of their own stakeholder group. Here there can be considerable reflection on what might be important to the other groups, and it allows for a discussion of what it will be like to work with those groups at the 'co-design' stage. Preparation for this is important: groups can discuss how they will work, what they are worried about and what they hope to gain. Via these processes, EBCD generates consensus *and* allows for crucial differences in perspective. One co-production study in a London mental health service measured its success in terms of each party not feeling they had to shift on key positions, but finding recognition of their perspective in the final result (Gillard et al., 2010). The work must proceed with a focus on what everyone agrees to be important, but often there is considerable surprise about how similar everyone's concerns are, once differences have been respected.

The co-design event: opening up new spaces for dialogue

When bringing together each participant group for the first time in the co-design event, the aim is to support individuals to express their perspective and to hear the perspectives of others, so that they can collaborate to design improvements to their environment. This has to be carefully planned and managed to ensure that these potentially mistrusting and unequal groups can come together in an atmosphere of mutual respect. The aim is to open up a new space, which takes people out of their usual territorial position. The result can be very positive, and can help develop alternative formulations about how to constellate the shared physical and psychosocial environment. In one example, at Oxleas, the co-design process led to the instigation of daily community patient-experience meetings on an inpatient ward. This in turn helped reduce formal complaints by effectively helping staff understand how their behaviour and attitudes were being perceived by service users (Springham & Robert, 2015).

The co-design event can be seen as an example of the contact hypothesis (Allport, 1954) in practice. The hypothesis, which has been robustly supported (Pettigrew & Tropp, 2006), states that intergroup contact will reduce hostility or prejudice. Four conditions are necessary: common goals, intergroup cooperation, support from authorities and the equal status of parties (Pettigrew & Tropp, 2005). Well-meaning attempts to bring groups together may actually cause more harm than good if these conditions are not met (see Hewstone & Swart, 2011). In EBCD, the feedback groups ensure there are common goals. The principle of co-design, implying partnership, encourages cooperation between groups and senior support from management authorities should be sought from the beginning. There are, as has been argued, inequities between service users and health care providers: service users may be vulnerable due to stigma and distress, and staff members may draw authority from organisational power structures. However, the contact hypothesis literature suggests that, even when there is initially inequality between groups, creating equal status during the contact (the co-design event) is enough to promote positive intergroup attitudes (Schofield & Eurich-Fulcer, 2001; see Pettigrew & Tropp, 2005).

The co-design event provides a space that is at least somewhat freed from the normal constraints of the inpatient environment. In this new landscape, service users, staff and carers are asked to suspend their typical roles, relationships and expectations in order to creatively re-design the inpatient space. The co-design event encourages spontaneous and collaborative interaction. To support participants, and to disrupt the existing culture of the ward, certain practicalities need to be in place. A physically pleasing space (on 'neutral territory', preferably off-site), appropriate refreshments, some easy-to-access emotional support, a reasonable allotment of time, a clear plan and achievable goals for the day are elements that go some way towards meeting the requirements for a successful contact intervention. If the event has gone well, on moving back into the inpatient space, participants show an increased capacity to see beyond the categories of 'staff', 'service user' or 'carer', to take the other's perspective and to interact more humanely, responsively and flexibly.

This process is more likely to be supported where there is an established and stable group that is committed to pursuing projects of this kind. At Oxleas, this was a pre-existing service user and carer research group ('ResearchNet'). The beneficial outcomes of EBCD in mental health environments, particularly the relational changes, are more likely to be maintained when this type of collaboration can be

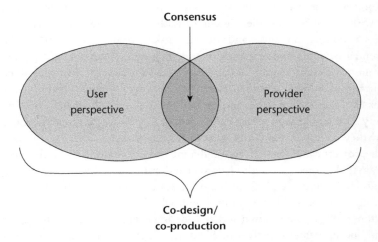

FIGURE 5.3 The differentiation of consensus versus co-production methodologies, where differences of perspective are utilised alongside points of agreement.

revisited on a regular basis. Unlike in physical health care, where a co-designed change can be implemented and easily maintained, many of the things that make a difference in mental health care are cultural and relational (Figure 5.3). Changes are hard won, and easily lost without continued attention, due to staff and service user turnover and the likelihood that people will fall back into ingrained patterns over time.

Using EBCD safely

Using EBCD in mental health services requires additional thought. We have adapted EBCD in various ways, so that it can be used successfully and safely in a mental health context. This has involved drawing on research ethics and peer research frameworks to ensure the work is done respectfully and without risk of harm. As shown, mental health services are not viewed favourably by service users and carers (Mind, 2011) and there are power dynamics that need acknowledgement. Recruitment to an EBCD project needs to be carefully managed. Service users must not feel coerced into taking part, nor feel they face barriers to participation. Participants must be able to give informed consent at the start, and assent during the project should also be carefully monitored. Some service users may have experiences that limit their willingness or capacity to engage with particular aspects of an EBCD project, for example being recorded (e.g. due to paranoia) or taking part in group events (e.g. due to social anxiety). Co-design teams must find ways to avoid causing distress and to encourage inclusivity. There may additionally be practical and social barriers to participants' engagement, such as shift patterns, wellness, discharge plans, childcare, etc. to accommodate.

In standard EBCD, one of the key aspects of the process is the filming of interview footage to be shared at the co-design event. There are a number of potential issues with this in the inpatient mental health context. Service users may have histories of trauma and abuse, and there is a risk of re-traumatisation in collecting experiential accounts, and in sharing them with others. Issues of confidentiality and anonymity, and consideration of the legacy and ownership of the material must be thought through. While a service user may be willing to share a distressing account of their experiences during the project, they may change their mind later in their recovery. We would suggest that those leading the co-design projects are cautious in how they collect accounts and what they do with them.

Our projects came up with two different ways to manage these challenges: In the CWMHT project, we audio recorded and transcribed the original experiential accounts, following a typical qualitative research approach. We then asked for service user and carer volunteers from the feedback groups to create more bespoke short films with us to be shown at the co-design event. We wanted to capture the 'real-life' positives and negatives that had been highlighted in the interviews, and give those staff who had not had already heard the findings the chance to gain a better understanding of service user and carer views, but we wanted to ensure this happened in a safe way. We held new interviews with the volunteers that still focused on the volunteers' experiences of inpatient care, but were less open-ended than the original interviews. The aim was to gather filmed material relating solely to the prioritised touchpoints. Each interview lasted approximately half an hour, and each was edited down to a 2-minute clip in the form of a condensed narrative. We were mindful that some of what volunteers said in these interviews might not feel safe to share in front of a large audience, and so we edited out personal details or anything that seemed unnecessarily exposing. We chose extracts that did not feel too controversial, but that linked to the priority areas. For example, a carer talking about how she had been frantic with worry when her son went missing. After many calls, she eventually located him in the local inpatient service. We linked this to our priority area of 'communication' because it was clear that a call saying that her son was safe would have prevented a great deal of anxiety. We previewed the clips with the volunteers to make sure that they were still happy for them to be shown. To help the audience, we also added onscreen titles to link the narratives to the priority areas. At Oxleas, initially no one wanted to make films, however once the service user design group got together to define the bounds of consent and data protection, and agreed to make and edit the films themselves, it was decided they would go ahead. Ownership throughout the production of the material ensured that people felt safe. In fact, they felt proud of the films, and saw high levels of commonality between their experiences. Having control over the process and the support provided by the group, including the chance to revisit issues as necessary, helped people to feel they could engage safely and on their own terms.

The co-design event can also become a source of distress for service users, carers and staff. Meeting with each other can be intimidating and anxiety provoking, but can also be deeply affecting. Great care was taken to prepare service users, families and staff very carefully for what to expect. We were conscious of the current context of inpatient care in the UK (e.g. Crisp et al., 2016), and that relationships between staff, service users and carers may be strained. Although most staff hold positive views towards service users, there is evidence reporting that some mental health professionals hold negative attitudes toward service users (see Wahl and Aroesty-Cohen, 2010) and can display the same negative stereotypes as the general public (Nordt, Rossler, & Lauber, 2006). As working in inpatient care can be very stressful (e.g. Ward, 2011), there can be widespread demoralisation (Crisp et al., 2016) and many staff can feel pressured by issues such as high bed occupancy, lack of training and lack of experienced leadership (Garcia et al., 2005). For these reasons, at CWMHT, there was a quiet room and support available for anyone who needed it, regardless of what role they held in the service. In this case, it was a member of staff who made use of these resources.

Making changes in mental health spaces

In mental health, there is a significant gap between the hopes of service users and their families, and the nature of services. To a degree, this may be due to the mixed 'care-coercion' model, and the shortage of effective medical interventions for many common difficulties (despite the continued dominance of the medical model). Thus a degree of expectation management is required. Appropriate aims must be established and the remit of the project must be clear. A local co-design project will not rewrite the Mental Health Act, provide more funding for therapists, nor will it challenge cultural-level stigma, for example. However, it can reasonably aim to improve the environment in which services are delivered, and the way in which they are delivered. It may improve the relationships between the various groups involved. There may also be some anxiety about experiential evidence: in our experience, the issues raised and improved through EBCD do not contradict evidence-based practice. They tend to complement good practice, or enable it to be enacted.

It can be a challenge to make sure that actions planned at the co-design phase are actually implemented. It helps if there is 'ownership' of the project from within the service. It helps too if there is a group that meets regularly to monitor progress, and if that group contains service users and families, as well as senior representatives from the host organisation who can make things happen. In both settings, when management were more closely involved they found it a moving experience. They described how normal reporting structures tended to edit out the experience of staff and users. Sometimes, the presence of an external collaborator, such as a researcher or evaluator can also be helpful. At points in both projects, we found meetings were cancelled due to genuine emergencies on the ward. It was at this point that service users became rather demoralised, as this mirrored their experience of feeling burdensome or undeserving of attention when more demanding things were happening. Likewise it was hard for staff to ignore emergencies to attend EBCD meetings, when they were liable to be blamed if things escalated on the ward. Having protected time set aside for regular meetings is supportive of all parties.

Conclusions

Environments dedicated to acute mental health care require our attention. They are frequently discomforting and are often disliked by all parties. However, making changes to mental health inpatient spaces is challenging and requires acknowledgement of the complexity of the environment. Inpatient wards are more than their material and spatial characteristics; they are relational, affective and atmospheric cultures. One way to improve mental health inpatient spaces is through use of the adapted EBCD described in this chapter. This approach is particularly successful when it can be implemented as part of a rolling programme of collaborative improvement work. In this context, EBCD can have a lasting impact on the culture of an inpatient environment, as well making changes at a more concrete level.

Success can be evaluated by monitoring whether the actions agreed at the co-design event have been implemented. Often it is surprisingly easy to think of broad indicators, (for example, number of complaints, or use of coercive measures such as restraint), which could be audited pre- and post-implementation, to judge whether actions have had an effect on the wider environment. There may also be ways of evaluating changes in the relationships *between* stakeholder groups, depending on the context of the project. Second, however, projects can lead to unexpected changes at an experiential level for individuals and groups. It is these changes that appear to be the most powerful, but the hardest to evaluate. Qualitative exploration of the impact of EBCD projects would be valuable. The success of EBCD projects is dependent on project leaders having the skill set required, as well as access to the resources they need and buy in from senior management and key stakeholders. Competencies with group work, a level of clinical understanding and an 'insider' status are necessary for project leaders.

EBCD for mental health is still in its earliest stages and EBCD more generally is still an emerging field. It is not yet clear what the core elements of the process are or exactly which psychosocial mechanisms are at play. One danger is that EBCD methodology is co-opted for use in non-collaborative approaches (Mulvale, Miatello, Hackett, & Mulvale, 2016). However, what has been published about EBCD to date suggests that it can be a powerful mechanism for service improvement, making services more acceptable to service users, carers, and staff. EBCD methodology thus has the potential to increase well-being for all concerned. However, challenges encountered in our work adapting EBCD for use in the mental health arena do illustrate the importance of implementing the approach with the right support, resources and care.

Acknowledgements

With particular thanks to Ami Woods (Oxleas) and Elizabeth Newton (CWMHT), as well as all the participants – service users, carers and staff.

Note

1 The argument that follows is largely focused upon how an existing inpatient environment might be improved, but the processes, of course, can also be used to think about how alternative forms of 'safe places' might be co-designed.

References

Allport, G. W. (1954). *The nature of prejudice*. Reading, MA: Addison-Wesley.
Bate, P., & Robert, G. (2006). Experience-based design: From redesigning the system around the patient to co-designing services with the patient. *Quality and Safety Health Care, 15*, 307–310.
Bate, P., & Robert, G. (2007). Toward a more user-centric OD: Lessons from the field of experience-based design and a case study. *Journal of Behavioral Science, 43*, 41–66.
Berkun, S. (2004). *Programmers, designers and the Brooklyn Bridge*. Retrieved from www.scottberkun.com/essays/essay30.htm.
Berry, K., & Haddock, G. (2008). The implementation of the NICE guidelines for schizophrenia: Barriers to the implementation of psychological interventions and recommendations for the future. *Psychology and Psychotherapy: Theory, Research and Practice, 81*, 419–436.

Corandson, D. (2005). Landscape, care and the relational self: Therapeutic encounters in rural England. *Health Place*, *11*(4), 337–348.

Coulter, A., Locock, L., Ziebland, S., & Calabrese, J. (2014). Collecting data on patient experience is not enough: They must be used to improve care. *British Medical Journal*, *348*, 2225.

Crisp, N., Smith, G., & Nicholson, K. (Eds.). (2016). *Old problems, new solutions: Improving acute psychiatric care for adults in England*. Commission on Acute Adult Psychiatric Care. Retrieved from http://media.wix.com/ugd/0e662e_aaca63ae4737410e9e2873dfde 849841.pdf.

Department of Health (2004). *Improving the patient experience – sharing success in mental health and learning disabilities: The King's Fund's Enhancing the Healing Environment Programme 2004–2008*. London: TSO.

Donetto, S., Tsianakas, V., & Robert, G. (2014). *Using experience-based co-design (EBCD) to improve the quality of healthcare: Mapping where we are now and establishing future directions*. London: King's College London.

Fenner, P. (2011). Place, matter and meaning: Ending the relationship in psychological therapies. *Health & Place*, *1*, 851–857.

Foucault, M. (2006). *Madness and civilization: A history of insanity in the age of reason*. London: Vintage Books. (Original work published 1964.)

Garcia, I., Kennet, C., Quarishi, M., & Durcan, G. (2005). *Acute care 2004: A national survey of adult psychiatric wards in England*. London: Sainsbury Centre for Mental Health.

Gesler, W., 1993. Therapeutic landscapes: Theory and a case study of Epidauros, Greece. *Environment and Planning D: Society and Space*, *11*(2), 171–189.

Gillard S., Turner K., Lovell, K., Norton, K., Clarke, T., Addicott, R., . . . Ferlie, E. (2010). 'Staying native': Coproduction in mental health services research. *International Journal of Public Sector Management*, *23*(6), 567–577.

Haigh, R. (2002). Acute wards: Problems and solutions. Modern millieux: Therapeutic community solutions to acute ward problems. *Psychiatric Bulletin*, *26*, 380–382.

Haigh, R., Harrison, T., Johnson, R., Paget, S., & Williams, S. (2012). Psychologically informed environments and the 'enabling environments' initiative. *Housing, Care and Support*, *15*(1), 34–42.

Hewstone, M., & Swart, H. (2011). Fifty-odd years of inter-group contact: From hypothesis to integrated theory. *British Journal of Social Psychology*, *50*, 374–386.

Hickman, G., Newton, E., Boden, Z., Fenton, K., Thompson, J., & Larkin, M. (2015). The experiential impact of hospitalisation on families of young people with early psychosis. *Clinical Child Psychology and Psychiatry*, *21*(1), 145–155.

Johnson, R., & Haigh, R. (2010). Social psychiatry and social policy for the 21st century – new concepts for new needs: The 'psychologically informed environment'. *Mental Health and Social Inclusion*, *14*(4), 30–35.

Keown, P., McBride, O., Twigg, L., Crepaz-Keay, D., Cyhlarova, E., Parsons, H., . . . Weich, S. (2016). Rates of voluntary and compulsory psychiatric in-patient treatment in England: An ecological study investigating associations with deprivation and demographics. *British Journal of Psychiatry*, *209*(2) 157–161.

Kinderman, P. (2014). *A prescription for psychiatry: Why we need a whole new approach to mental health and wellbeing*. London: Palgrave Macmillan.

The King's Fund. (2012). *Experience-based co-design toolkit*. Retrieved from www.kingsfund. org.uk/projects/ebcd.

Lelliot, P., Bennett, H., McGeorge, M., & Turner, T. (2006). Accreditation of acute in-patient mental health services. *Psychiatric Bulletin*, *30*, 361–363.

Mid Staffordshire NHS Foundation Trust. (2013). *Report of the Mid Staffordshire NHS Foundation Trust Public Inquiry*. London: TSO.

Mind. (2011). *Listening to experience: An independent inquiry into acute and crisis mental healthcare*. London: Mind.

Morrison, A., Bowe, S., Larkin, W., & Nothard, S. (1999). The psychological impact of psychiatric admission: Some preliminary findings. *Journal of Nervous and Mental Disease, 187*, 250–253.

Mulvale, A., Miatello, A., Hackett, C., & Mulvale, G. (2016). Applying experience-based co-design with vulnerable populations: Lessons from a systematic review of methods to involve patients, families and service providers in child and youth mental health service improvement. *Patient Experience Journal, 3*(1), 117–129.

National Institute for Health and Care Excellence. (2012). *Service user experience in adult mental health: NICE guidance on improving the experience of care for people using adult NHS mental health services*. London: British Psychological Society and The Royal College of Psychiatrists.

Nordt, C., Rossler, W., & Lauber, C. (2006). Attitudes of mental health professionals toward people with schizophrenia and major depression. *Schizophrenia Bulletin, 32*, 709–714.

Pettigrew, T. F., & Tropp, L. R. (2005). Allport's intergroup contact hypothesis: Its history and influence. In J. F. Doviio, P. Glick, & L. A. Budman (Eds.), *On the nature of prejudice: Fifty years after Allport* (pp. 262–277). Oxford: Blackwell.

Pettigrew, T. F., & Tropp, L. R. (2006). A meta-analytic test of intergroup contact theory. *Journal of Personality and Social Psychology, 90*, 751–783.

Repper, J., & Perkins, R. (2003). *Social inclusion and recovery: A model for mental health practice*. Kent: Balliere Tindall.

Robert, G. (2013). Participatory action research: Using experience-based co-design (EBCD) to improve the quality of health care services. In S. Ziebland, J. Calabrese, A. Coulter, & L. Locock (Eds.), *Understanding and using experiences of health and illness* (pp. 138–149). Oxford: Oxford University Press.

Schofield, J. W., & Eurich-Fulcer, R. (2001). When and how school desegregation improves intergroup relations. In R. Brown & S. L. Gaetner (Eds.), *The Blackwell handbook of social psychology: Intergroup processes* (pp. 475–494). Malden, MA: Blackwell.

Springham, N., & Robert, G. (2015). Experience based co-design reduces formal complaints on an acute mental health ward. *British Medical Journal Quality Reports, 4*(1), doi: 10.1136/bmjquality.u209153.w3970.

Wahl, O., & Aroesty-Cohen, E. (2010). Attitudes of mental health professionals about mental illness: A review of the recent literature. *Journal of Community Psychology, 38*(1), 49–62.

Ward, L. (2011). Mental health nursing and stress: Maintaining balance. *International Journal of Mental Health Nursing, 20*, 77–85.

World Health Organisation (1953). *Expert committee on mental health: Third report*. Geneva: WHO.

6
SENSORY SPACE IN CHILD AND ADOLESCENT MENTAL HEALTH INPATIENT CARE

Nathan Parnell and Bernice Rooney

Sensory approaches

Sensory approaches were one of the predominant methods to address both physical and emotional aspects of humanity. Specifically for mental health or emotions, sensory approaches can be dated back to as far as 6000BC, with Egyptians utilising aromatherapy for religious and medicinal purposes (Thomas, 2002) and Greeks using music (Watkins, 1997) and botany (Keller, 2014) for positive effects on mood, anxiety and healing. Within the present day, sensory modulation is broadly defined as

> the capacity to regulate and organise the degree, intensity and nature of responses to sensory input in a graded and adaptive manner. This allows the individual to achieve and maintain an optimal range of performance and adapt to challenges in daily life.
> *(Miller, Reisman, McIntosh, & Simon, 2001)*

The predominant use of sensory-based rooms or methods to address the above have been popular in developmental disabilities such as Autism Spectrum Disorder (ASD) following the recognition that sensory dysregulation can lead to significant behavioural and mood changes (Ben-Sasson et al., 2007; Case-Smith & Bryan, 1999; Houghton et al., 1998; Tomchek & Dunn, 2007).

Recently, research has shown that those with diagnosed mental health problems such as depression, anxiety and trauma have sensory needs they may not be aware of, or may not be addressed, that subsequently contribute to mental well-being (Chalmers, Harrison, Mollison, Molloy, & Gray, 2012; Liss, Timmel, Baxley, & Killingsworth, 2005). Although there is a significant gap in sensory research when compared to traditional evidence-based approaches such as cognitive behavioural therapy (CBT), psychoanalysis and family work, research has shown these methods to be beneficial to many mental health problems. In conjunction with further treatment, adults with depression and trauma have shown reduced aggression and positive affect responses to sensory based approaches (Chalmers et al., 2012; Lee, Cox, Whitecross, Williams, & Hollander, 2010), with the current sparse research in older adolescents also showing similar results (Champagne & Sayer, 2003). Further, as individual differences and reactions to varying therapy models and theories are being brought to light (Fonagy & Roth, 2006) this not only highlights that evidence-based practices need bolstering, but that there could be further potential for an eclectic approach to therapies to account for variation in treatment response.

Although there are a number of important aspects of sensory approaches, one predominant focus is the space in which it is carried out. In order to achieve the aim of self-modulation, the space in which this takes place needs to be malleable to the individuals' sensory preferences while maintaining the ability to change as these preferences develop. Further, the predominant lead of sessions also stem from the individuals themselves, creating an equal or user-led session that somewhat differs from traditional and professionally led recovery therapies (Champagne & Sayer, 2003). Despite these considerations, there is little attention paid to these spatial and interactional aspects of sensory approaches, with the majority of research focusing on the functional aspects of sensory therapies. Further, the slender research that has been conducted on general sensory approaches outside of ASD has been predominantly conducted with adults.

To start to address both of these gaps, this chapter will focus on how this particular space – usually used for relaxation and exploration of the senses – is used within a place that is paradoxically identified with significant distress; an acute mental health ward for adolescents. The acute ward is a place where significant emphasis is placed on the individual through therapies and structured recovery plans to aid in negotiating this distressing time. As outlined in the coming sections, although there are many significant components to sensory modulation, the sensory space is explored within this chapter as a different area that switches some of the focus from the individual to the physical, social and symbolic space, while also considering how this influences the adolescent journey through relational aspects of their environment and engagement with mental health professionals.

Inpatient space and mental health

Despite the importance of space, environments can be difficult to manage when other expectations of care are prioritised in the field of mental health. Within the NHS, the predominant focus of recovery in mental health problems is on the individual rather than the setting itself. The space in which these individuals are admitted and reside – particularly for those admitted to inpatient wards – are secondary in terms of therapeutic value relative to the presenting symptoms and risk.

As such, logically there may be a significant gap between research into evidenced-based therapies and the space that individuals receiving therapy occupy. Although the person is rightly a significant focus of risk management and recovery during the start and throughout admission, there is evidence to suggest the space they occupy, how they use this and what it means to them, are important in influencing how a person negotiates such a distressing time (Curtis, Gesler, Fabian, Francis, & Priebe, 2007).

For health geography, individuals such as Gesler (1992) and Curtis (2010) note the idea that places and health are mutually entwined to the point that the experience of these landscapes or places can impact on or are important to health. Within this idea, therapeutic landscapes that connect these dimensions of space and health are proposed (Curtis, 2010). Although wide-reaching landscapes encompassing power/resistance, material poverty and so forth are put forward, of interest is the therapeutic landscape of physical and mental well-being – the idea that space and settings are connected to emotional response. Within this perspective on space, both Curtis (2010) and Gelser, Morag, Curtis, Hubbard, and Francis (2004) further note the idea that the physical, social and symbolic dimensions of environments put forward are important, with each coinciding along the life course of individuals to influence their mental well-being. As such, the interactions between the person and these three changing settings are thought to be important in influencing an individual's health outcome and experience. Further, due to the complexity of the aforementioned factors, it is noted that these are best viewed through a framework devised by Cummins, Curtis, Diez-Roux, and Macintyre (2007), in that combining the above factors feed into one half of a dichotomous perspective of space and its relation to mental health – a relational perspective on space. Conversely the other half of this theory – a conventional perspective – the relational perspective is one of fluidity within spaces; with dynamic definitions of space and place; variability in contextual meanings of spaces; and boundaries being replaced with emerging and changing divisions within space being developed by social power relations and cultural meaning.

The other half of the framework is the conventional perspective. Within this, space is viewed as something with definitions that are static; contextual features of space consistent within groups; and an overall segmented and boundaried view to varying spaces. When considering the organisations that help care for individuals experiencing distress and mental health problems, such as the NHS, parallels can be drawn within this framework of space conceptualisation. Considering the inpatient ward specifically, each area is designed to promote recovery and manage risk. Physically, bedrooms are standard and uniform with minimal materials for risk management. Assigned rooms for family time, therapy and education are commonplace. What individuals eat, where they eat and what they eat with are all monitored and assigned to rooms and places. Socially, each area is occupied by staff depending on observational tasks and activities and the topic of conversation is monitored depending on the age of adolescents present. Symbolically, this may logically change the meaning of each space within the ward as a by-product.

Although these actions may be necessary to mitigate and manage risk, the overarching segmented approach seems to put a typical ward in line with what seems to be a translational microcosm of conventional space; standardised and defined boundaries for activities and daily life that are contextually static.

Specific to the mental health context, Curtis et al. (2007) illustrate this feature within a qualitative study looking at hospital design and ex-service user perspectives. Themes including security and surveillance through division of space (uniform rooms and offices for sleeping and observations); respect and empowerment (carceral symbolism through fences and physical location of the ward and environment); and territoriality, privacy and social interactions (need for more private space in assigned areas) all emerged from the narratives provided. Although positive aspects of the environment did emerge, those noted seem to be aligned with a more conventional space perspective. Interestingly, it was also found that the importance of the physical aspects of the environment of hospitals designer, planners and architects, whereas the narrative within service user perspectives on hospital design were situated in the social and symbolic aspects of space, highlighting a disconnect between what was deemed physically necessary and what was deemed socially and symbolically important for those occupying and moving through that space during admission.

The impact on experiences was noted through the narratives of those previously admitted to the ward. Individual variations emerged from these themes; some individuals stated that the environment was welcoming and friendly, they had provided a valuable input into some design aspects of the environment and they had privacy to be in their room despite risk management aspects such as vision panels in the doors. There were, however, significant negative interpretations of the environment and spaces, including the carceral symbolism associated with individuals experiencing mental health problems as 'deviants' needing to be kept separate from society, and the need for more private spaces. This evidently had bearings on their experiences and overall demonstrated how hospital space influences health and lived experiences through physical, and subsequent social and symbolic space interpretations, specifically oriented toward respect and empowerment, psychological comforts, self-expression and a link to the community.

Albeit rooted in minimal evidence thus far, given the evident clinical influence and policy implications, this research might have for inpatient spaces, it is important to continue to look into alternative ways to address health and explore how these aspects shape individual experiences during such a distressing time. One further aspect of note from Curtis et al. (2007) and Gelser et al. (2004) however, are the challenges faced when translating this research into practice, particularly when making hospital design more congruent with what has been explored in previous research on the primary physical and risk management needs of a new unit. As this dominant discourse may take time to over turn, it may be pragmatic to step back and explore some key initial steps – as they appear existing spaces – and how they might be reviewed in order to start to align current research with existing aspects of inpatient space.

How may sensory spaces differ?

Given the research on space and its influence on mental health, one would assume that interest in such spaces would be prevalent. Further, the overriding need to keep someone safe and revive/resume their pathway through admission is paramount within the first period of admission, therefore providing spaces that are conducive to this primary need would be the logical choice for designing any room within an inpatient ward. One aforementioned key word, however, is pathway; admission is a journey of emotions and behaviours. On one end of the spectrum is the initial experience of distress and accompanying problems depending on the diagnosis or situation; the other is the point at which admission is no longer deemed necessary; and in the middle is the ever-changing transition period from these two points including periods of risk, progress and improvement.

In contrast to this journey that young people experience from admission to discharge, the 'conventional' space in which they occupy on a ward does not significantly change with them. Barring personal observations and leave, the same general rules and spaces apply to each individual whether they are recently admitted or ready to be discharged. This static space contrasted with the individual journey may be somewhat at odds with their experiences; their journey of admission has progressed, adaptation of therapies have been made, social interactions and input from staff vary, yet they are still afforded the same spaces that they occupied when they were first admitted and experienced extreme distress. In the same vein that it is necessary for risk to be managed and life to be preserved, it may well be reasonable to suggest that as the risk decreases and the journey towards leaving the clinical environment is nearing, the space they occupy – at least in part – could also reflect this flexibility towards their health, through flexibility in the environment.

In relation to this, Curtis et al. (2007) noted within the theme of expression and retention of identity and autonomy that those service users who suggested activities that are desirable therapeutically, were more informal than the structured occupational therapy activity schedule and had implications for hospital design. The theme of empowerment and respect within the same paper further explores the service user perspective which is related to the degree to which people are encouraged to participate in the decisions about hospital design and the activity regime, with this not only enabling greater empowerment but also autonomy. Staff who were interviewed on their perspectives of hospital design also recognised that the individual receiving therapy is just as important as the evidence informing it given 'they are the ones receiving it'.

Although uncommon, one sensory project reflects the importance of the flexibility of space as well as the empowerment that it affords to service users. Chalmers et al. (2012) adapted the physical environment of several rooms in their research with sensory resources, including their seclusion room within the ward, demonstrating that specific rooms within the ward can hold varying contexts and flexibility to the purpose and meaning of the room. The accompanying freedom of user-led sessions to pick and choose how they use the room led to positive changes within the individuals admitted to the ward. Although this study does not directly follow up on those perspectives, this initial change of context from seclusion room to sensory-friendly environment is an example of the flexibility in reflecting progress in the journey through admission. Further, the option of being user-led further reinforces this through choice rather than risk-management decisions, affording the individuals empowerment to choose how their session is directed towards addressing their symptoms. Subsequently, the meaning of the room has changed to reflect their emotional journey; they are not being restrained in a room originally built for that purpose, but it has been adapted to reflect their progress from potential deprivation of liberty, to a sense of freedom within a confined space, to solely influencing their own recovery.

In essence, the above example is portrays how some perceived 'conventional' spaces within a ward that usually have static contexts and definitions – such as a seclusion room – can be transferred into a flexible and dynamic space of a somewhat relational nature. Importantly, the adjunctive benefits of this have little evidence base, yet seem prominent; potential to improve outcomes of those admitted to an inpatient ward; empowerment for the individual to solely influence and somewhat take ownership of a session that may have therapeutic positive effects on behaviours and mood; and in the long term, it was noted to be a potential vessel for new empowering approaches within psychiatry, which require further evidential support.

Together, sensory-based approaches and the concurrent factors on space and empowerment are of interest and have been slowly growing over recent years. However, there are few studies which have examined any such factors in depth, in order that we might fully understand how sensory methods can be applied within current inpatient settings.

Our sensory space

The space outlined in this chapter arose from a young person admitted to an adolescent inpatient ward. Utilising clinical and non-clinical information from young people, and breaking down the supposition that the professional is the one holding all of the answers to navigating this pathway is the reason the room first started.

A young person diagnosed with autism admitted to an adolescent inpatient unit for affective and behavioural problems was seen to be jumping from stacked chairs. After initial staff conversations, it became apparent that the reason behind this was the sensation of falling as opposed to any self-injurious behaviour. After discussions with management around obtaining sensory resources to aid this need in a safe way, it was made apparent that an entire room could be developed.

When the proposal was submitted to obtain funding for the room, there was little research on pre-emptive methods to reduce aggression and subsequent seclusion and restraint with sensory methods. Existing research has shown sensory methods can reduce anxiety/arousal and the need for seclusion and restraint within adult services, and the room itself was proposed in the hope that it would add to the small amount of momentum behind sensory methods within adolescent psychiatric care.

The idea of the room itself was derived to provide a different space for young people on the ward. One of the main ways to achieve this was to allow them to develop the proposal collaboratively with staff. Physically, this was a space that was designed by those who would be using the space; socially it would be used as a group setting for young person-led relaxation or sensory activities; symbolically, this meant the two aforementioned approaches may then set this space aside from the uniformly NHS-designed spaces of the ward and be a more flexible and dynamic setting.

The original space was adapted from the 'quiet room', which consisted of several soft chairs and footstools. The main function of the room was to provide a space for young people to sit, with staff, when they were finding education sessions, group activities or meetings too distressing. While the room was used sparingly, it often led to escalations in distressed behaviour and young people requesting to return to 'their own space' – usually their bedroom – on the ward. When considering the impact Curtis et al. (2007) noted that regarding effective territorial spaces and the need for service users to have a space where they do not feel observed by staff or constrained by their behaviour, it seemed apparent that the desire to return to 'their own space' would be desirable in this situation. Consequently, when looking at developing a public space that could be flexible and personalised to an individual preference, this space appeared to be the most appropriate.

Before work on the room began, the young people on the ward were invited to a sensory awareness session. This comprised of basic information around sensory awareness, preferences and encouraging exploration of some handmade items (stress balloons/corn-starch putty) and small sensory toys (tangle ties/aroma-dough). Alongside this, an additional session for staff was included in the teams' 'away day'; including a presentation on sensory preferences and several hands-on activities. Additional discussion times were created during education sessions and the weekly young person business meeting, so that young people and staff could explore purpose-made sensory items through specialist sensory catalogues and a discussion of their ideas. These sessions were vital in gaining insight into what sensory items, methods and topics may help them and other young people in their situation. From these discussions, some young people created 'their ideal sensory room' using images from the catalogues and images they had drawn. The images created and subsequent discussions subsequently directed the development of the room; further sessions based on young people's preferences and interests in purpose-made sensory items – such as bubble tubes and fibre optic lights – lead to practical sessions around making home-made versions of these, and how these could be used to develop sensory awareness. Young people kept these items for use on the ward, and during further sessions, discussed what had been helpful or unhelpful about the items. Figures 6.1 and 6.2 show images of before and after room change, for an idea of how the room subsequently changed.

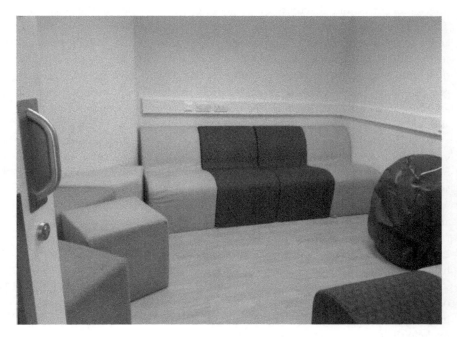

FIGURE 6.1 Before room change.

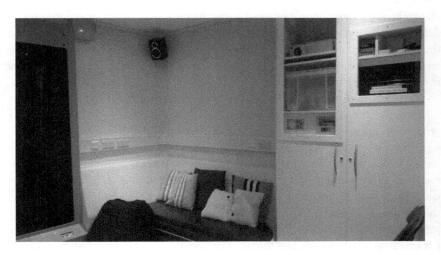

FIGURE 6.2 After room change.

Theory to practice

In practice, these group sessions were led by the young people attending and consisted of activities and discussions around their chosen sensory preference. Depending on the preferences of the group, several activities can take place in one session or an initial activity can be developed to include further elements. To do this, sets of hands-on activities were created using a range of sensory items and equipment in the room. This provided an opportunity for young people and staff to gain some basic information around sensory modulation and recognise their unique sensory preferences. Often individuals who have attended sensory groups before or have previous experience with sensory modulation will request an initial activity. When possible, the young person/people explain the activity and will start off the session.

In the initial stages of the space being used for both group and individual work, young people were also asked to rate their anxiety, restlessness, agitation and distress on a scale of 0–10, 0 being not at all and 10 being high. Alongside this, staff were asked to rate each young person in the group before and after the session using the same rating scale. These before and after measures were included in the proposal and running of the room to look at whether anxiety and arousal were significantly reduced subjectively within young people and objectively within staff ratings after each session. In addition to this, young people were provided an opportunity to make comments or suggestions for the continued use of the space, methods and structure of the sessions, which, for the purpose of this chapter, is the main focus of exploration here. Below are some excerpts from the feedback relating to the insights provided into the experiences, responses and suggestions the young people made in the group sessions and space, such as "I can't do relaxation things".

Feedback from the previous week led to a discussion around the meaning of 'relaxing' and 'relaxation'. Most young people associated it with comical sketches from television about people in a psychiatric hospital doing yoga or an interpretive dance with tambourines. As a group, the young people and staff 'set the scene' of the room; projecting an image of a forest on the wall; picking woodland noises; and choosing a green coloured light setting, saying: "I am a tree! [. . .] The Sensory room makes me a tree".

With the room set, there was a collaborative attempt to act out this notion of relaxation seen on TV, leading to everyone being in fits of giggles and making a group agreement that it wasn't 'their way of relaxing'. This then led on to a discussion about what each individual did when they wanted to relax at home. Choices were to listen to loud music and dance, make a den/fort or sleep. These were then explored in subsequent groups with young people bringing their own music or items to be used in the group. The symbolic meaning of both the space itself and the means in which it is engaged with were addressed here through the young people's autonomy and empowerment to direct the session into an area that they felt represented relaxation. The theme of respect and choice around users' perspectives in the decision-making process seemed key to the further development of empowerment and autonomy, in contrast to choices being based exclusively on risk management (Curtis et al., 2007; Chalmers et al., 2012): "The sensory room relaxes me so much [. . .] I heart cocooning myself and just 'being', love hearing people do things around me and not having to take part". In line with this, it is important to note that engagement is not always about the participation in the activity, sometimes the act of being with a group of people and not taking part mirrors life outside of the hospital. Opposed to clinical settings, which emphasise continuous engagement and observation in aid of managing risk and monitoring progress – with both the individual and group work – there has been a clear expectation that using the space is not mandatory but a 'choice' made by the individual. While the majority of the therapeutic groups set joint ground rules at the start of each session, the sensory group extended this to include any sensory input from activities, for example scent or lighting effect in the room. If it is not possible to continue the current activity without this element, the group picks a new activity. This is unlike most groups where, if the individual is finding an element of the group or mostly structured activity distressing – particularly if being facilitated by a manual – they are given the option to either remain in the group or return to the ward. When considering the therapeutic goal of a structured activity being derived from a pre-set agenda versus the aim of the sensory group – that seeks to develop with the group – adaptation of the space was important for all involved to explore sensory awareness and modulation in their desired expression: "My nose and taste buds were having a mini orgasm #smellgasm".

During the formation of a group, how each individual expresses their responses to an activity or sensory input is vital. As stated, for some this might be passive engagement in the group, but for others the use of descriptive and personalised language is central to their exploration of sensory awareness. While offensive or derogatory language is clearly not acceptable, often the young people use language not characteristic of conversations with staff. For the facilitating staff, this can be a difficult line to tread but often allows for the development of a social link within discussions about current activities and life outside of the hospital. With the need for an environment to reflect the flexibility found in a young person's progression from admission to discharge, there is a parallel to their sense of identity and readiness to express this.

In addition, the subsequent transition away from member of a community to that of individual in a hospital can, at times, consequently sever the link to a previous social life and support system outside of hospital (Curtis et al., 2007). To further champion the idea of this sensory space being flexible and to continue fostering a link to life outside of the hospital, staff and young people collaborated on several transformations of the space to mark community celebrations. This included young people and staff creating props, decorations and accessories to turn the room into a Comic Relief 'set the scene photo booth' (Figure 6.3). Young people encouraged staff to come and get their picture taken in their chosen style and setting for a small donation to Comic Relief. The young people took time to explain to staff how to use the sensory equipment to create their desired scene and helped snap the final photos.

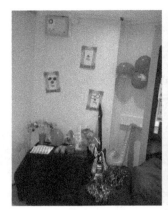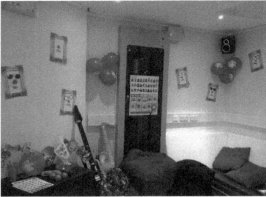

FIGURE 6.3 Comic Relief photo booth.

A further example of a sensory room is shown in Figure 6.4, which shows a China town themed room. In order to celebrate Chinese New Year young people and staff created traditional decorations, food and gifts to give to family and friends. To explore this celebration further, some young people went to China Town in central London to experience the decorations and collect traditional ingredients for the cooking group. Young people and staff used this information to turn the sensory room into a venue in which they could celebrate together.

Some comments from young people were: "Dimmer lights in this room make me feel calmer", and "Having the lights really low was super relaxing. It was good to just sit for a while".

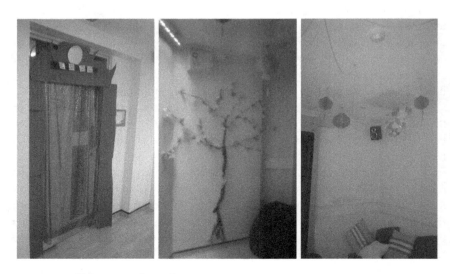

FIGURE 6.4 China town themed room.

Lastly, the most frequent comment about the sensory room was the flexibility of the environment compared to the rest of the ward; in particular, the young people's capacity to independently direct the brightness of the lights. In contrast, because of the need for observations and risk management on the ward, most young people experience no point at which all the lights are switched off – during the night, hall lights are on but reduced and a flashlight is used during night observations. From previous research (Curtis et al., 2007) the balance between supervision and freedom from supervision is an ongoing issue that will continue to direct how space is developed in psychiatric care. As expressed above, small flexibilities within spaces can impact how an individual engages with that space and therefore the overall situation.

Reflective space

Overall this chapter has looked at how a sensory space for young people in an inpatient unit can be an important influence on how an individual negotiates this distressing time. A form of sensory space that is flexible and malleable is able to position itself in contrast to the conventional areas of an inpatient ward. Due to this relational microcosm, the physical, social and symbolic dimensions of space interacting with each other, and the individual, seemed to emerge as an important influence on young people's experiences. Physically, this space was designed by those who use it; socially it has been used for user-led relaxation, sensory awareness and self-modulation work; symbolically, this seems to have set it aside from the uniformly 'conventional' static space characteristic of an inpatient ward.

The collaborative development of physical environment seemed to afford the young people an opportunity to not only have a significant impact on design, but links to the empowerment and respect themes emerging in previous research (Curtis et al., 2007). The effort from both staff and young people to listen to their needs providing a narrative of equality, seemingly enabling them to get the most therapeutically out of the space provided, both in design and in use. Following this, the choice of use or non-use seemed to also reflect their choice in participation of their time in the ward. As mentioned, a significant proportion of admission is focused on the individual themselves to help them through this journey. The sensory space, however, also reflected a focus away from the individual and on to the space itself, which emerged as important for some, as a way to feel in control of their environment and link to the outside world.

Socially, self-expression seemed to link with the language attributed to the space. Although appropriateness and professionalism is warranted within settings such as inpatient wards – particularly for adolescents – the social and symbolic aspect of this space meant that they could use language that wouldn't necessarily be in line with formal activities that occur in an inpatient space, and more aligned with links to friendship talk or social aspects outside of this environment. Given the transition from member of a community – and the subsequent status and responsibility of social life – to that of inpatient and the focus on risk management, an environment that can champion this link back to the social life outside of hospital is paramount. The flexibility of the physical environment seemed to also emphasise this link and challenge the carceral perspective that can occur in inpatient settings (Curtis et al., 2007). By symbolically bringing the community into the physical space of the ward through events, this seemed to foster the above expression and further set this space aside as a relational space that promotes the social and community bond that may be disrupted when admitted.

Following on, the focus between the individual and the symbolic meaning of the space to them seemed to be prominent and key to the young people's experience. The key impact of the flexibility of the space in affording individuals' empowerment of choice to use this space, and how to use the room, along with the potential for subsequent autonomy in their journey through this choice, was a main factor in both the development and continuing structure of this sensory space. From the start of this project, throughout its development and to its current practice, the space has been developed to fully immerse young people in decision making and choice of interaction with the space as well as the content covered in the groups. Further, the user-led group style has aimed to offer something different from the traditional professionally led therapies (Champagne & Sayer, 2003). Parallel to this, the sensory space has attempted to address the contrast between the journey young people experience, and the static 'conventional' space this takes place in while they occupy a ward. Similar to previous research, by focusing on the young people's choices around their engagement with the space, as opposed to choices being solely based on risk management, primary health or interventional needs, the sensory space has looked to mirror the flexibility and progress of an individual through flexibility in their environment (Chalmers et al., 2012; Curtis et al., 2007).

Considering the implementation of the room and the impact it can have, its use has to be taken into consideration within the set of challenges previously noted by Curtis et al., (2007) and Gesler et al. (2004). Shifts in an established pattern of physical focus on space are difficult to manage, however, it has been shown to be possible given the correct steps forward through previous research and this sensory room. Further suggestions from Champagne and Stromberg (2004) have been noted that methods such as sensory-based approaches can shift toward more collaborative care. Although it is still necessary to initially manage risk through primarily through the physical aspects of the inpatient environment and space, the impact of sensory methods within a physical space offers may be one of the small steps that can facilitate a move towards the outlined shift in previous projects to provide, among other factors, a space that is reflective of the pathway through admission (Curtis et al., 2007; Champagne & Stromberg, 2004). Through providing a relational microcosm and adapting existing spaces first, this step has shown the potential for considering further methods of collaborative care.

Overall it appears that the sensory room may be in line with a relational space that contrasts with the conventional inpatient environment. Importantly, instead of competing with traditional hospital ward spaces, it may be useful to view this sensory space as a transitional environment space that reflects the emotional and after behavioural aspects of admission. The input from young people here seems to resonate with the idea that this environment may positively shape experience during this difficult time via facilitating empowerment, choice, autonomy, links to the community and many other positive aspects shown previously. It is evident that this area – both sensory and spatial research – requires further exploration in order to fully grasp its potential. There is, however, promise from this chapter and previous work that suggests sensory methods – alongside many other interventions and practices – not only in itself may it be beneficial for use in mental health services and with adolescents, but the space that it affords, and how this is used when placed in an environment associated with distress, can also contribute to shaping young people's experiences during a very difficult time.

Acknowledgements

We would like to thank the Maudsley Charity for providing the grant money to fund this project. We would also like to thank the staff and management at the adolescent unit for their acceptance and support of the sensory room and the members of our previous team for their flexibility, support and guidance of this project while carrying out our duties. We would also like to thank the young people at the unit, as without their input, strength to work through their journey and subsequent participation, this room, and indeed this chapter, would not exist.

Conflicts of interest

Nathan Parnell and Bernice Rooney were the grant holders from the Maudsley Charity which helped to develop and contribute to this sensory space within the adolescent unit. They were both employed by the NHS trust at the time of the grant award.

References

Ben-Sasson, A., Cermak, S. A., Orsmond, G. I., Tager-Flusberg, H., Carter, A. D., Kadlec, M. B., & Dunn, W. (2007). Extreme sensory modulation behaviors in toddlers with autism spectrum disorders. *American Journal of Occupational Therapy*, 61(5), 584–592. Retrieved from http://search.proquest.com/docview/231972114?accountid=11862.

Case-Smith, J., & Bryan, T. (1999). The effects of occupational therapy with sensory integration emphasis on preschool-age children with autism. *American Journal of Occupational Therapy*, 53, 489–497.

Chalmers, A., Harrison, S., Mollison, K., Molloy, N., & Gray, K. (2012). Establishing sensory-based approaches in mental health inpatient care: A multidisciplinary approach. *Australasian Psychiatry*, 20(1), 35–39.

Champagne, T., & Sayer, E. (2003). The effects of the use of the sensory room in psychiatry. Retrieved from www.ot-innovations.com/pdf_files/QI_STUDY_Sensory_Room.pdf.

Champagne, T., & Stromberg, N. (2004). Sensory approaches in psychiatric settings: Innovative alternatives to seclusion and restraint. *Journal of Psychosocial Nursing and Mental Health Services, 42*(9), 34–44.

Cummins, S., Curtis, S., Diez-Roux, A. V., & Macintyre, S. (2007). Understanding and representing space in health research. *Social Science and Medicine, 65*(9), 1825–1838.

Curtis, S. (2010). *Space, place and mental health*. Farnham, UK: Ashgate.

Curtis, S., Gesler, W., Fabian, K., Francis, S., & Priebe, S. (2007). Therapeutic landscapes in hospital design: A qualitative assessment by staff and service users of the design of a new mental health inpatient unit. *Environment and Planning C: Government and Policy, 25*, 591–610.

Fonagy, P., & Roth, A. (2006). *What works for whom: A critical review of Psychotherapy research* (2nd ed.). New York, NY: Guilford Press.

Gesler, W. (1992). Therapeutic landscapes: Medical issues in light of new cultural geography. *Social Science and Medicine, 34*(7), 735–746.

Gesler, W., Morag, B., Curtis, S., Hubbard, P., & Francis, S. (2004). Therapy by design: Evaluating the UK hospital building program. *Health and Place, 10*, 117–128.

Houghton, S., Douglas, G., Brigg, J., Langsford, S., Powell, L., West, J., . . . Kellner, R. (1998). An empirical evaluation of an interactive multi-sensory environment for children with disability. *Journal of Intellectual and Developmental Disability, 23*(4), 267–278. doi: 10.1080/13668259800033761.

Keller, H. (2014). The evolution of aromatherapy. In J. Buckle, *Clinical aromatherapy: Essential oils in healthcare* (p. 2). St Louis, MO: Elsevier Health Sciences.

Lee, S. J., Cox, A., Whitecross, F., Williams, P., & Hollander, Y. (2010). Sensory assessment and therapy to help reduce seclusion use with service users needing psychiatric intensive care. *Journal of Psychiatric Intensive Care, 6*(2), 83–90.

Liss, M., Timmel, L., Baxley, K., & Killingsworth, P. (2005). Sensory processing sensitivity and its relation to parental bonding, anxiety, and depression. *Personality and Individual Differences, 39*(8), 1429–1439. doi: http://dx.doi.org/10.1016/j.paid.2005.05.007.

Miller L. J., Reisman J. E., McIntosh D. N., & Simon, J. (2001). An ecological model of sensory modulation: Performance of children with fragile X syndrome, autistic disorder, attention-deficit/hyperactivity disorder, and sensory modulation dysfunction. In S. Smith-Roley, E. I., Blanche, & R. C. Schaaf (Eds.), *Understanding the nature of sensory integration with diverse populations* (pp. 57–88). San Antonio, TX: Therapy Skill Builders.

Thomas, D. V. (2002). Aromatherapy: Mythical, magical, or medicinal? *Holistic Nursing Practice, 17*(1), 8–16.

Tomchek, S. D., & Dunn, W. (2007). Sensory processing in children with and without autism: A comparative study using the Short Sensory Profile. *American Journal of Occupational therapy, 61*, 190–200.

Watkins, G. R. (1997). Music therapy: Proposed physiological mechanisms and clinical implications. *Clinical Nurse Specialist, 11*(2), 43–50.

PART II
Community spaces
Beyond the therapy room

7
SUSTAINING SPACES

Community meal provision and mental well-being

Rebekah Graham, Darrin Hodgetts, Ottilie Stolte and Kerry Chamberlain

Societal challenges such as wealth concentration, underemployment, increased living costs and the retrenchment of publically funded services are most keenly felt by socio-economically vulnerable people (Hodgetts & Stolte, 2015). Lives under austerity are characterised by low incomes, inadequate housing, food insecurities, growing debt and social exclusion (Hodgetts, Chamberlain, Tankel, & Groot, 2013). Such social determinants of health (Raphael, 2011) work in concert to create day-to-day living situations that are draining and divisive (Hodgetts, Chamberlain, Groot, & Tankel, 2014). Experiences of material deprivation and stress undermine people's psychological and physical health (De Vogli & Owusu, 2014; Wilkinson & Pickett, 2015). Increased austerity contributes to increased substance misuse, suicide, homicide, mental distress and anxiety for many (Mattheys, 2015; Quaglio, Karapiperis, Woensel, Arnold, & McDaid, 2013). Austerity programmes have relentlessly stripped away income and social supports, placing people under increasing material and psychological strain (Bramall, 2013; Stuckler & Basu, 2013). Demand for mental health services is increasing at a time when resources for such services are decreasing with further negative consequences for people's health (O'Hara, 2014; Quaglio et al., 2013).

The precariat comprises an emerging social class of denizens, who live insecure lives with restrained socio-economic resources, reduced rights and decreased hope of social mobility (Standing, 2011). Members of this precariat survive on inadequate state benefits, low wages and degrading, dangerous, disrupted and 'flexible' (under)employment (Standing, 2014). Precariat lifeworlds are textured by uncertainty, despair and limitations of agency. These precarious lives are characterised by perilous access to the basic necessities in life and psychological supports that often buffer people against austerity (Hodgetts et al., 2013, 2014). Such cityscapes of hardship and fragmentation, or landscapes of despair, are textured by the neoliberal dismantlement of social infrastructure (Dear & Wolch, 1987; Knowles, 2000). Precarious lives are not experienced in a vacuum, but exist within this wider landscape of despair, with topographies of poverty manifesting in histories of institutional violence and exclusion, rendering members of the precariat as 'people out of place' (Bauman, 2004; Cresswell, 1996). In this context, experiences of alienation and dislocation (Hodgetts, Hayward, & Stolte, 2015; Marx, 1867/1974), stigma (Newnes, Holmes, & Dunn, 2001), discrimination (Corker et al., 2013), isolation (Ootes, Pols, Tonkens, & Willems, 2013) and social exclusion (Parr, 1997) are commonplace for mental health service users.

Contemporary landscapes of despair intensify the need for access to spaces in which members of the precariat can find basic resources such as food as well as respite, understanding and support. Despite ongoing pressure to conform to neoliberal ideals of the atomised, self-interested individual, people continue to enact social practices that manifest a relational or communitarian ethos in social life. Central to such practices are reciprocal social relationships evident in informal work, peer advocacy, time-banking and bartering (Pickering, 2003), which cultivate local generosity and responsibility for the well-being of others (Bargh, 2007). Such practices manifest an ethics of interconnected humanity that comprises a challenge to the atomised individual that is at the heart of the neoliberal project (Hodgetts et al., 2013).

This chapter explores such practices in the construction of an *enclave of care*, where we document how marginalised groups can respond to adversity through a collective initiative. We consider how a community meal not only provides a constant, reliable source of food, but also provides a judgement-free space for members of the precariat that affords respite from the pressures associated with the broader landscape of despair (Stolte & Hodgetts, 2015). We show how, within increasingly penal and punitive everyday landscapes (Waquant, 2008), members of the precariat co-create an enclave of care where they can gain respite, dignity, a sense of belonging and sustenance. To explore these issues, we draw on Lefebvre's (1991) work on the dialectics of place to explore how emplaced social practices or routine shared activity structures (Hodgetts et al., 2015) serve to texture and transform the community meal into an enclave of care that produces inclusive and humane experiences, strengthens social networks and contributes towards the construction of a sense of self-worth and belonging (Fortier, 1999; Williams, 1999). This is particularly important for the meal participants, many of whom are mental health outpatients and are all too aware of their marginalisation in the broader landscape of despair.

The community meal as enclave of care

Situated within central Hamilton, a modest-sized city in New Zealand, Gateway Church provides a weekly hot, hearty and filling two-course evening meal. The church hall, with its well-equipped kitchen, and bathroom facilities are used for church activities throughout the week, however, on Wednesdays it 'belongs' to the community meal (Figure 7.1 (left) shows an exterior view of the rear of the

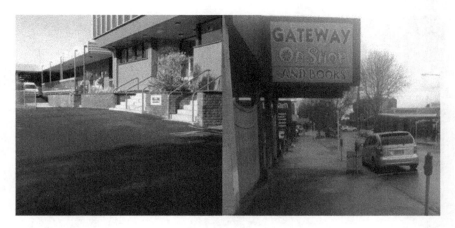

FIGURE 7.1 Exterior spaces of the meal and charity shop.

church). The meal is located within the church hall. Although, the faith-based ritual of 'saying grace' is observed, the space of the meal is not overtly religious, nor is it employed as an evangelical tool for proselytising attendees. The meal relies on both public donations and the sale of second-hand goods in the charity shop. The shop, located within easy walking distance on a nearby street (Figure 7.1 (right) shows a street view of the charity shop, looking towards the church) also doubles as an office, meeting room and informal 'drop-in' centre for local people.

The first author (Rebekah) employed an ethnographic approach to explore the funding, set-up and organisation of the meal, which she attended weekly for 12 months. Rebekah spent time shadowing Bobbie, the meal organiser and leading social worker, became involved in funding activities and helped to prepare the meal. While attending the meal, Rebekah talked with meal attendees and organisers, made extensive field notes, took photographs (as appropriate and as consented by participants), observed social interactions and engaged in a series of formal interviews and shop-along excursions with seven precariat families. These sources inform our analysis, and provide a comprehensive overview of the meal as well as detailing specific emplaced interactions within this space. In this chapter, we focus on the meal and the experiences of diners to understand the construction of this enclave of care.

Journeying into the central city from their homes in the less affluent outer suburbs by public bus, carpooling or even by sleeping rough at the entranceway, a group of up to eight volunteers arrive prior to 7:30 am and by 9:00 am the church hall has been transformed into a dining room (see Figure 7.2). The seating arrangements are reminiscent of those to be found in a *wharekai* (dining hall) at a modern-day *marae* (Māori communal complex for the conduct of everyday life). The arrangement of the tables and chairs in this manner evokes a culturally familiar space for many participating meal attendees from which they can draw strength and renew their sense of belonging and connectedness (Mead, 1934/2003;

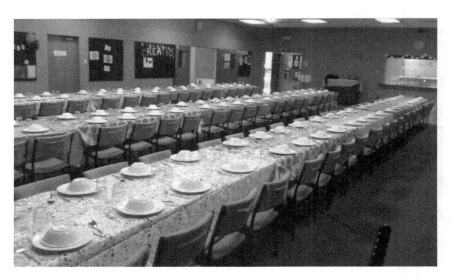

FIGURE 7.2 Main dining area of the Gateway community meal, looking towards the entrance and servery area.

King, Hodgetts, Rua, & Whetu, 2015). These volunteers set up and then dress the trestle tables with colourful tablecloths, china crockery, stainless-steel cutlery, glasses, smart stainless-steel water carafes and matching salt and pepper shakers. These small, inexpensive touches transform an ordinary church hall into a humanising dining space, elevating the provision of food into a sociable meal. As we demonstrate through our analysis, such small acts texture the hall as an enclave for respect, dignity and inclusion.

In the kitchen, volunteers engage in food preparation, peeling potatoes, chopping pumpkins and preparing favoured desserts, while talking about mundane topics of conversation (see Figure 7.3, depicting volunteers, kitchen and food preparation). For this food preparation team, being able to engage in taken-for-granted forms of social interaction provides relief from a landscape textured by exclusion. The banter and interactions occurring as the volunteers perform mundane tasks are reminiscent of scenes from a *marae* kitchen. These simple food-related acts encompass past traditions in the present, anchoring people in time and space and reaffirming a sense of belonging, connectedness and contribution (King et al., 2015). This sense of connection is evident in reflections from the volunteers who present their involvement in the meal as a meaningful and fun activity through which they can *manaaki* (care for) other people:

> I class [meal preparation] as a service . . . [I come] to serve others. To use my own tongue [Māori language], to tautoko [to support, acknowledge, engage and dialogue with other]. To help without requiring or expecting any form

of financial gain. To help for nothing. I enjoy hanging around here . . . I've got a good crowd to work with . . . You look back at what's been done and see that little bit of goodness and that little bit of help.

(Buddy)

[I like] the craziness that we get up to. It's basically doing something for the poor of Hamilton who can't afford food.

(Roxy)

These quotes highlight the value of caring for others that the volunteers, who are themselves members of the precariat, find in the day's activities. Such accounts challenge neoliberal characterisations of welfare recipients as indolent abjects.

The volunteers take command of and reconstruct the space through small acts, such as Buddy bringing music to play throughout the day: "I bring my own own music . . . it livens up [people and the space] . . . I help where I can and share what I have. I have the music so I share it". By bringing along music, Buddy becomes more than a recipient of charity; he becomes an active participant in the texturing of the space. The food preparation ritual transforms these individuals from discarded members of society (Bauman, 2004) into contributing, valued members of a community of care. This democratising process is particularly salient given the context of a broader landscape of penal welfare (Waquant, 2008) within which the

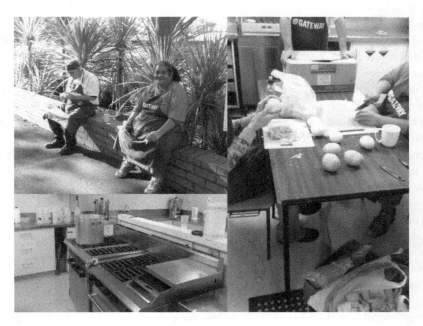

FIGURE 7.3 Photographs depicting kitchen facilities, food preparation and break time.

emphasis is on controlling members of the precariat and reducing their perceived laziness and dependency.

Context is important in understanding the prosocial nature of the meal enclave. The volunteers who set the scene for the meal are often considered out of place (Douglas, 1966) in public places and 'moved along' in accordance with the aesthetic sensibilities, preferences and rules of more affluent social groups (Stolte & Hodgetts, 2015). Through the construction of an enclave of care for people who are deemed out of place, the construction of the meal space acts as an ordered transgression against oppression. The actions of the volunteers destabilise commonly held and abjectifying characterisations that are imposed on the precariat by neoliberal protagonists and institutions. In this context, the actions of the volunteers constitute re-enactments of citizenship by people who are often positioned as 'failed citizens' (Standing, 2011). The creation of a fleeting space of respite generates the sense of purpose, identity and citizenship crucial for mental well-being (Parr, 2000).

The community meal: care, dignity and respite

The scene is set and people arrive for dinner. Some diners walk to the meal, some come by public transport, others pile into cars. Coins are donated (or not) in a cup by the entrance, people find a seat, some save spaces for family and friends. At 5:30 pm, grace or *karakia* (Māori prayer) is said, after which the meal is served. The meal servers comprise a group of middle-class volunteers who arrive at the end of the working day, and take over from the precariat volunteers who cook the food. Diners take up their dinner plates and wait patiently in line (Figure 7.4). The actions of the meal servers in this space are influenced by Bobbie's ethos and her emphasis on Christian values. As Bobbie reflects, "you're serving the meal to Jesus. If that person was Jesus, would you just throw the food on the plate any old how? No, you wouldn't, would you? You would place it nicely, with a smile." Here, Bobbie demonstrates an awareness of mundane acts of care that materialise through the provision of food and invokes a broader ethic of care. After being served, people return to their seats, eat the meal and converse with one another (Figure 7.4). Clean, cold water is provided in tall stainless steel carafes. Many people also indulge in seconds. Meal servers collect the dirty plates, cutlery and unused items. Sometimes too efficiently, leaving people without spoons to eat dessert, which invokes humorous and good-natured banter. After the main meal, dessert is served along with hot drinks. People relax, read the local newspaper, enjoy a cup of tea and leave to go home at their leisure. Volunteers remove the dirty plates and cutlery to the kitchen, clean the brightly patterned tablecloths, pack away the trestle-tables, stack the chairs, vacuum the floor and wash the exterior patio.

The meal is not just about feeding hungry people. It is also intended to provide nourishment in humanising ways to restore the dignity of attendees who live precarious lives within the broader neoliberalised and uncaring landscape. Contrasts between the meal space and key neoliberal locales within the broader landscape

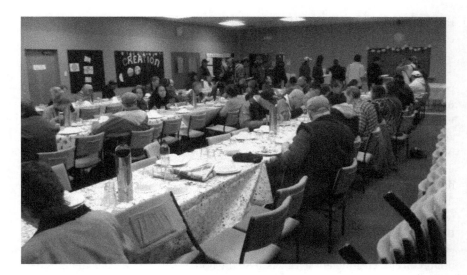

FIGURE 7.4 Main dining area in use on a Wednesday evening.

of despair are useful at this point to foreground the re-humanising and inclusive functions of the Gateway meal. Below, a meal attendee, Lea, contrasts the Gateway meal with another meal offered in a local car park:

> I like coming here [Gateway meal] because you can sit down and eat. At [other meal], it's just in a car park and there's nowhere to sit, so people just sit in the garden or the gutter to eat their food.

The car park meal provides food on paper plates with plastic utensils. People literally have to eat out of the gutter. This reflects not only the disposable nature of the food and cutlery, but also the people who consume it. The material implications of ideological systems coalesce into disposable plates and uncaring spaces, contributing towards a landscape of despair that erodes the well-being, dignity and value necessary for mental health. The significance of such details is easily overlooked by those for whom eating on proper plates and sitting at tables is a taken-for-granted everyday practice.

In contrast, in the Gateway space, the provision of proper table settings, welcoming smiles, non-judgemental inclusion, and a hot meal supports mental health (cf. Johnson, 2012). Dignity, respect and value are crucial components in the construction of the Gateway meal as an enclave for care. Small deeds, such as carefully placing mashed potatoes on an everyday object like a real dinner plate, have much broader significance. Many soup kitchens typically offer a hasty, harried feed, without the rituals associated with both meal preparation and consumption (Musarò, 2013). The lack of commonly used objects in the social construction of a legitimate meal – tables and chairs, cutlery and crockery – effectively dehumanises those in receipt of the food. While providing food to needy people is important, a lack of care in the provision of a meal risks reducing the status of the precariat to 'not-quite-human'.

The shared space of the meal increases positive interactions among diverse meal participants (Desjardins, 2004). At the meal, people are invited to participate as valued members of society who collectively create a dignifying enclave of care from which they can gain a sense of support and solidarity. The middle-class meal servers also gain through socially interacting with members of the precariat that they might otherwise never meet: 'the poor' become familiar faces with individual names. This 'betwixt and between' space of the meal (Sibley, 1995) holds the potential to dissolve the social distance between attendees by fostering a sense of support and 'being in this together'. For example, Maree described how, when hearing a person make derogatory remarks about a 'lazy bum' in the street, her children rebuked the speaker, saying, "No, he's not. He goes to Gateway. He's actually a really nice guy." This 'crossing over' from excluded outsider to known friend exemplifies the importance of creating enclaves whereby the border between insider and outsider, legitimate and illegitimate is blurred. The shared space of the meal increases positive interactions amongst diverse meal participants (Desjardins, 2004), fostering a sense of support and 'being in this together', which challenges instances of exclusion and delegitimisation within the broader cityscape.

The broader landscape of despair manifests an abjectifying climate of blame and disgust (Tyler, 2008), where the (dis)stress of precarious lives is often internalised as a personal failing (Smail, 1996; Walker, Johnson, & Cunningham, 2012). The meal enclave provides a space for diners to externalise such (dis)stress, and to discuss strategies of resistance to victim-blaming narratives and penal institutional practice. The understanding and support attendees offer each other is invaluable in the management and preservation of their mental health. Dinner conversations are often generic in nature, but they also reflect the everyday experiences of navigating the city as a member of the precariat. One meal participant Lea walks for 45 minutes to eat her only meal of the day, while enduring derogatory remarks from passers-by. In contrast to this humiliation, at the meal Lea is treated as an enjoyable dinner companion who participates in conversational topics. Because mental health issues have common currency among diners, conversations also include references to encounters with mental health professionals. For example, during one particular evening, Molly recounted her frustration at having her experiences of medication use dismissed by mental health professionals: "I'm not doing so well. I can feel a bit of a downer coming on . . . I know when I'm getting low . . . I can tell." Her comments at the dinner table were readily understood, and met with nods of agreement, by those seated nearby. A lively discussion ensued whereby other dinner attendees shared their stories of being patronised, condescended to or otherwise ignored by health care staff. Emplaced support such as this reflect the sense of solidarity that is cultivated in the meal space, which also contributes to the promotion of the mental health of people living with mental health issues (Wicks, Trevena, & Quine, 2006). The certainty that her experiences of being alienated

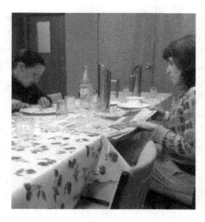

FIGURE 7.5 Reading the newspaper after dinner.

from her own mental health issues were shared by others, externalised the distress she felt, working to generalise her experiences to an increasingly uncaring system.

The ordinary practices woven throughout the meal humanise and dignify diners. One such example is the reading of a local newspaper during the meal. Previously, in Figure 7.4, which was taken during the meal, a folded copy of the paper lies on the table, while its owner queues for dessert. As shown in Figure 7.5, Roxy is engrossed in reading the paper after eating her meal. It is commonplace for attendees to read this newspaper while waiting for the meal, during dinner, with a hot drink after dessert or to take it away for later reading.

Easily overlooked, simple practices such as reading a newspaper and engaging in mundane social interaction are synchronous with the texturing of the meal space, transforming an ordinary church hall into a domesticated locale for dwelling, belonging and respite. The newspaper itself is a familiar object that populates the space, and reading it connects the user to the wider landscape, invoking ideals of citizenship and participation for diners as members of an imagined audience (Csikszentmihalyi & Rochberg-Halton, 1981). A sense of self and belonging comes to the fore through these emplaced practices (King et al., 2015) that involve the use of material objects (Heidegger, 1927/1962). In addition, the value of 'being together' (Heidegger, 1927/1962), as materialised in the emplacement of the newspaper, is easily overlooked when one does not experience exclusion on a daily basis. As such then, the meal provides a 'space for being' where members of the precariat can engage in the enjoyment of a meal, and its attendant social practices, without fear of disruption or of being 'moved along'.

The meal is also an opportunity to relax and enjoy a meal without the pervasive concerns and worries of everyday life, particularly the ever-present worry of stretching food budgets to meet the household's needs (Carne & Mancini, 2012). As Ginny puts it, "It's like a night off, it's the one day I don't have to think about cooking . . . it's hard work making everything from scratch". This break from the relentlessness of daily food preparation and cleaning up is cherished, as is the physical and mental respite. We see glimpses of this also in the following comment from Bev, a retiree: "I like going [to the meal]. I like everything they make – sausages, macaroni cheese, stew. I like not having to do the dishes . . . I don't tell my kids that I go. They'd have fit!" Bev is able to draw strength from this space of respite, which also acts as a buffer on return to the (dis)stress of everyday life. The process of coming together and eating a meal, without associated worries and concerns provides participants with a sense of belonging, dignity and solidarity with fellow diners, and is fostered through human connections in this enclave (Fenger & van Paridon, 2011). Sharing a communal, family-style dinner, along with the shared experiences of being together, offers respite from, and a space for, sharing experiences of precarious and insecure lives.

As an important cultural practice that can enable social engagement (Sobal & Nelson, 2003), communal eating satisfies a need for union with others, with conviviality establishing and reinforcing social ties (Mintz & Bois, 2002; Simmel, 1910/1993). Coming together to eat can transform a mundane meal into an occasion of social renewal, support and care (Sobal & Nelson, 2003). These aspects of the meal are evidenced in the myriad of mundane taken-for-granted social interactions that texture the space: people saving seats for friends, a cheerful greeting, gentle enquiries after one's health, conversations over dinner, the promise to 'see you next week' as people leave. Diners report liking to sit in a particular place so as to engage in social interactions with those around them, as Bob said, "some people, they're always having a bad week . . . but yeah, we have good conversations down that end [of the table]".

Conclusion

There is something very familiar, yet profound, about communal eating that makes the positive emplaced aspects of a community meal realisable. The meal brings people together in a basic human activity, while simultaneously relieving pressure on limited budgets and creating a participatory event that people can 'go out' to in a consumer society where, due to a lack of resources, their participation is often limited and devalued. Our research into this dynamic communal space that is communally constructed by members of the precariat, illustrates how during austere times people can co-create enclaves within which they are able to gain dignity and respect, and to engage with others in ways that promote mental wellness. Many urban spaces are experienced as hostile spaces by members of the precariat (McGrath & Reavey, 2015), and are subsequently either avoided as much as possible (Pinfold, 2000), or utilised in ways that render their presence 'invisible' to members of the public (Knowles, 2000). In contrast to these experiences, in the meal space all are welcome, treated with dignity and their well-being is of chief concern. Here, denizens can become citizens again, attendees can interact with others on their own terms and they can gain respite from the prejudices of more affluent groups that negatively texture their everyday lives in the neoliberal city.

The sociocultural norms that regulate and texture the meal space are those of the families who attend, not those of the wealthy philanthropic donor class who commonly like to dictate how, when, where and in what way charity occurs. Here, 'beggars can be choosers', and members of the precariat are not treated as people out of place.

For members of the precariat, food and poverty are intricately interconnected, with food poverty affecting social inclusion (Fitchen, 1988; Garden et al., 2014). As noted by Musarò (2013, p. 150), "food spaces without friends, festivity and social connectivity become spaces of alienation, distress and loneliness". An inability to eat with others not only results in social isolation, but also a loss of the (collective) identities that are shared during such meals (Warde, 1997). The provision of an evening meal is particularly salient, given that evening meals have special meaning as a shared meal (Sobal, 2000), are viewed as an important time to be with friends and family (Blake, Bisogni, Sobal, Jastran, & Devine, 2008) and enact important sociocultural values (Charles & Kerr, 1988; Murcott, 1982). This is particularly relevant for those who live alone on limited means (Holm, 2001), and whose participation offers a chance to eat with people experiencing similar circumstances. The meal is textured as a space that enhances the potential for building cohesive community bonds (Turner, 1977; Watkins & Shulman, 2010). The practices of resourcing, preparing and sitting down together to eat a meal using small objects of inclusion such as proper cutlery and china plates, transforms participants back from denizens into valued citizens (Simmel, 1910/1993).

In considering issues around the humanising potential of food, this chapter deviates from the dominant focus in research into food insecurity, which typically examines 'healthy' food provision for the poor (e.g. Pelham-Burn, Frost, Russell, & Barker, 2014), improving nutrient intakes of attendees (e.g. Dachner, Gaetz, Poland, & Tarasuk, 2009), and reducing food waste (e.g. Freedman & Bartoli, 2013). These issues are clearly important. However, such research ignores the broader human dimensions of community meals, and the spaces for care that can be created through the collective provision of food with dignity. For members of the precariat, particularly those who live alone with mental health issues, communal food preparation and consumption is an important social and humanising event (King et al., 2015), which helps to cultivate a sense of participation, inclusion (Dowler, Kneafsey, Cox, & Holloway, 2009), belonging (Musarò, 2013), recognition as a community member (Jansen, 1997), as well as the preservation of mental health (Mattheys, 2015). Sharing a meal can provide a deceptively simple way of cultivating social inclusion, fostering community, enacting solidarity, and positive social interactions (Watland, Hallenbeck, & Kresse, 2008). The community meal explored in this chapter reflects how collective efforts can result in the co-construction of human enclaves of care for members of the precariat to be together in a way that promotes dignity, inclusion and wellness (King et al., 2015).

The meal is an inclusive and sustaining space that actively works to support mental health. This enclave of care fosters agency, solidarity and a sense of community, externalises despair, creates a space to be and counteracts the internalised distress of poverty. Such enclaves of care are particularly significant given the landscape of despair and hardship that textures the everyday reality of many meal attendees. Here, at the meal, mundane food-related practice acts as a humanising force, and is itself an act of resistance to dominant discourses. The process of providing a meal is part of a global pattern of resistance to neoliberalism and oppression that involves socially transformative practice (Bargh, 2007; Preston & Aslett, 2013).

Considering the broader implications of our work, the promotion by successive neoliberal governments of measureable, uniform solutions to multifaceted issues has seen locally responsive and socially transformative programmes, such as this provision of a weekly meal, relegated to the side-lines of social service delivery (Giroux, 2010; Preston & Aslett, 2013). Yet, it is these 'unregulated' local and community-led initiatives that enact humane and dignified responses to poverty that are too often absent from programs focused on achieving measureable outputs and reducing social spending. Indeed, configuring the poor as 'dependents' who require managing is one tactic in persuading the public that alleviating the hardship and suffering of poverty is to remove a whip that, when cracked, will motivate people to work harder and be less indolent. As our chapter illustrates, it is the reverse that is true: when considered as valued citizens within an enclave of care, members of the precariat take great pride in working and participating as equals (Hodgetts et al., 2015). It is worth noting here that European countries such as Finland and Sweden, which have historically had strong social supports and who increased their social welfare spending, including investing in family care programmes, mitigated the adverse effects on mental health experienced by more neoliberal countries (Karanikolos et al., 2013). An increase in social welfare spending saw reduced mortality from both suicide and diseases related to social circumstances, as well as improved mental health outcomes (Karanikolos et al., 2013). Considering mental health in particular, increased social welfare spending is a key feature in reducing the despair felt by members of our society. The provision of social welfare in conjunction with humanising and dignifying social services protects vulnerable people, preventing further social and economic harm. In the meantime, the creation of enclaves of care is one possible way of keeping people alive until such time as our governments adjust their policies to become more humane.

References

Bargh, M. (2007). *Resistance: An indigenous response to neoliberalism*. Wellington, NZ: Huia.
Bauman, Z. (2004). *Wasted lives: Modernity and its outcasts*. Cambridge, UK: Polity Press.
Blake, C. E., Bisogni, C. A., Sobal, J., Jastran, M., & Devine, C. M. (2008). How adults construct evening meals: Scripts for food choice. *Appetite*, *51*, 654–662.
Bramall, R. (2013). *The cultural politics of austerity: Past and present in austere times*. London: Palgrave.
Carne, S., & Mancini, A. (2012). *Empty food baskets: Food poverty in Whangarei*. Whangarei, NZ: Child Poverty Action Group.

Charles, N., & Kerr, M. (1988). *Women, food and families*. Manchester: Manchester University Press.

Corker, E., Hamilton, S., Henderson, C., Weeks, C., Pinfold, V., Rose, D., . . . Thornicroft, G. (2013). Experiences of discrimination among people using mental health services in England 2008–2011. *British Journal of Psychiatry, 202*(55), 56–63. doi: 10.1192/bjp.bp.112.112912.

Cresswell, T. (1996). *In place/out of place: Geography, ideology, and transgression*. Minneapolis, MN: University of Minnesota Press.

Csikszentmihalyi, M., & Rochberg-Halton, E. (1981). *The meaning of things: Domestic symbols and the self*. Cambridge, UK: Cambridge University Press.

Dachner, N., Gaetz, S., Poland, B., & Tarasuk, V. (2009). An ethnographic study of meal programs for homeless and under-housed individuals in Toronto. *Journal of Health Care for the Poor and Underserved, 20*(3), 846–853. doi: 10.1353/hpu.0.0167.

De Vogli, R., & Owusu, J. T. (2014). The causes and health effects of the Great Recession: From neoliberalism to 'healthy de-growth'. *Critical Public Health, 25*(1), 15–31. doi: 10.1080/09581596.2014.957164.

Dear, M. J., & Wolch, J. R. (1987). *Landscapes of despair: From deinstitutionalization to homelessness*: Oxford: Polity.

Desjardins, M. (2004). Teaching about religion with food. *Teaching Theology & Religion, 7*(3), 153–158. doi: 10.1111/j.1467-9647.2004.00205.x.

Douglas, M. (1966). *Purity and danger: An analysis of the concepts of pollution and taboo*. New York, NY: Routledge.

Dowler, E., Kneafsey, M. R., Cox, R., & Holloway, L. (2009). 'Doing food differently': Reconnecting biological and social relationships through care for food. *Sociological Review, 57*(S2), 200–221.

Fenger, M., & van Paridon, K. (2011). Towards a globalisation of solidarity? In M. Ellison (Ed.), *Reinventing social solidarity across Europe* (pp. 49–70). New York, NY: Policy Press.

Fitchen, J. M. (1988). Hunger, malnutrition, and poverty in the contemporary United States: Some observations on their social and cultural context. *Food and Foodways, 2*, 309–333. doi: 10.1080/07409710.1987.9961923.

Fortier, A.-M. (1999). Re-membering places and the performance of belonging(s). *Theory, Culture & Society, 16*(2), 41–64. doi: 10.1177/02632769922050548.

Freedman, M. R., & Bartoli, C. (2013). Food intake patterns and plate waste among community meal center guests show room for improvement. *Journal of Hunger & Environmental Nutrition, 8*(4), 506–515. doi: 10.1080/19320248.2013.787380.

Garden, E., Caldin, A., Robertson, D., Timmins, J., Wilson, T., & Wood, T. (2014). *Family 100 research project: Speaking for ourselves*. Auckland, NZ: Auckland City Mission.

Giroux, H. A. (2010). Bare pedagogy and the scourge of neoliberalism: Rethinking higher education as a democratic public sphere. *Educational Forum, 74*, 184–196. doi: 10.1080/00131725.2010.483897.

Heidegger, M. (1962). *Being and time* (Trans. J. Macquarrie & E. Robinson). London: SCM Press. (Original work published 1927.)

Hodgetts, D., Chamberlain, K., Groot, S., & Tankel, Y. (2014). Urban poverty, structural violence and welfare provision for 100 families in Auckland. *Urban Studies, 51*(10), 2036–2051. doi: 10.1177/0042098013505885.

Hodgetts, D., Chamberlain, K., Tankel, Y., & Groot, S. (2013). Researching poverty to make a difference: The need for reciprocity and advocacy in community research. *Australian Community Psychologist, 25*(1), 35–48.

Hodgetts, D., Hayward, B., & Stolte, O. (2015). Medicinal commodities and the gift of a caring mother. *Journal of Consumer Culture*, *15*(3), 287–306. doi: 10.1177/1469540513 498611.

Hodgetts, D., & Stolte, O. (2015). Homeless people's leisure practices within and beyond urban socio-scapes. *Urban Studies*. Online first. doi: 10.1177/0042098015571236.

Holm, L. (2001). The social context of eating. In U. Kjaernes (Ed.), *Eating patterns: A day in the lives of Nordic peoples* (pp. 159–198). Lysaker, Norway: National Institute for Consumer Research.

Janson, W. (1997). Gender identity and the rituals of food in a Jordanian community. *Food and Foodways*, *7*(2), 87–117.

Johnson, K. (2012). Challenges for critical community psychology. In C. Walker, K. Johnson, & L. Cunningham (Eds.), *Community psychology and the socio-economics of mental distress* (pp. 267–284). London: Palgrave Macmillan.

Karanikolos, M., Mladovsky, P., Cylus, J., Thomson, S., Basu, S., Stuckler, D., . . . McKee, M. (2013). Health in Europe 7: Financial crisis, austerity, and health in Europe. *Lancet*, *382*, 1323–1331. doi: 10.1016/s0140-6736(13)60102-6.

King, P., Hodgetts, D., Rua, M., & Whetu, T. T. (2015). Older men gardening on the marae: Everyday practices for being Māori. *AlterNative: An International Journal of Indigenous Peoples*, *11*(1), 14–28.

Knowles, C. (2000). Burger King, Dunkin Donuts and community mental health care. *Health & Place*, *6*, 213–224.

Lefebvre, H. (1991). *The production of space*. Cambridge, MA: Blackwell.

McGrath, L., & Reavey, P. (2015) Seeking fluid possibility and solid ground: Space and movement in mental health service users' experiences of 'crisis'. *Social Science & Medicine*, *128*, 115–125.

Marx, K. (1867/1977). *Capital: A critique of political economy* (vol. 1). New York, NY: Vintage Books.

Mattheys, K. (2015). The coalition, austerity and mental health. *Disability & Society*, *30*(3), 475–178. doi: 10.1080/09687599.2014.1000513.

Mead, G. H. (2003). *Mind, self and society from the standpoint of a social behaviorist*. Chicago, IL: University of Chicago Press. (Original work published 1934.)

Mintz, S. W., & Du Bois, C. M. (2002). The anthropology of food and eating. *Annual Review of Anthropology*, *31*, 99–119. doi: 10.1146/annurev.anthro.32.032702.131011.

Murcott, A. (1982). On the social significance of the 'cooked dinner' in South Wales. *Social Science Information/sur les sciences sociales*, *5*(1), 677–696. doi: 10.1177/053901882021004011.

Musarò, P. (2013). Food consumption and urban poverty: An ethnographic study. *Italian Sociological Review*, *3*(3), 142–151. doi: 10.13136/isr.v3i3.65.

Newnes, C., Holmes, G., & Dunn, C. (2001). *This is madness too: Critical perspectives on mental health services*. London: PCCS Books.

O'Hara, M. (2014). *Austerity bites: A journey to the sharp end of cuts in the UK*. Bristol: Policy Press.

Ootes, S. T. C., Pols, A. J., Tonkens, E. H., & Willems, D. L. (2013). Where is the citizen? Comparing civic spaces in long-term mental healthcare. *Health & Place*, *22*, 11–18. doi: 10.1016/j.healthplace.2013.02.008.

Parr, H. (1997). Mental health, public space, and the city: Questions of individual and collective access. *Environment and Planning D: Society and Space*, *15*(4), 435–454. doi: 10.1068/d150435.

Parr, H. (2000). Interpreting the 'hidden social geographies' of mental health: Ethnographies of inclusion and exclusion in semi-institutional places. *Health & Place*, *6*(3), 225–237. doi:10.1016/S1353-8292(00)00025-3.

Pelham-Burn, S. E., Frost, C. J., Russell, J. M., & Barker, M. E. (2014). Improving the nutritional quality of charitable meals for homeless and vulnerable adults. A case study of food provision by a food aid organisation in the UK. *Appetite*, *82*(1), 131–137. doi: 10.1016/j.appet.2014.07.011.

Pickering, K. (2003). The dynamics of everyday incorporation and antisystemic resistance: Lakota culture in the 21st century. In W. A. Dunaway (Ed.), *Emerging issues in the 21st century world-system: Crises and resistance in the 21st century world system*. East Westport, CN: Praege.

Pinfold, V. (2000). 'Building up safe havens . . . all around the world': Users' experiences of living in the community with mental health problems. *Health & Place*, *6*(3), 273–288.

Preston, S., & Aslett, J. (2013). Resisting neoliberalism from within the academy: Subversion through an activist pedagogy. *Social Work Education*, *33*(4), 502–518. doi: 10.1080/02615479.2013.848270.

Quaglio, G., Karapiperis, T., Woensel, L. V., Arnold, E., & McDaid, D. (2013). Austerity and health in Europe. *Health Policy*, *113*, 13–19. doi: 10.1016/j.healthpol.2013.09.005.

Raphael, D. (2011). A discourse analysis of the social determinants of health. *Critical Public Health*, *21*(2), 221–236. doi: 10.1080/09581596.2010.485606.

Sibley, D. (1995). *Geographies of exclusion: Society and difference in the West*. London: Routledge.

Simmel, G. (1993). Sociology of the meal. In D. Frisby & M. Featherstone (Eds.), *Simmel on culture* (pp. 130–136). London: Sage. (Original work published 1910.)

Smail, D. (1996). *The nature of unhappiness* (2nd ed.). London: Constable.

Sobal, J. (2000). Sociability and meals: Facilitation, commensality and interaction. In H. L. Meiselman (Ed.), *Dimensions of the meal: The science, culture, business, and art of eating* (pp. 119–133). Gaithersburg, MD: Aspen.

Sobal, J., & Nelson, M. K. (2003). Commensal eating patterns: A community study. *Appetite*, *41*(2), 181–190.

Standing, G. (2011). *The precariat: The dangerous new class*. London: Bloomsbury Academic.

Standing, G. (2014). *A precariat charter: From denizens to citizens*. New York, NY: Bloomsbury Academic.

Stolte, O., & Hodgetts, D. (2015). Being healthy in unhealthy places: Health tactics in a homeless lifeworld. *Journal of Health Psychology*, *20*(2), 144–153. doi: 10.1177/1359 105313500246.

Stuckler, D., & Basu, S. (2013). *The body economic: Why austerity kills*. London: Penguin.

Turner, V. (1977). Variations of the theme of liminality. In S. Moore, & B. Myerhoff (Eds.), *Secular ritual* (pp. 36–52). Assen/Amsterdam: Van Gorcum.

Tyler, I. (2008). 'Chav mum chav scum'. *Feminist Media Studies*, *8*(1), 17–34. doi: 10.1080/14680770701824779.

Walker, C., Johnson, K., & Cunningham, L. (Eds.). (2012). *Community psychology and the socio-economics of mental distress: International perspectives*. New York, NY: Palgrave Macmillan.

Warde, A. (1997). *Consumption, food and taste*. Manchester: Sage.

Watkins, M., & Shulman, H. (2010). *Toward psychologies of liberation*. London: Palgrave Macmillan.

Watland, K. H., Hallenbeck, S. M., & Kresse, W. J. (2008). Breaking bread and breaking boundaries: A case study on increasing organizational learning opportunities and fostering communities of practice through sharing meals in an academic program. *Performance Improvement Quarterly*, *20*(3–4), 167–184.

Waquant, L. (2008). *Urban outcasts: A comparative sociology of advanced marginality*. Cambridge, UK: Polity Press.

Whelan, J., & Lindberg, R. (2012). Still hungry and homeless. *Parity, 25*(6), 1.
Wicks, R., Trevena, L. J., & Quine, S. (2006). Experiences of food insecurity among urban soup kitchen consumers: Insights for improving nutrition and well-being. *Journal of the American Dietetic Association, 106*(6), 921–924. doi: 10.1016/j.jada.2006.03.006.
Wilkinson, R., & Pickett, K. (2015). Income inequality and social dysfunction. *Annual Review of Sociology, 35*, 493–511. doi: 10.1146/annurev-soc-070308-115926.
Williams, A. (Ed.). (1999). *Therapeutic landscapes: The dynamic between place and wellness.* Lanham, MD: University Press of America.

8
BURSTING BUBBLES OF INTERIORITY

Exploring space in experiences of distress and rough sleeping for newly homeless people

Laura McGrath, Tassie Weaver, Paula Reavey and Steven D. Brown

Homelessness, space and mental distress

Homelessness is an increasing problem in the UK, which intersects in multiple ways with experiences of mental distress. Within the term 'homeless' are contained people in a variety of living situations, including those living in temporary accommodation (hostels, couch surfing, B&Bs) as well those sleeping rough. The latter category is the least common, but on the rise. Between 2010 and 2017, rough sleeping more than doubled in England and Wales, with just under a quarter of total rough sleepers concentrated in London (MHCLG, 2018). Loopstra et al. (2016) argue that the combination of recession and austerity has pushed homelessness upwards, with cuts in welfare spending on social care, housing services and income support for older people most clearly associated with this rise. Of new rough sleepers, around 70 per cent have a mental health diagnosis (NHS Confederation, 2012). This is not just a UK phenomenon; a 2009 population based study in the United States similarly found mental health diagnoses to be three to four times more prevalent in the homeless population (Shelton, Taylor, Bonner, & van den Bree, 2009). This relationship is multifaceted. Both mental health problems and homelessness are argued to be inter-related outcomes of lives characterised by adversity, trauma and abuse (Kim, Ford, Howard, & Bradford, 2010). The relationship is also bidirectional; a distress and mental health crisis can lead to people leaving their homes, while homelessness, with its accompanying insecurity and potential for trauma, can also precipitate, deepen or trigger further mental health problems.

In this climate of rising numbers of homeless people, it is noticeable that several researchers have also pointed to the inherent hostility of the urban spaces that many rough sleepers negotiate. Hodgetts, Radley, Chamberlain, and Hodgetts (2007), for instance, discuss the ways in which public space is increasingly designed to subtly exclude homeless people through: "the design of park benches that people cannot sleep on and the hiring of security guards to remove vagrants from train stations or shopping districts" (2007, p. 722). Knowles (2005), in her study with people with mental health problems living in homeless hostels, found that participants had to spend their days in public spaces defined by consumption and capitalism, from which they were both implicitly and explicitly excluded. She found her participants were often able to remain in certain low-status consumer spaces, generally food courts and fast food restaurants, for long periods of time on the condition that they did not trouble other customers; in other words: "remaining *invisible* is the price of using public space" (p. 224). This echoes Parr's (2008) argument that our public spaces are 'purified' of difference, including visible distress (McGrath & Reavey, 2013, 2015), homeless people (Hodgetts et al., 2007; Hodgetts et al., 2008) and street drinkers (Dixon, Levine, & McAuley, 2006). The visibility of difference in mainstream space is hence widely argued to be "a matter of public concern", with difference seen to "infect, spoil or taint" (Hodgetts et al., 2007, p. 722) public space, and hence become a focus of control and risk management practices.

Such practices of public space can in turn be seen as part of a wider public/ private "grand dichotomy" (Weintraub, 1997, p. xi) differentiating between forms of a wide range of phenomena, including: 'internal' experiences of the self versus 'external' social behaviour; family life versus political and workplace life; and even 'publicly' funded versus 'privately' owned organisations. More 'public' forms of socio-spatial practice (Lefebvre, 1991; Massey, 1994) hence might entail the presentation of a productive, rational self, capable of work (Foucault, 1965; Walker & Fincham, 2011) while more 'private' forms might include the expression of intimacy, emotion and sexuality (Mallet, 2004). Dislocating behaviour or activities that are usually 'private', such as intimate activities of sleeping and homemaking, into public space can be seen as "transgressing the moral geography of everyday behaviour" (Dixon et al., 2006, p. 197). Furthermore, a key 'hidden', or privatised experience in Western society, has been argued to be mental distress (McGrath & Reavey, 2013; Parr, 1997, 2008). Those people who are both homeless and experiencing mental distress can hence be seen to potentially doubly violate the normative practices of public space.

For those inhabiting space as a homeless person therefore, there is a difficult line to walk in retaining an acceptable invisible presence within public space. Hodgetts et al. (2010) describes homeless people as adopting a 'chameleon-like' functioning, adapting behaviour and physical appearance to the subtle shifts in the expectations and allowances of the public spaces that they inhabit. Dangers are also contained in homeless life, whether from violence or threats to health, so remaining safe is also a key concern for homeless people, particularly women (Radley, Hodgetts, & Cullen, 2006) Considering the precarities of living in public space, it is perhaps surprising that Hodgetts et al. (2007) consider the relative community and agency as embodied in the practices and communities of street homeless people compared to the isolated, low-quality and insecure housing that may be offered as an alternative.

Less explored, arguably, are the experiences of people who are newly homeless, and so have not yet established the patterns of homeless living described by Hodgetts and colleagues (2006, 2007, 2010). It is these experiences that we will discuss in this chapter, exploring how people who are newly homeless, without the strategies in place that help to maintain an acceptable invisible presence in public space. The question remains of what kinds of spaces people with no history on the streets, but living with experiences of distress, might seek, form and negotiate within the landscape outlined here. Considering the importance of questions of public and private, interior and exterior, and the creation of micro spaces of safety, we will draw here on Sloterdijk's (2011, 2014, 2016) theory of spheres, as a route to understanding some of the complexities in new rough sleepers' experiences. It is worth explaining some of the key features of this theory before moving on to describing the study and findings.

Sloterdijk's (2011, 2014, 2016) epic *Spheres* trilogy outlines his theory of space and subjectivity. He argues that human experience is fundamentally located and constituted through relationships. Whether on intimate, social or cultural scales, he argues that people together build shared spaces, or spheres, which define the boundaries of their world. On the most intimate scale, Sloterdijk talks about how through intimate relationships we create 'bubbles' of shared space, meaning, affect and habit. He argues:

> The sphere is the interior, disclosed, shared realm inhabited by humans [. . .] Because living always means building spheres, both on a small and a large scale [. . .] Living in spheres means creating the dimension in which humans can be contained.
>
> *(Sloterdijk, 2011, p. 28)*

The image of the bubble here is twofold. First, it captures the spatial nature of Sloterdijk's conception of subjective experience. Second, it captures the primary proposed function of building spheres, that of providing a layer of protection or separation from the rest of the world. Sloterdijk argues that through building bubbles and spheres, from the smallest scale of two friends sharing a coffee in the corner of a cafe, to a shared world religion that frames the world in a particular way, people protect and immunise themselves against the coldness and vastness of the world:

> For humans being-in-spheres constitutes the basic relationship – admittedly one that is infringed upon from the start by the non-interior world, and must perpetually assert itself against the provocation of the outside, restore itself and increase. In this sense, spheres are by definition also morpho-immunological constructs. Only in immune structures that form interiors can humans continue their generational processes and advance their individuations.
>
> *(Sloterdijk, 2011, pp. 45–46)*

The metaphor of 'immunology' is here used to describe how a shared space necessarily includes some element of exclusion; how the creation of interiority contains and necessitates an exterior. Elsewhere, Sloterdijk refers to the shared space as a 'climate'. Our climate on earth contains the conditions for living, but also has a protective element; our atmosphere shields us from the ravages of outer space: intense cold, the heat of the sun and potentially deadly asteroids. In creating shared spaces of meaning, habit, affect and culture, therefore, Sloterdijk argues that humans work together to keep at bay the vast emptiness of existence. In this chapter we will explore how newly homeless people negotiate the hostile climate of public space, to seek out protective immunological bubbles in which they can exist in relative safety.

The study

This study aimed to explore the role of space in experiences of new rough sleepers who also had experiences of mental distress. The study was designed adopting a multimodal approach combing both visual and narrative data; an approach successfully employed in previous psychological explorations into both experiences of homelessness (Hodgetts et al., 2006, 2010; Knowles, 2005; Wang, Cash, & Powers, 2000) and experiences of distress (McGrath & Reavey, 2013, 2015, 2016). Photo-production was used as a tool to engage participants in the research, and to offer an alternative means of expression to complement the narrative (Reavey & Prosser, 2012). In order to empower an otherwise marginalised group, it was important during this research for participants to be collaborators rather than just respondents (Wang et al., 2000). As suggested by Reavey (2012), visual methods such as photo production can encourage participants to reflect on their emotions and experiences in particular settings. This was certainly found to be true in this research, where this method was successful in facilitating participants' reflections on both the spaces captured, and also spaces and places they were not able, or did not want to, visit. For example, some participants were reluctant to photograph anything at all, however the request to do so stimulated reflection as to the reasons, prompting interesting and meaningful dialogue.

Participants were recruited from three assessment hubs for new rough sleepers. To be included in the study, participants needed to also self-report as having experienced, or be currently experiencing, mental distress. The ages of the participants ranged from 24 to 51 years of age. There were 20 participants altogether, 13 men and 7 women. Ethical approval was gained from the host university before commencing the study, and the agreement of the services was also secured. The second author was also a member of staff in the service at the time.

Once participants had been recruited, they were given a disposable camera. Participants were asked to take photographs over the following 48 hours that captured spaces and places that were meaningful to them or within which they spent time. Ideas and examples were discussed and instructions regarding the usage of the camera, including ethical considerations such as ensuring anonymity of other service users. The cameras were collected, photos printed, and follow-up interviews were then conducted in the assessment hubs the following day. This truncated timetable was necessary due to the quick turnover of clients in the hubs; the service aims to have clients move on within 48–72 hours. Photo production proved to be a valuable tool in creating a relationship and rapport between the researcher and participant in advance of the interview. That the researcher had met participants on two occasions prior to the interview (once during recruitment and again when collecting the camera) allowed for a sense of familiarity, encouraging a more relaxed interview and perhaps deeper engagement from the participant.

Analytical approach

The interviews were transcribed verbatim. The photographs were primarily understood as prompts that helped to elicit accounts of the various places in which difficulties were experienced, and hence given meaning by the participant in the context of the interview, rather than treated as data to be analysed independently (Reavey & Prosser, 2012). The photographic material was organised by each participant, who then responded to interview questions, in the light of discussing each photograph in turn. Our reading of the audio material was guided by the overall research question of how the participants experienced and lived in the spaces and places described. The concern with space was generated directly by our ongoing theoretical position, which directly connects distress with spaces and settings, shaping and mediating them and creating the possibilities for action (see Brown & Reavey, 2014, 2015; McGrath, 2012; McGrath & Reavey, 2013, 2015, 2016; Reavey, 2010).

After notating and coding the material with these questions in mind, the data were re-organised into themes, as well as considered in the light of literature that could help to contextualise the analysis. A process-oriented thematic decomposition (Stenner, 1993) approach was used to analyse the data. This thematic decomposition was achieved by following the stages of analysis that are commonly found in many forms of qualitative research (Willig, 2008). We familiarised ourselves with the data via repeated readings of the transcripts, generating initial codes by paying close attention to the meaning of the talk, followed by matching the initial codes together to form candidate themes and sub-themes. Each of the authors was involved in discussions around whether the theme titles and definitions adequately captured the meaning of the data. Our analysis can be seen as 'theoretical', as the data were read and notated from the beginning of the process of analysis in terms of how the space was constructed and accounted for by participants, using the theoretical position outlined above. Nevertheless, the interpretation produced was also 'inductive', in the sense that the final reading produced was based on a close reading of the material, and not on previously fixed ideas about what the final themes would be. An interpretation also involved exploring the implicit meaning of the material, rather than a more descriptive, 'semantic' reading. The validity of the findings was ensured, using conventional qualitative procedures, including group analysis by key researchers and peer review, to ensure the analysis was sufficiently grounded in the data (Creswell & Miller, 2000).

Bursting bubbles: escaping the confines of isolated interiority

The reasons described by participants for becoming homeless were multiple. Several described problems or breakdowns in intimate and family relationships as key, as is commonly found in the literature (Shelton et al., 2009). Several participants were also homeless following release from institutions – both prison and psychiatric wards. A number of participants also described their homelessness as stemming from their mental distress. This section will focus on some of those participants, who described a crisis of containment, a need to escape or overflow. One participant, for instance, commented on what drove her to leave home:

> It was just like, I don't know what came over and I said right, I've got to leave. I can't cope, I can't cope. Right I just can't cope, I'm gonna leave, I'm gonna leave. All I did was to just grab my little bits and bobs that I needed, phone the landlord, handed my keys back and everything. All the goodness of mind was in there. I said I don't wanna know . . . Because I just, for me it's like, almost like choking. I just needed to get out. I just couldn't cope. I just could not cope.

Here, the participant locates her drive to be homeless with an overwhelming feeling of being 'choked' in the space of her home. Her distress here becomes overwhelming, seemingly over-spilling the contours of her living space to such an extent that she can no longer remain within the space of home and also 'cope' with her distress. This experience of internal spaces as confining, and an intensifier of distress can be a feature of mental health crisis, as we have explored previously (McGrath & Reavey, 2015). Another participant described a similar experience:

> Well I can't work, so therefore you can't put yourself into it, because you find while you're working your brain's occupied, but being stuck in a room while you've got all these other things going on, it just makes, I think it's just a point of it all ganging up on you, you just can't deal with it, while when you're working you normally have these problems and you deal with it in your head. I'd explain it like a solitaire, you know, with four aces. You prioritise and you put them there and once you've dealt with it you swipe it away, so that's how I've always dealt with it, but I can't seem to deal with it. With everything else going on I just can't seem to think straight.

This participant describes his distress here becoming overwhelming, dominating his experiences rather than being able to 'swipe away' or minimise these aspects of his experience through distraction in work and other activities. This highlights an important point about the living conditions of many of the people we interviewed. Before becoming homeless, many had already experienced a crisis of some kind, whether a family breakdown or job loss. This meant that they had often been forced into more confined, isolated living arrangements. Exacerbating the distress here is a reduction in the different spheres of his life; his distress has nowhere to go while he is 'stuck in a room' rather than being active in the world. Another participant described a similar experience:

> I suppose I'm just used to only going to my bedroom for sleep but obviously everything else you do in the other rooms. But when you're stuck in a room and you're eating in that room because it's a family house, so you're eating in your room, you're doing everything in that same room, you become isolated. It's like a prison cell, and when you're losing your physical ability to go out and things, it becomes, it does become a prison cell where you feel like you're limited and all you've got is these four walls to look at.

While another similarly commented:

> It's been like this for the last four years, I've been in a room, TV, bed, that's it. Sitting there, staring at four walls, errr, feeling, errr, useless. There's nothing I can do about it, I just, there's so much inside myself, just not going out . . . sometimes just sitting there and not even eating sometimes. Just sleep.

These experiences together point to a particular issue with the isolated 'prison-like' living conditions common among those on the lowest rungs of the housing ladder. Supported housing, hostels, lodging and multiple occupancy housing all tend to reduce people's living spaces to a single room. All aspects of people's lives are folded together into this single space, with the 'four walls' described as encapsulating their confinement. As Latour (2005, p. 72) argues, material objects can "allow, afford, encourage, permit, suggest, influence, block, render possible, forbid" actions, interactions and experiences. Here, the 'four walls' of their small living spaces seem to both reflect back the participants' isolation upon them, reducing their capacity to make connections with the world. These experiences are described as compounded by the intensity of their distressing experiences. As we have previously argued (McGrath & Reavey, 2015) some intense experiences of distress can be exacerbated in confined spaces, leading people to seek to distribute the intensity of their experiences through movement, social interaction and open spaces.

What these participants can be seen as describing is a crisis of interiority, intimacy and home. Described here are incidents of uncontainable intensity being experienced within a space of compacted, cut-off isolation. Sloterdijk (2011) argued that all bubbles that we create as spaces of intimacy and interiority 'work towards bursting'. The experiences of distress, of "not being able to cope" or of having "too much inside myself" to be confined in such small, isolated spaces are here described as being implicated in leaving these spaces and becoming homeless.

A skinless existence: exposure, shame and visibility in rough sleeping

Once homeless, participants described in many ways the opposite experience: one of being over-exposed, vulnerable, almost "skinless" (Sloterdijk, 2011, p. 36) to the world. Compounding a physical sense (and reality) of danger, participants described deep senses of shame, and craving invisibility in public space:

Participant: I felt so low. I felt, I felt like nothing to be honest with you, I felt, sometimes I just felt to myself that I used to be a good person like most people, an average person, a working-class person, and now I've got nothing. Sometimes I just used to think is it worth me living?
Interviewer: How did it feel if people just walked past you? Do you prefer people to walk past or do you want people to stop?
Participant: Well I don't want anybody to see me most of the time, I just cover my head with my sleeping bag until somebody taps me on my shoulder or my leg and says are you alright? Most of the times I just cover my face.
Interviewer: You say you cover your face? Is that because you're embarrassed?
Participant: Ashamed.

An intense level of shame is here described as being felt through being visibly homeless in public space. Evidence of the emotions felt in response to their new social status manifested throughout the interviews with recurrent language such as "humiliation", "worthlessness", feeling "so low . . . like nothing", "embarrassment", "failure", "shame", and feeling "victimised". Shame and humiliation are felt violations of moral or social standards (Tracy, Robins, & Tangney, 2007); these feelings can be seen as embedded in the rough sleeper's position in space. The inherent hostility of public space to those experiencing homelessness and distress (Hodgetts et al., 2007; Knowles, 2000; McGrath & Reavey, 2016) can be seen to be felt here by our participants, who experience their dislocation in space as a violation of a moral standard.

These general feelings of being out of space, were described as being compounded by occupying familiar spaces, now in changed circumstances:

> I was sleeping on a little bench, and then the mosquitos were biting me, there was a sense of shame because when I was younger I was popular in that area. So, you know I felt like every time I saw a car with music playing, maybe there are people . . . like even now I feel a bit ashamed, but sometimes you have to go through hardship before you can appreciate good things.

Here the participant described the particular shame of potentially being seen or spotted by people who they know, and who have known them in other periods of their life. Another participant, for instance, described sleeping rough in the area where he had grown up, meaning "My Dad saw me once, that was, that weren't very nice." In this context, it was noticeable that many of those sleeping rough for the first time moved a considerable distance from their homes. Contrary to research on 'entrenched' rough sleepers, who often congregate in communities or central sites, our participants described seeking invisible and distant sites when leaving their homes. As we will explore more thoroughly in the next section, several participants, for instance, described moving into the woods at the edge of London. Another participant, meanwhile, described sleeping in a stairwell, up on the ninth floor to avoid detection, as so high up, people are less likely to use the stairs:

> This first picture is in a tower block. This is on the ninth floor. Over here is a stairway as you can see, a bit of the stairway, and over here is the landing. So what I tend to do is put my sleeping bag right on the bottom of that landing bit and just sleep there [. . .] where it's on the eighth floor people tend to use the lift a lot. [. . .] it's warm, you don't get cold as much as you would out on the park bench or in the bushes.

Another participant described taking pains to make himself invisible even within public space:

Participant: It was umm . . .a bush which is facing like a floating Chinese or a Japanese restaurant [. . .] I was right across the road from there so I could actually see the restaurant all the time. [. . .] It's like really dark there and I'm a black person so [laughing] sorry . . . so they really can't see me if you know what I mean. You get the gesture of it.
Interviewer: Is that the main thing that you're thinking about when you're rough sleeping; where can I go so that people can't see me?
Participant: Yeah. It's always gotta be a dark corner, that's where I feel safer.

The participant here describes finding the darkest corners where due to his skin colour, he describes becoming invisible within the public space of the park. This, as well as hiding in the woods or under stairwells, can be seen as a strategy to combat the "skinless" (Sloterdijk, 2011, p. 32), exposed experience of sleeping rough. Other participants described finding places to sleep within industrial estates, locked at night, while another spent some time sleeping in a car locked in a garage. Within the urban environment opportunities to disappear in this way are limited, and involve considerable creativity and skill. This experience of living without a bubble, in Sloterdijk's terms, is here described to be deeply felt and provide a further impetus for newly homeless people to hide.

Bubbles of interiority: creating home and security in exposed spaces

Caught between homes that stifle and public spaces that reject, our participants described multiple strategies for re-creating bubbles of interiority within such hostile spaces. As touched upon above, one of the key spaces described by participants for engaging in this process was the forest, and other hidden, green spaces. As well as being used to hide in, green, particularly wooded, spaces were discussed as important healing and comforting spaces for some participants. One female participant, in particular, described her camp in the forest, a tent in the middle of a bush, as a place of relative freedom:

Participant: God I miss my fox and my tent you know. I need peace.
Interviewer: Sometimes you think it would be better to go back?
Participant: Go back to the tent and just go in and see my fox again and feed it in the middle of the night you know, just have the birds tweeting and the deers in the morning and just, yeah I do miss the privacy and the kind of freedom.

This account is striking in comparison to the paucity of the living spaces described in the first section. Central to Sloterdijk's (2011, 2014, 2016) analysis is that our most intimate experiences and bubbles of space are fundamentally relational; in common with much developmental psychology, he saw the foundational relationship not as the individual, but as the dyad. Rather than a world closed in on itself, the forest here provides connection, with foxes, deer, birds; an experience of dyadic interiority facilitated by relationships with nature.

In common with several participants in this study, Sharon had found a temporary home here in Epping Forest, on the edge of London. Ashon (2017) describes this space as 'enantiodromic', as a space that contains opposites; it is both urban and rural, both an escape and an enclosure. As Ashon writes, the forest is an outside space that turns you in upon yourself; in contrast to the expansion of the mountain or meadow, forests constrain your view, hide you and discombobulate your sense of space and time. In much of literature and myth, from *A Midsummer Night's Dream*, through *Red Riding Hood* to *The Hunger Games*, forests occupy such a contradictory position; a place of both possibility and danger, where rules are suspended, senses heightened, relationships reformed and alternatives explored (Ashon, 2017; Harrison, 2009).

For our participants, seeking spaces of safety within the 'skinless' existence of being newly homeless, the dual nature of the forest as being both outside and enclosed seem to provide tools to create bubbles of interiority within outside spaces:

Participant: It was like a neat little base, you have to go like right in.
Interviewer: So they couldn't see you there?

Participant: No. I was hidden [. . .] I was literally surrounded so I know nothing could get to me. I did it for safety, so if anyone would move I would hear the cracking and there would be no access to me. Nobody found me. You have to walk too deep in. Nobody would have seen me, nobody would have gone that far in because there are thorn bushes.

The enclosure of the forest is here described as being used to the participant's advantage, as creating a natural barrier between her and the more exposed urban environment. In creating interiority within outside space, these participants can be seen to be finding ways to settle both their need to escape the confines of oppressive interiority seen in the first section, while also be safe within the 'skinless', exposed and shaming urban outside spaces.

A second strategy for settling this dilemma was that some participants described utilising familiar or safe institutional spaces in a similar way to Claire and Sharon describe using forest spaces. One participant, for instance, described bedding down in the doorway of his mental health service:

I was so like tired and I just wanted to sleep and I was shattered and like, I was looking over my shoulders, you know, but when I got to the Spires then I just slept outside their building. [. . .] I think it was early Monday morning because Spires opened, this guy come up to me and I was fast asleep. 'You alright?' I thought yeah, he went, "I've just come out from prison" . . . and it was very very early in the morning, you know, even the street lights were still on, and I thought ok, and then he just went, sat next to me, put his arm round me and I went umm . . . take your arm off me please, he went "sure, no problem, do you want me to go home, I can bring you a cup of tea or something?"

Another described her favoured location for rough sleeping as being in the doorway of a church:

I always slept outside the church because I felt safe. It was quiet up there, I mean it's basically, it was my safest option because I didn't want to go down the West End because, don't get me wrong, I had a little bit of hassle. I can handle myself to an extent but I must admit, I don't go down the West End or down Camden because I'm anti-drugs, [. . .] It was down the road from where I used to live. It was down the same road, just on the opposite side. It was quiet, umm, I knew, I knew people that lived in the area. Even, I mean, they even tried, I mean when I was there, they even tried to come either with cups of tea, like proper cups, that's where I got this one from (points to cup), and I've kept it.

Both participants here can be seen to be using the familiarity of either the mental health service or the church as a way to create a bubble of interiority within outside space. The glimmers of domesticity described in both of these quotes are encapsulated in the 'cup of tea' brought from acquaintances in the area or the service. For these two participants, continued connection with past relationships are used to create the same feelings of (relative) safety, security and connection that other participants describe in the forest. These bubbles of safety are created through drawing on past relationships and institutions, but can be seen as performing the same function, of creating interiority within the skinless world of homeless living; they here immunise their personal microclimates against the hostility of public space.

Conclusions

In this chapter we have outlined some of the key ways in which newly homeless people in London describe negotiating the relationship between space and mental health, and the strategies that they use to navigate the hostile spaces available to rough sleepers. These experiences highlight the multiple paucities of urban space; the inadequacies of many home spaces and also the harshness of urban public space. Participants described seeking a balance between stifling interiority and exposing exteriority.

For several participants, experiences of stifling interiority were described as playing a role in precipitating homelessness, in line with previous research on seeking movement and fluidity in mental health crisis (McGrath & Reavey, 2015). These intensive, claustrophic bubbles of interior space can be seen as 'bursting' (Sloterdijk, 2011) dramatically with the rupture experience of homelessness. While arguably seeking freedom, what many participants described as encountering in public space was a 'skinless' hostility, danger and shame (Dixon et al. 2006; Hodgetts et al., 2010; Knowles, 2000). Responding to these experiences of exposure, participants described various strategies to re-create bubbles of interiority in exterior space: whether through creative use of urban space; utlising the interior/exterior duality of wooded spaces (Ashon, 2017); or connecting with institutions and past relationships.

It is worth noting that these different strategies had variant outcomes for the participants. The participant who lay down outside their mental health service, spent only one night sleeping rough. Sharon, buried deep in Epping Forest, on the other hand, spent 12 weeks sleeping rough before encountering services once she had moved closer to the edge of the forest. Of course, this is partly through choice; Sharon explicitly compares her experience in the forest positively to being in the homeless service, and it is claustrophobia in home spaces that has pushed several of these participants into homelessness in the first place. It is certainly questionable whether a hostile environment would provide the same experience of simultaneous containment and expansion that Sharon describes in the forest. Nevertheless, it is worth considering that remaining invisible is such a driver in these newly homeless people with mental health problems, that this includes remaining invisible from any services attempting to help them.

References

Ashon, W. (2017). *Strange labyrinth: Outlaws, poets, mystics, murderers and a coward in London's great forest*. London: Granta Books.
Brown, S. D., & Reavey, P. (2014). Vital memories: Movements in and between affect, ethics and self. *Memory Studies, 7*(3), 328–338.
Brown, S. D., & Reavey, P. (2015). *Vital memory and affect: Living with a difficult past*. Abingdon: Routledge.
Creswell, J. W., & Miller, D. L. (2000). Determining validity in qualitative inquiry. *Theory into Practice, 39*(3), 124–130.
Dixon, J., Levine, M., & McAuley, R. (2006). Locating impropriety: Street drinking, moral order, and the ideological dilemma of public space. *Political Psychology, 27*(2), 187–206.
Foucault, M. (1965). *Madness and civilization*. New York, NY: Pantheon.
Harrison, R. P. (2009). *Forests: The shadow of civilisation*. London and Chicago, IL: University of Chicago Press.
Hodgetts, D., Hodgetts, A., & Radley, A. (2006). Life in the shadow of the media Imaging street homelessness in London. *European Journal of Cultural Studies, 9*(4), 497–516.
Hodgetts, D., Radley, A., Chamberlain, K., & Hodgetts, A. (2007). Health inequalities and homelessness considering material, spatial and relational dimensions. *Journal of Health Psychology, 12*(5), 709–725.
Hodgetts, D., Stolte, O., Chamberlain, K., Radley, A., Groot, S., & Nikora, L. W. (2010). The mobile hermit and the city: Considering links between places, objects, and identities in social psychological research on homelessness. *British Journal of Social Psychology, 49*(2), 285–303.
Hodgetts, D., Stolte, O., Chamberlain, K., Radley, A., Nikora, L., Nabalarua, E., & Groot, S. (2008). A trip to the library: Homelessness and social inclusion. *Social & Cultural Geography, 9*(8), 933–953.
Kim, M. M., Ford, J. D., Howard, D. L., & Bradford, D. W. (2010). Assessing trauma, substance abuse, and mental health in a sample of homeless men. *Health & Social Work, 35*(1), 39–48. https://doi.org/10.1093/hsw/35.1.39.
Knowles, C. (2005). *Bedlam on the streets*. London: Routledge.
Latour, B. (2005). *Reassembling the social: An introduction to actor-network-theory*. Oxford: Oxford University Press.
Lefebvre, H. (1991). *The production of space*. Oxford: Blackwell.
Loopstra, R., Reeves, A., Barr, B., Taylor-Robinson, D., McKee, M., & Stuckler, D. (2016). The impact of economic downturns and budget cuts on homelessness claim rates across 323 local authorities in England, 2004–12. *Journal of Public Health, 38*(3), 417–425.
McGrath, L. (2012). *Heterotopias of mental health care: The role of space in experiences of distress, madness, and mental health service use*. London: South Bank University.
McGrath, L., & Reavey, P. (2013). Heterotopias of control: Placing the material in experiences of mental health service use and community living. *Health & Place, 22*, 123–131.
McGrath, L., & Reavey, P. (2015). Seeking fluid possibility and solid ground: Space and movement in mental health service users' experiences of 'crisis'. *Social Science & Medicine, 128*, 115–125.
McGrath, L., & Reavey, P. (2016). 'Zip me up, and cool me down': Molar narratives and molecular intensities in 'helicopter' mental health services. *Health & Place, 38*, 61–69.
Mallet, S. (2004). Understanding home: A critical review of the literature. *The Sociological Review, 52*(1), 62–89.
Massey, D. (1994). *Space, place and gender*. Cambridge and Oxford: Polity Press.

Ministry of Housing, Communities and Local Government. (2018). *Rough sleeping statistics autumn 2017, England*. London: MHCLG.

NHS Confederation. (2012). *Mental health and homelessness: Planning and delivering mental health services for homeless people*. London: NHS.

Parr, H. (1997). Mental health, public space, and the city: Questions of individual and collective access. *Environment and Planning D: Society and Space, 15*(4), 435–454.

Parr, H. (2008). *Mental health and social space: Towards inclusionary geographies?* Oxford: Blackwell Publishing.

Radley, A., Hodgetts, D. & Cullen, A. (2006). Fear, romance and transience in the lives of homeless women. *Social and Cultural Geography, 7*(3), 437–461.

Reavey, P. (2010). Spatial markings: Memory, agency and child sexual abuse. *Memory Studies, 3*(4), 314–329.

Reavey, P. (2012). *Visual methods in psychology: Using and interpreting images in qualitative research*. London: Routledge.

Reavey, P., & Prosser, J. (2012). Visual research in psychology. In H. Cooper, P. M. Camic, D. Long, A. Panter, D. Rindskof, & K. Sher (Eds.), *The APA handbook of research methods in psychology* (vols 1–3, pp. 185–207). Washington, DC: American Psychological Association.

Shelton, K. H., Taylor, P. J., Bonner, A., & van den Bree, M. (2009). Risk factors for homelessness: Evidence from a population-based study. *Psychiatric Services, 60*(4), 465–472.

Sibley, D. (1995). *Geographies of exclusion: Society and difference in the West*. Hove: Psychology Press.

Sloterdijk, P. (2011). *Bubbles, spheres volume I: Microspherology*. Retrieved from https://philpapers.org/rec/SLOBSV.

Sloterdijk, P. (2014). *Globes, spheres volume II: Macrospherology*. Los Angeles, CA: Semiotext(e).

Sloterdijk, P. (2016). *Foams, spheres volume III: Plural spherology*. Los Angeles, CA: Semiotext(e).

Stenner, P. (1993). Discoursing jealousy. In E. Burman and I. Parker (Eds.), *Discourse analytic research: Repertoires and readings of texts in action* (pp. 94–132). London: Routledge.

Tracy, J. L., Robins, R. W., & Tangney, J. P. (2007). *The self-conscious emotions: Theory and research*. New York, NY: Guilford Press.

Walker, C., & Fincham, B. (2011). *Work and the mental health crisis in Britain*. Chichester, UK: John Wiley & Sons.

Wang, C. C., Cash, J. L., & Powers, L. S. (2000). Who knows the streets as well as the homeless? Promoting personal and community action through photovoice. *Health Promotion Practice, 1*(1), 81–89.

Weintraub, J. (1997). The theory and politics of the public/private distinction. *Public and Private in Thought and Practice: Perspectives on a Grand Dichotomy, 1*, 7.

Willig, C. (2013). *Introducing qualitative research in psychology*. London: McGraw-Hill Education (UK).

9

CARING SPACES AND PRACTICES

Does social prescribing offer new possibilities for the fluid mess of 'mental health'?

Carl Walker, Orly Klein, Nick Marks and Paul Hanna

Introducing a controversy

In 1981 Barbara Smith explored the ways in which the disease 'black lung', or 'coal workers' pneumoconiosis' came to prominence as a struggle for the recognition of an occupational disease. As a medical construct, the changing definitions of the disease could be traced to major shifts in the political economy of the coal industry and would represent a bitter controversy over who would control the definition of that disease. Mol and Berg (1998) note that there were two versions of black lung – the black lung that translated the interests of the mining companies and the black lung that reflected the position of the miners. In her account, Smith (1981) warned health advocates in other areas that they too may have to change the definitions of the diseases they try to eradicate by changing the social relations that produce them.

Such an idea, however, stands in contrast to the classic knowledge foundations of medicine where unity is the norm against which variety must be measured and discarded. Here diversity is taken to be a temporary state that can be overcome and dismissed through such things as randomised control trials, evaluations studies, protocols and the standardisation of terminologies (Mol & Berg, 1998).

The Psy professions are one such arena that show just such a fixation on unity. Psychiatry has been critiqued in particular for developing fixed diagnoses that categorise thoughts, deeds and whole persons as deviant (Newnes, 2011). Moreover it has been suggested that the activities and diagnoses of the Psy disciplines have, in the process of privileging professional understandings of mental distress, reduced the dignity of 'lay' human selfhood (Rapley, Moncrieff, & Dillon, 2011) where human beings in the West no longer have any sense of agency in the understanding and amelioration of their psychological distress.

Described as 'a conspiracy against the laity' (Newnes, 2011), the dominance of psychiatric ideas has meant that 'mental' remarks have become the preserve of the

Psy professions despite 'ordinary people having perfectly sufficient descriptions of themselves' (Rapley et al., 2011, p. 5). Through this activity, the medical profession has been accused of monopolising forms of knowledge and treatments and, as such, creating a united front against 'outsiders' such as patients, the state and insurance companies (Mol & Berg, 1998).

Newnes (2011) has suggested that this has led in many cases to the removal of people from socially valued sources of support and the diminution of support networks in the community that can work to prevent the existence and escalation of crises, and that hold people until de-escalation, without medication or violence (Emmanouelidou, 2012).

This chapter seeks to premise this controversy as a platform from which to explore the relatively recent phenomena of social prescribing, or community referring. Drawing on recent empirical work from around the UK (Walker, Hanna, & Hart, 2017) we will explore the social and relational practices that occur in the informal community settings and spaces that are used in social prescribing, and then examine some of conceptual and practical implications for how we understand and perform mental health and its attendant care practices.

Enclosing the 'Psycommons'

Furedi's (2014) therapeutic turn of history has established the 'therapeutic culture' as the dominant Western cultural idiom through which people can make sense of their predicaments. He suggests that such a turn enables and encourages victims of past wrongs to frame their claims in the language of psychology. Here an array of circumstances, relationships and events exhibit potential for therapeutic encounters, with counselling positioned as the answer to almost every type of personal and social problem; including boredom, loneliness, over excitement, rejection, unattractiveness, workplace change and marital infidelity (Moloney, 2013). The widespread use of therapeutic jargon and techniques for 'better relating' have made it harder for many people to use their own intuitions to see how their feelings arise from what is going on in their lives (Moloney, 2013).

Denis Postle (2013) suggests that the idea of 'the commons' can be useful to explore such claims. The commons is the great variety of natural, physical, social, intellectual and cultural resources that make our everyday survival possible (Nonini, 2007). They are assemblages, groups and ensembles of resources that human beings hold in common and that we draw upon for our everyday living. However, what can be understood as 'common resources' are fiercely contested.

Postle (2013) has discussed the 'Psycommons' as the universe of rapport and relationships between people that we draw from to navigate through our daily lives. Herein lies ordinary wisdom, insights and understandings on a whole range of 'issues of living'– this Psycommons is thus the rich stock of psychological knowledge that people have access to.

According to Postle (2013) it is a territory that, like many other forms of commons, has been encroached upon and enclosed. In this case, largely by the Psyprofessions of psychiatry, psychology, counselling and psychoanalysis. These professional institutions have, through their privileged discourses and legitimising systems of professionalisation, fenced off and claimed ownership of an increasing proportion of the Psycommons and extracted value from them through monopoly rents.

It could, however, be argued that such enclosing practices have largely failed to understand the way that misery and suffering results from complex and embodied arrays of social experiences that are embedded within specific historical, cultural, political and economic settings (Cromby, Harper, & Reavey, 2013; Farmer, 1997; Walker et al., 2017).

There is a tendency for Western contemporary psychological theory and practice to create artificial boundaries between the intrapsychic and the socio-economic, such that we tend to speak of and act upon 'individual people' and their 'individual problems'. However, the complex nature of distressing experiences means that much of the routinised misery inflicted upon, and experienced by people, is invisible (Kleinman et al., 1997) both to the sufferer and to the professional who works with or on them. It is not necessarily distress but being unable to account for distress, sadness or worry that marks some out as potentially appropriate for mental health interventions (Cromby et al., 2013).

All manner of large-scale social forces and discreet local social experiences can be translated into personal distress and misery (Farmer, 1997) and life choices and ways of knowing the world are structured through experiences of social class, abuse, gender, race, disability, exclusion and grinding poverty (West Midlands Psychology Group, 2012). To explain the nature of suffering requires individual biographies to be embedded in this larger matrix of culture, history and political economies, which, when understood through the biomedical lens of the Psy institutions, are often rendered imperceptible. 'Amaze' are a Brighton-based parent carer-led community organisation who support parent carers of children with complex needs. Donna, a parent who has used the service, highlights the socially embedded nature of her mental distress and treatment:

> Of course, many of the parents, myself included, have serious depression. I was very depressed when my son was diagnosed and yes, when the school summer holidays and vacations are coming up all our parents from the support group say, "OK, it's time to be alone again". Laughs. So it is a lot of stress, many antidepressants, it is normal to be on antidepressants.
>
> *(Donna, parent carer from Amaze)*

It has been suggested that what has been made knowable as symptomatic behaviour, can also be explained by forms of social deprivation. Some 60–70 per cent of people experiencing visual or auditory hallucinations have been subject to physical or sexual abuse as a child and distress is consistently associated with markers of social inequality such as unemployment, low income and impoverished education (West Midlands Psychology Group, 2012). People abused as children are 9.3 times more likely to hear voices and people who have endured three types of abuse, sexual, physical and bullying have an 18-fold higher risk of hearing voices suggesting the link is causal.

Moreover, social exclusion and relationship breakdowns can cause neurological changes that are experienced as real pain (Dillon, Johnstone, & Longden, 2012). The structural violence that lies at the heart of so much suffering all too often defeats those who try to capture it (Farmer, 1997). Most recent attempts to do so by the mainstream Western Psy institutions have resulted in various political, economic and social forces being translated into personal distress and disorder (Farmer, 1997). It is with this in mind that Young (1992, p. 272) notes that: "Some people suffer not because a tyrannical power intends to keep them down but because of the everyday practices of well-intentioned liberal society".

With these many critiques in mind we come to the broader purpose of this chapter. Despite the introduction above, this chapter does not seek to position itself as one more challenge to the foundations of classic psychiatry. Nor indeed is the intention to suggest alternative forms of care to replace current Psy dominance. This chapter is first and foremost about *mess*. It is about the mess of distress and the care practices that emerge in different informal social and community settings that only occasionally speak to the enclosures of the Psy territories.

The intention here is not to follow the path of prescriptive approaches to care ethics (Barnes, 2012) that seeks to shape mess. To design yet another doctrine through which to displace the current biomedical and diagnostic focus of the mainstream care models. This chapter won't prescribe the essence of what good care looks like for those experiencing distress.

Rather it follows Pols' (2015b) empirical ethics of care to think through the different and sometimes conflicting notions of what constitutes good care within the practices made possible in different settings. This is based on the idea that chronic 'disease' is not a singular natural or biomedical event but is shaped by practices, technologies and people. A particular experience lived through different practices emerges as a different entity, because it is treated differently with real consequences (Pols, 2015b).

Social prescribing

Recent decades have seen a year-on-year increase in the provision of individually oriented mental health interventions, including psychiatric medication and psychological therapy (Harper, 2016). Psychiatric medication still tends to be the default in mental health with 92 per cent of servicers having taken medication. Ilyas and Moncrieff (2012) report that prescriptions for antidepressants have risen exponentially between 1998 and 2010, and they note that the total amount spent on all psychiatric drugs, adjusted for inflation, rose from over £544m in 1998 to £881m in 2010. Similar figures are not available for individual psychotherapy but last year 1,250,126 people were referred and 815,665 people began receiving therapy under the Improving Access to Psychological Therapies initiative (Health and Social Care Information Centre, 2015).

It is against this backdrop that we are seeing a growth in what is known as social prescribing or community referring. Social prescribing can be loosely understood as the practice of linking service users in primary care with sources of support within the community, usually following a form of assessment. In Worthing for instance, a project called 'Going Local' intends to build and test a "completely new way of working between Primary Care, the councils and communities" (JobsGoPublic, 2016). And while one could question the claim to innovative practice, it is fair to state that it certainly represents something of a departure from the standard therapy/medication dominance outlined above.

Broadening the debate to the UK as a whole, the evaluations of the social prescribing pilots thus far appear to have some benefits. They appear to provide GPs, the typical UK gatekeeper to more specialist forms of medical treatment, with a non-medical referral option. Such an approach is understood to be useful because Clinical Commissioning Groups (CCG) who commission services, GP practices and the wider NHS are understood to benefit from the opportunity to reduce demand on costly hospital episodes in the longer term, provide wider preventative benefits likely to emerge over a longer period and because service users and carers benefit from an alternative approach to support (Dayson, 2014).

Recent research suggests that social prescribing is useful for those who are considered to have 'mild to moderate mental health problems', and that such practices have been adjudged positively from those referring (Krska, Taylor, & Morecroft, 2012) and have a positive impact on the waiting list for conventional treatments (Krska et al., 2012). This has included a significant reduction in the number of GP appointments and prescriptions for anxiolytics (Palmer, Dalzell-Brown, Mather, & Krska, 2010). However, there were reported issues in terms of voluntary sector capacity (Friedli, Jackson, Abernathy, & Stansfield, 2009).

Our local pilot version describes Going Local as 'social prescribing', or 'community connecting', the purpose of which is to connect social and community based help and support – as opposed to just medical responses – to individuals presenting to their GPs with social, emotional or practical needs. Underpinning much of the discourse on social prescribing is an idea of 'fixing' specific mental health problems with different methods. And this brings us back to our initial controversy, that of the dominance of Psy models of distress and their potential limiting of people's agency in the understanding and amelioration of their distress.

We are going to suggest that, despite the largely biomedical rhetoric that still underpins the social prescribing concept, when we move distress out into the community different things happen to it and to the people referred. Things start to change shape, certainties are lost and new ideas are forged. Statuses change, practices alter and the typical roles of the care giver and receiver start to change (Mol, Moser, & Pols, 2010). Evidence from our research in recent years suggests we start to see mess emerge.

Mess, suffering and materiality

Law (2004) suggests that alcoholic liver disease is located and enacted in a wide range of different locations including general hospitals, alcohol advice centres, the Samaritans, the Salvation Army, GP consultation rooms, pubs, off-licences and homes. For Law (2004), it is a fractional object, differently enacted through varying practices in multiple sites. Not differently *described* or *constructed* but enacted, that is, it changes shape and sometimes its name too.

Likewise, Annemarie Mol (2002) foregrounds practices so that objects like 'diseases' are not passive things to be seen from different perspectives. Instead they come into being and disappear with the practices within which they are manipulated. That is, objects can be differently enacted in different practices and in the different sites that these practices occur. She talks of an approach that rejects the absence of the body's physical reality and foregrounds practicalities and events; what is done in practice. 'Bike Minded' is a cycling charity from Bristol that offer group cycling for individuals with mental health issues. The following account suggests that an orientation toward non-clinical practices can have implications for how people see themselves and their distress:

> It just takes their mind off their mental health. They get a ride and they just sort of feel like a cyclist you know with a group of cyclists. I think I just, I don't think of them as people with mental health problems really, I just think of them as people.
>
> *(John, Bike Minded service user and volunteer)*

The spaces we occupy and the objects that surround us participate in the enactment of self at any given time (Reavey & Brown, 2009). If we understand distress as an acquired and embodied way of being in the world (West Midlands Psychology Group, 2012), not an idea that someone holds but a legacy of encounters with a social world that can manifest in misery (Mezzina et al., 2006), then we can start to think about it as multiply realised across a variety of spatial locations. Mol and Law (1994) suggest that some social spaces take a fluid form. We would suggest that the spaces in which psychological distress moves can behave rather like a fluid and that distress is a fluid, changeable object moving in a fluid space.

In given locations a specific version of distress is clearly visible, understood and formed, for instance in medical settings, pharmacies, therapy rooms and in workplaces where missing days require legitimation of a specific version of distress. If we think of distress as having the capacity to be enacted as on thing in some places and something else in another, this makes it intrinsically messy. The certainties and diagnoses that hold it fixed in one network start to drift beyond the things that hold it together.

The multiple ways in which Western mental health paradigms have sought to deal with the mess of psychological distress – the inherent instability and ambiguity – has been through the development of largely administrative systems that lead to the diagnoses of people (Dodier, 1998). In so doing the individual 'patient' is enacted into a population that allows a health professional to know enough about their situation to act upon it. Mostly regardless of other particularities, they will be treated like other members of that population and, in so doing, the frame of mental health is always administrative rather than truly 'clinical'. And while these disorders may change over time, according to this perspective they don't effectively change in one single time point over different social contexts.

For instance the patient whose distress is diagnosed as clinical depression is a patient 'with' clinical depression regardless of whether they are sat at home, at their desk at work, inside a psychiatrist's office or at a local art class. They may experience these places differently, they may act differently in these contexts but in effect they remain patients with clinical depression across space. Here, distress as the object of interest is relatively unchangeable in a given time point.

We would say, however, that distress as an object is not as unchangeable as is routinely held in biomedical psychiatry. As it moves from the centre to the periphery of the biomedical network, for instance from the psychiatrist's or GP's office to a local social club, the truths that form it become progressively less reliable (Walker et al., 2017).

People experiencing distress will, as a matter of course, encounter other social spaces. Some of these social spaces will not require such a diagnostic process, some may require it, but the administration process may be to fix the person and their distress in different ways using non-diagnostic criteria. In many of these spaces there will be no Psy professionals and treatments and so detecting specific diagnoses is not urgent or important.

In some locations distress is enacted a certain way and with certain implications, at other parts of the fluid space it will be enacted differently with different implications (Walker et al., 2017). A volunteer at a bike maintenance workshop for people with mental health difficulties said that 'alternative spaces' with non-clinical goals can offer something to people, a new-found sense of purpose through an alternative focus from that of 'recovery':

> The workshop is a completely different place so the atmosphere was different so we could talk about different stuff (other than recovery) and it seemed to everyone that they were just talking about other things you know. A lot of them said, like, I just like coming here you know it is just nice to be here, it is just somewhere different, you know?
> *(Bob, volunteer in a bike maintenance workshop)*

At a peer support group for parents of children with complex needs, parents spoke of a comradeship and solidarity that allowed for an emergent change in their collective and individual identities and status. There was a sense of a space that had opened up where voices previously silenced through practices of stigma and lack of empathy, were replaced by a sense of shared purpose and belonging in the group:

I really enjoyed the people, the people were, were fabulous, there was a real sense of belonging, of, people not, not being afraid to be there and to share their emotions and then their knowledge and talk about experiences, that was good.

(Nichola, parent carer)

Care practices and space

Psychological experience is spatially distributed in the sense that different self-identifications can emerge in and across settings and the environments that surround us participate in our very constitution at a given time (McGrath & Reavey, 2015). Spaces offer zones of possibility, that can be experienced as sanctuary and relaxing, and also threatening and oppressive; the kinds of community spaces invoked by social prescribing networks can be both (McGrath & Reavey, 2015).

We are not seeking to make value-based arguments for one type of space being any 'better' than the other (although such a pursuit may well have merit) but rather to explore the different possibilities that emerge in and from these informal spaces. With this in mind we undertook research exploring both the instrumental and often intangible experiences that emerged in such settings as a cycling project for people diagnosed with mental health problems, an advocacy service for the parents of children with complex needs, a community centre for unemployed families, a community choir and a fishing group for young people.

What emerged, variably, were spaces, settings, projects and groups that appeared to accommodate well, the fluidity of distress. They often allowed fluid distress to be non-visible or visible in different ways. They fixed few if any rigid boundaries around people's distress. Indeed it is worth noting that in many such informal spaces, the activities therein were not considered relevant to either 'care' or 'mental health'. Unlike biomedicine, which often seeks to hold distress in rigid spaces within rigid networks of relations, definitions, roles, expectations and narratives, these spaces did so far less or at least did so in ways that were not usually centered on the concerns of medicine.

The Brighton Unemployed Families Centre Project is an open space and tea bar/café. Every weekday and for the whole day, anyone can come along and use the Internet, have a cup of tea, rest, socialise, get advice on benefits and housing or do an art or yoga or education class with others. It also has a free crèche. Such an open environment, with many ways of using space, was suggested to be important for centre users in transitioning from feelings of hopelessness, despair and low self-worth, to a sense of capability. Unlike previous experiences with health and employment authorities, people who worked in the space said that their identities were not fixed before the person using the service entered the service. As Sally noted:

> Well I think, I think it gives them a space, a safe space and I think it's, you can come and be without having any stigma of being 'it's just a service for people with mental health problems' because we don't, we're not that.
>
> *(Sally, former volunteer and worker)*

Our case studies of informal spaces highlighted that what can be so useful for mental distress is actually hugely variant in nature. It could be a singing group, a cycling group, an organisation to support parents of children with complex needs and/or a sedative. It could be an advocacy and information service for people using benefits, debt guidance, employment advocacy or advice on local facilities for a disabled family member, or just sitting down with other people in a space that isn't your house.

Duff (2012) speaks of enabling places, that is, the privileging of a relational account of place that acknowledges the resources for the 'everyday work of recovery'. This includes the diverse objects, assets and benefits that circulate in and through local communities. These include intangibles like companionship, empathy, atmosphere, hope and non-judgementalism and more tangible things like practical support, advice and advocacy that were regularly spoken about during our research.

The practices enacted in these spaces were enabled in the main by 'non-professional' people who were oriented not around diagnosis, treatment and recovery, but around what was discussed as connectedness, humanity, benevolence, support and safety. Without (or at least with less) goal-oriented programmes, there was potential for people to talk about themselves and their distress in different ways, or not at all, and to experiment with social roles and imagine alternative futures and trajectories (Pols & Kroon, 2007).

People spoke of a sense of 'being in place' that appeared to include their relationships with other people and groups. Some participants suggested that this sense of 'being in place' offered different options for status and identity than they had ever experienced during mainstream biomedical settings (Walker et al., 2017).

Medical professionals *and* the people who inhabit informal community spaces can be seen as bringing different social worlds into being, with very clear implications for how people understand themselves and their distress (Pols, 2006). When patients arrive in a community setting they are 'incoming citizens' who engage in everyday practices and recreational activities (Pols, 2015a). Different possibilities emerge, for instance regarding ideals strived for, values enacted, or routines implemented (Pols, 2015b).

If we are to think through which possibilities are enabled through social prescribing (and lest we remember that this is a process still made possible through the administrative gatekeeping of general practice) then it is useful to focus on the way that social practices are ordered across space and time, and which conditions enable certain outcomes, forms of knowledge and citizenship. In such spaces, experience may best be understood, not as outcomes of professional expertise and consequences of individual actions, but as ongoing fluid processes in which a variety of different routines, social relations and activities are made possible.

What is enabled by the social prescribing paradigm might be understood, in most cases, as quite different from those of the more conventional biomedical realm. There is something emergent and collective about the care that is practiced. These contexts make possible different forms of knowledge. Here knowledge is not a professional asset that can be moved between organisations or professionals, but instead emerges as people engage in practices with other people, courses of action, spaces and activities. This again has implications for how we recognise and value care practices. In such settings there are multiple care practices. Some can be done, told, known and visible while others remain invisible, silent and implicit (Singleton, 2010). One of the volunteers at Bike Minded discussed the importance of a relatively intangible idea like 'sense of duty' and how it can manifest a feeling of belonging:

> [A] sense of belonging, a sense of having, being obliged . . . that confers some kind of a duty, having duty is an interesting thing, it kind of ties you to something, you have chosen that activity but it's still you, you're attached to something.
>
> *(Steven, Bike Minded volunteer)*

Parent carers from a peer support group, for the parents of children with complex needs discussed the importance of 'atmosphere' in being able to experience a space as helpful:

> But, yea, I think it's a lot more it's not informal, it's a friendly relaxed atmosphere so you are far more likely to sort of talk in depth and a little bit more openly and candid about.
>
> *(Pauline, parent carer)*

> It was informal, it was relaxed. I think informal to me, to me personally I feel informal is good cos I don't like feeling like I am back in the classroom but I feel that informal makes people more relaxed, more willing to open up and talk about things than if you're sitting behind a desk.
>
> *(Nichola, parent carer)*

If such practices are only talked about in medical terms that are not appropriate to them, however, they may not be well captured or understood (Singleton, 2010). If care can only be understood as 'care' if practiced by the correct people (for example, psychologists, therapists or psychiatrists), then we miss the practices that happen both in *informal* and *formal* settings (Walker et al., 2017). The current dominance of the knowledge and measurement practices of positivistic bio-cognitivism not only misses care practices and the knowledges articulated in various informal settings, but it also does scant justice to the spaces of Psy practitioners themselves.

It is with this in mind that we now think through how we name the care practices being valued. How is it that, for instance, volunteering in a community arts programme might be considered *therapeutic* for some people experiencing psychological distress (Chinman & Wandersman, 1999) and what are the repercussions of recognising such an activity as a *therapeutic* thing? Central to understanding this requires a reimagining of what constitutes a 'therapeutic space'.

The term 'therapeutic landscape' has had prominence in recent years in health geography (Doughty, 2013). As part of this shift there has been an emphasis on the notion that ordinary places have potential for well-being – places like the home, local community amenities or the garden (Doughty, 2013; Milligan & Bingley, 2007; Williams, 2002). However, the term therapeutic must be understood as having different modalities. It is a medical term and also a lay term and it takes forms that represent and value what lies between.

One therapeutic, is the medical therapeutic of experts and mental health. This encompasses a range of interrelated medical activities and devices including diagnoses, treatments, psychiatrists, psychologists, psychotherapy, pharmacology, experts, research, scientific evidence and NICE (National Institute of Clinical Excellence). It is a term owned by, enclosed and defined, by the practitioners of medicine (Walker et al., 2017). However, events outside the immediate spaces of Psy have also come to be understood through therapeutic terminology.

A far from exhaustive list might include reading, singing, walking, volunteering, drawing, yoga or having a holiday. One might talk about the 'therapeutic capture' of such everyday activities in different ways. They might be understood as the latest exemplars of Psy enclosure or they might be understood as a modernising and demedicalising movement of Psy ideas and practice. Either way the therapeutic assigned to such activities is one that is currently considered less legitimate than the therapeutic assigned to the standard practices of biomedicine. Here, social and cultural 'things' can be therapeutic but are always *less so* than biomedical and professional 'things'. Indeed a cursory glance at the stepped care model of IAPT programmes (Improving Access to Psychological Therapies) and the privileging of some forms of evidence over others in NICE guidelines highlights the inherently hierarchical nature of what is understood as therapeutic. To be 'properly medically therapeutic' involves experts, diagnoses, therapies, evidence-based medicine and research.

Academics interested in ethics of care often mobilise prescriptive models for what constitutes 'good care' (Pols, 2015b). Pols' (2015b) empirical ethics of care moves from this position in order to make it possible to analyse the different and sometimes conflicting notions of what good care is within care practices. In our case, with social prescribing into informal spaces, such an approach opens up possibilities for valuing the different types of care that traditional biomedical views of care fix in relatively rigid hierarchies.

If we are to activate an empirical ethics of care approach to account for and compare care practices, then *therapeutic* may not do a robust job of accounting for the practices inherent in the informal spaces of social prescribing or community referral. Although to characterise the activities of a wide array of referral places in one or two sentences will almost inevitably do them scant justice, it is reasonable to say that the practices in these spaces are often not primarily oriented toward helping people to get better from an illness. In this sense they are not therapeutic.

Rather they are rather more disparate, flexible and bespoke and adhere closer to practices of humanity, compassion, benevolence, support, safety and connectedness.

If we seek to develop social materialist models of distress that incorporate historically situated, fluid and embodied experiences, then it may improve the tools at our disposal, to move away from variants of 'therapeutic' when describing the practices and activities of people in everyday settings.

Conclusions

Should we wish to know about and attribute value to the fluid, innovative care practices that routinely emerge in informal community settings then methods sensitive to such fluidity are needed (Pols, 2010). Well-being and distress may be better understood not as internalised qualities of individuals but instead as sets of effects produced in specific times and places; complex assemblages of relations not only between people but also between people and places, material objects and less material components like atmospheres, histories and values (Atkinson, 2013).

Like the informal spaces of social prescribing, 'formal' Psy spaces are themselves not the uniform, rigid and boundaried straw men that are typically constituted in critical debates on distress (and that we have to a degree reproduced). These spaces themselves are fluid. Perhaps less so than other social spaces, but there is fluidity in the spaces of Psy, with great variation in the degree to which practitioners constitute the objects of distress and great variation, in how they do or do not mobilise the enclosing, fixing and constituting biomedical apparatuses of distress (Walker et al., 2017).

The current ways that we name, understand, negotiate, value and measure care and distress are at present poorly equipped to understand the complex arrays of settings, practices, citizenships, knowledges and enactments of distress that are currently understood as informal mental health care. If care practices and distress are only talked about in terms that are not appropriate to their specificities, they will be submitted to rules and regulations that are alien to them (Mol et al., 2010). The social prescribing paradigm, as with more formal mainstream mental health care, is still largely governed by biomedical versions of people, care and distress and that produce a world where, as in fairytales, there tend to be happy endings. A focus on care practices might start a move away from such rationalist versions of the human being into altogether more nuanced terrain.

References

Atkinson, S. (2013). Beyond components of wellbeing: The effects of relational and situated assemblage. *Topoi, 32*, 137–144.

Barnes, M. (2012). *Care in everyday life: An ethic of care in practice.* Cambridge, UK: Policy Press.

Chinman, M. J., & Wandersman, A. (1999). The benefits and costs of volunteering in community organisations: Review and practical implications. *Non-profit and Voluntary Sector Quarterly, 28*(1), 46–64.

Cromby, J., Harper, D., & Reavey, P. (2013). *Psychology, mental health and distress.* Basingstoke: Palgrave Macmillan.

Dayson, C. (2014). *Evaluation of the Rotherham social prescribing pilot*. Retrieved from www4.shu.ac.uk/research/cresr/ourexpertise/evaluation-rotherham-social-prescribing-pilot.
Dillon, J., Johnstone, L., & Longden, E. (2014). Trauma, dissociation, attachment and neuroscience: A new paradigm for understanding severe mental distress. In E. Speed, J. Moncrieff, & M. Rapley (Eds.), *De-medicalising misery II: Society, politics and the mental health industry*. London: Palgrave Macmillan.
Dodier, N. (1998). Clinical practice and procedures in occupational medicine: A study of the framing of individuals. In M. Berg & A. M. Mol, *Differences in medicine*. Durham, NC: Duke University Press.
Doughty, K. (2013). Walking together: The embodied and mobile production of a therapeutic landscape. *Health & Place, 24*, 140–146. doi: 10.1016/j.healthplace.2013.08.009.
Duff, C. (2012). Exploring the role of 'enabling places' in promoting recovery from mental illness: A qualitative test of a relational model. *Health and Place, 18*, 1388–1395.
Emmanouelidou, A. (2012). Drawing money from empty coffers: Self-help and social solidarity as a recovery answer to psychiatric pain. *Journal of Critical Psychology, Counselling and Psychotherapy, 12*(1), 7–13.
Farmer, P. (1997). On suffering and structural violence: A view from below. About suffering: Voice, genre and moral community. In A. Kleinman, V. Das, & M. Lock, *Introduction: Social suffering*. Berkeley, CA: University of California Press.
Friedli, L., Jackson, C., Abernathy, H., & Stansfield, J. (2009). *Social prescribing for mental health: A guide to commissioning and delivery*. London: Care Services Improvement Partnership.
Furedi, F. (2014). Is it Justice? Therapeutic history and the politics of recognition. In E. Speed, J. Moncrieff, & M. Rapley, *De-medicalising misery: Society politics and the mental health industry*. Basingstoke: Palgrave Macmillan.
Harper, D. (2016). Beyond individual therapy. Retrieved from https://thepsychologist.bps.org.uk/volume-29/june/beyond-individual-therapy.
Health and Social Care Information Centre. (2015). *Psychological therapies: Annual report on the use of IAPT services*. London: Health and Social Care Information Centre.
Ilyas, S., & Moncrieff, J. (2012). Trends in prescriptions and costs of drugs for mental disorders in England, 1998–2010. *British Journal of Psychiatry, 200*(5), 393–398.
JobsGoPublic. (2016). Retrieved from www.jobsgopublic.com/job/community-referrer-cd-16-15234/atom.
Kleinman, A., Das, V., & Lock, M. (1997). *Social suffering*. Berkeley, CA: University of California Press.
Krska, J., Taylor, J., & Morecroft, C. (2012). *Evaluating the role of the wellbeing sefton coordinator*. Sefton, UK: NHS Sefton.
Law, J. (2004). *After method*. London: Routledge.
McGrath, L., & Reavey, P. (2015). Seeking fluid possibility and solid ground: Space and movement in mental health service uses' experience of 'crisis'. *Social Science & Medicine, 128*, 115–125.
Mezzina, R., Davidson, L., Borg, M., Marin, I., Topor, A., & Sells, D. (2006). The social natures of recovery: Discussion and implications for practice. *American Journal of Psychiatric Rehabilitation, 9*, 63–80.
Milligan, C., & Bingley, A. (2007) Restorative places or scary spaces? The impact of woodland on the mental well-being of young adults. *Health & Place, 13*, 799–811.
Mol, A. M. (2002). *The body multiple: Ontology in medical practice*. Durham, NC: Duke University Press.

Mol, A. M., & Berg, M. (1998). Differences in medicine. In M. Berg & A. M. Mol, *Differences in medicine*. Durham, NC: Duke University Press.

Mol, A. M., & Law, J. (1994). Regions, networks and fluids: Anaemia and social topology. *Social Studies of Science, 24*(4), 641–671.

Mol, A. M., Moser, I., & Pols, J. (2010). Care: Putting practice into theory. In A. Mol, I. Moser, & J. Pols (Eds.), *Care in practice: on tinkering in clinics, homes and farms*. Bielefeld: Verlag.

Moloney, P. (2013). *The therapy industry: The irresistible rise of the talking cure, and why it doesn't work*. London: Pluto Press.

Newnes, C. (2011). Toxic psychology. In M. Rapley, J. Moncrieff, & J. Dillon, *Demedicalising misery: Psychiatry, psychology and the human condition*. Basingstoke: Palgrave Macmillan.

Nonini, DM. (2007). *The global idea of the commons*. New York, NY: Berghahn Books.

Palmer, S., Dalzell-Brown, A., Mather, K. & Krska, J. (2010). Evaluation of the impact on GP surgeries of the Citizens Advice Bureau health outreach service. Sefton, UK: NHS Sefton.

Pols, J. (2006). Washing the citizen: Washing, cleanliness and citizenship in mental health care. *Culture, Medicine & Psychiatry, 30*, 77–104.

Pols, J. (2010). Telecare: What patients care about. In A. Mol, I. Moser, & J. Pols (Eds.). *Care in practice: On tinkering in clinics, homes and farms*. Bielefeld: Verlag.

Pols, J. (2015a). Analysing social spaces: Relational citizenship for patients leaving mental health care institutions. *Medical Anthropology*. doi: 10.1080/01459740.2015.1101101.

Pols, J. (2015b). Towards an empirical ethics in care: Relations with technologies in Health care. *Medical Health Care and Philosophy, 18*, 81–90.

Pols, J., & Kroon, H. (2007). The importance of holiday trips for people with chronic mental health problems. *Psychiatric Services, 58*(23), 262.

Postle, D. (2013). The richness of everyday relationships. *Therapy Today, 24*(3), 262–265.

Rapley, M., Moncrieff, J., & Dillon, J. (2011). Carving nature at its joints? DSM and the medicalisation of everyday life. In M. Rapley, J. Moncrieff, & J. Dillon, *Demedicalising misery: Psychiatry, psychology and the human condition*. Basingstoke: Palgrave Macmillan.

Reavey, P., & Brown, S. D. (2009). The mediating role of objects in recollections of adult women survivors of child sexual abuse. *Culture & Psychology, 15*(4), 463–484.

Singleton, V. (2010). Good farming: Control or care. In A. Mol, I. Moser, & J. Pols (Eds.). *Care in practice: On tinkering in clinics, homes and farms*. Bielefeld: Verlag.

Smith, B. (1981). Black lung: The social production of disease. *International Journal of the Health Service, 11*, 343–359.

Walker, C., Hanna, P., & Hart, A. (2017). *Building a new community psychology of mental health: spaces, places, people and activities*. Basingstoke: Palgrave Macmillan.

West Midlands Psychology Group. (2012). Draft manifesto for a social materialist psychology of distress. *Journal of Critical Psychology, Counselling and Psychotherapy, 12*(2), 93.

Williams, A. (2002) Changing geographies of care: Employing the concept of therapeutic landscapes as a framework in examining home space. *Social Science & Medicine, 55*, 141–154.

Young, I. M. (1992). Five Faces of Oppression. In T. Wartenberg (Ed.), *Rethinking power*. Albany, NY: State University of New York Press.

10
SPACES OF 'SANCTUARY'
Unfolding older, mental health service users' experiences within the spaces of the home

Lesley-Ann Smith

Introduction

In terms of mental health, the home and garden[1] are important spaces to consider as research has indicated that older service users are more inclined to spend time within their household (or places of psychiatric care) than anywhere else due to physiological deterioration, financial constraints and psychological barriers (Tucker & Smith, 2014; Williams, 2002). In terms of service user's social practices, it could be seen as unconventional within the local neighbourhood to display catatonic behaviours, such as the waving of arms in a haphazard manner (Parr, 1999). Such unconventional behaviours can have socially problematic impacts by further isolating people who "are trying to become reintegrated into society" (Miller, 2004, p. 3). Here we are provided with some ways in which the occupation of community space can be constituted by the status, identity and the social role of ex-psychiatric patients (Parr, 1997). Socially visible issues such as these need to be taken into consideration when discussing 'home' spaces and distress in that the home may offer the opportunity to be privately 'insane' away from the politically and socially regulated orders of psychiatric practices and community spaces (Blunt, 2005; Parr, 1997; Pinfold, 2000). As McGrath & Reavey (2015) note, experiences in the more visible community spaces and potentially hidden private home spaces are pivotal in understanding the ways in which mental distress can be both performed and expressed.

This chapter will explore service user's embodied experiences and how these expressions are spatially distributed within home spaces including the outside garden space. This is a distinct move away from defining home spaces as merely consisting of an array of geometric rooms through which people simply physically move within, whereby psychological phenomena is analysed as a separate entity (Blunt & Varley, 2004; Dovey, 1985; Smith, 2012; Tucker, 2010a; Urry, 2005).

Here the relational forms of materiality and expression within home spaces together with the cartographical markers such as furniture will be explored in an attempt to gain a sense of how this space is temporally embodied (Brown & Tucker, 2010; Hurdley, 2006, 2007; Tucker & Smith, 2014). It is an exploration of how service users make sense of their everyday home life.

Furthermore, Imrie and Edwards (2007, p. 627) argue that for those people who already experience social marginalisation, such as service users, the home comprises a variety of "paradoxical and contradictory spaces". It is a space that can require the occupant to juggle with their distress while trying to maintain an element of normalcy and routine to add stability to daily life and provide a sense of agency. Home for service users can therefore be a space of safety and sanctuary or indeed a space of exhausting obstacles (real or imagined) to overcome (Smith, 2012). Consequently, it is this area that is of specific interest to gain a further insight into the strategies employed by service users in actualising their individual micro milieu and understanding the constituent nature of how a large portion of everyday service user life is produced and continually (re)produced (Blunt & Dowling, 2006; Low & Lawrence-Zuniga, 2003).

Home spaces as an ideology

Taking a somewhat idealised position, the cultural notions of home can endorse a spatiality of safety and private sanctuary, a place where we can 'breathe a sigh of relief' as negotiated social identities played out in community spaces are replaced by the need to focus on personal needs and wants and more widely as the place enveloping private family life (Blunt, 2005; Blunt & Dowling, 2006; Somerville, 1997). In contrast, Miller (2001, p. 15) notes, "If home is where the heart is, then it is also where it is broken, torn and made whole in the flux of relationships, social and material". Rather than being a private space away from prying eyes, home can indeed be a social space of constant negotiation with others and the self, it is a political landscape imbued with power and identity (Blunt & Varley, 2004; Brickell, 2012, Putnam, 1999). These positions highlight the tensions between how the seemingly private home space on one hand, can also be an arena for social performances on the other. Therefore, the home and its contents can become a very public territory ripe for scrutiny by others (Brickell, 2012; Doyle, 1992; Graves-Brown, 2000). For example, a quick tidy up or a more thorough clean up of the home before a visit is made by an outsider is not an unusual occurrence. The appearance of our home is an important way of presenting ourselves in terms of social and cultural desirability and respectability – it is not an abstract space filled with inanimate objects, it is wholly emotional, cultural and socially influential (Blunt & Dowling, 2006). Subsequently, it is the multiplex nature of this space in terms of the mutable relational nature between mental distress, embodiment, expression and materiality, which are important in this piece of work (Brown, 2001; Davidson, 2003; Tucker, 2006).

The ordering and coding of home and garden spaces

Wise (2000, p. 295) draws attention to the ways in which repetition (such as housework) and the stabilising of space by the use of physical markers (e.g. walls, furniture), personal territories are mapped out to create "a space of comfort amidst fear, in other words, home". Nevertheless, this does not mean that this space or indeed, practices of home endure as static entities of establishing one's personal sense of place, rather these elements are both transitional and wrapped up with strands of connectivity to the outside world (Knappett, 2002; Wise, 2000). In other words, the structural elements of home spaces are bound up with the processes of wider social norms and self-identity. It is these notions of how these spaces are (re)formed and (re)constructed as a result of interactions with inanimate objects that serve to create home as an affective territory.

Cloutier-Fisher and Harvey's (2009) research explored the lived experiences of older people moving from the wider community to a retirement community. They concluded that people draw from their past history, lived environmental experiences and self-identity in an attempt to situate and arrange their home space as constituting their 'own' embodied space. However, in reality, the process of interacting within the home environment is constantly evolving with the relational components in the wider world (Blunt & Dowling, 2006; Massey, 2004). Nevertheless, people seek to create cartographical markers such as placing personal photographs in an attempt to 'fix' their private spaces (Blunt & Varley, 2004; Urry, 2005).

These kinds of ordering, arrangement and containment of materiality and the stratification of people's roles with the home (the female as 'domestic goddess', for example) can emanate a sense of social order, morality and stability within home spaces (Curtis, 2010). However, there is a flip side here, namely disordered, 'dirty' home spaces, which are linked with immorality and idleness – those homes that do not conform to a structured organisation of content and expression (Clarke, 2001; Cox, 2012). Culturally, there are television programmes that largely focus on the home spaces of social deprivation and low functioning, such as *A Life of Grime* and *How Clean Is Your House?* and that present an array of negative social practices.

Within the set-up of *How Clean Is Your House?* we have two middle-class presenters who perform as life-style experts and offer advice to facilitate the (re)production of unkempt and culturally distasteful home spaces into a space of socially acceptable normality and morality. In other words, homes should be kept neat, ordered and clean. Here, home spaces are not part of a process of leaving visibly undetectable traces of bodily performance and movement (such as the shedding of dead skin and hair) (Thrift, 2004) but are more bound up with the visual evidence of human mess and murk. Imageries proliferate of dirty washing strewn across spaces, kitchen sinks full of dirty cutlery and decomposing food and toilets embellished with the stains of old faeces and urine. It would also be reasonable to suggest that the well-structured order and daily routine cleaning practices of moral home spaces can also act as an indicator of positive mental health whereby dirt and mess suggest low levels of social functioning (Bijl & Ravelli, 2000; Cwerner & Metcalfe, 2003). In this way, cleanliness and order can present the ideals of distinctive virtuous qualities of 'righteousness' when compared to the disordered and dirty elements associated with 'deviance' (Cieraad, 1999). Here we have a dichotomy of social positioning linked to behaviours imbued within the regulation of home spaces, which can in turn produces adages such as; 'a clean home is a happy home'. These kinds of constructions are reinforced by commercial advertisements linked with home spaces as well as the television programmes mentioned previously. In contrast, those homes where space is littered with dirt, grime and waste are linked to dysfunctional ways of living.

This can, at some level, support the constructed positions of service users as necessarily having poor levels of day-to-day functioning (Reynolds et al., 2000; Slade, Phelan, Thornicroft, & Parkman, 1996). Research has indicated that service users are largely unable to engage in 'normal' behaviours associated with cleaning and the ordering of space and objects within home spaces (Slade et al., 1996). In other words, mental health and home spaces may not be socially constituted within the same prevailing codings and parameters whereby the home is positioned as a cultural space flowing with integrity and organisation. To some extent, service users may reside on the boundaries of these particular constructions.

In terms of ordering and arrangements within garden spaces, Lefebvre (1999, p. 157) notes:

> This remarkable institution of the garden is always a microcosm, a symbolic work of art, an object as well as a place, and it has 'diverse' functions which are never merely functions . . . the garden exemplifies the appropriation of nature, for it is at once entirely natural – and thus a symbol of the macrocosm – and entirely cultural – and thus the projection of a way of life.

What Lefebvre is referring to in the above extract is the ways in which people do, or conversely, do not, manufacture and control that which is culturally positioned as a natural production of space. From a macro perspective, gardens have been constructed as a haven of relaxation within natural surroundings. There is a plethora of media advertising families enjoying the availability of this 'open' space peppered with selected shrubs, flowers, borders, rockeries and other adornments such as statues, swings and slides. Subsequently, on the face of it, this space is enveloped within the use of cultural artefacts associated with easy living. In addition, the garden can cross the divide from a private to a more public space where many gardens are wholly or partially visible to outsiders.

To obtain cultural approval, gardens should be preened, pruned, weeded and adorned with selected garden ornaments or, conversely, they can be left to the forces of nature, whereby the grass is kept long and all manner of plant life is able to exist (Curtis, 2010). In this way garden spaces can be more observably open to interpretation by others, which may or may not adhere to social expectations of normative living. This in turn, can lead to assumptions being made about the occupant(s) linked to this particular space. In other words, those that display elements of undesirable behaviours such as allowing a garden to overgrow with all manner of vegetation can be socially positioned as deviant in that their gardens are not 'produced' in line with the more dominant cultural perspectives of this manufactured space. Subsequently, the architectural landscaping, maintenance and cultural artefacts of a garden can be a window into the day-to-day lives of occupants (Cwerner & Metcalfe, 2003). Above all, the garden is also a space of morality, cultural performance and social competence and it is arguably a more public space than the confines of the home, rendering this space as open to public surveillance and scrutiny.

In terms of mental health, research has been conducted with service users both young and old to assess the impacts of gardening and psychological well-being (e.g. Parr, 2007). This way of introducing service users to gardening and sharing an allocated green space to grow vegetables and flowers is now a favoured therapeutic intervention, largely due to the positive results this activity provides. Findings suggest that collaborative gardening reduces feelings of social isolation together with lessening physical and psychological degradation (Milligan, Gatrell, & Bingley, 2004). These types of 'green' activities have now been formalised and function as part of a psychological treatment plan known as 'Ecotherapy' (Mind, 2015). These therapeutic interventions and research objectives primarily focus on the social and material elements of gardening within allocated pieces of land (Parr, 2007). Subsequently, the feelings of service users' positively embodying practices of engaging alone in 'green' work within their own garden spaces may well have different meanings and practices. It may be a place that can exacerbate feelings of loneliness and isolation as the continuous production of a 'natural' but 'well-composed' space such as the garden has little social and emotional meaning and does not offer strong connections with other people – in other words, the garden can become a wasteland both literally and symbolically. It can be an observable reflection of states of distress (Smith, 2012).

Research methodology

All participants attended various Mind charitable day centres within the East Midlands area. In total five day centres were visited and 21 participants (10 females and 11 males) took part within the interview research data collection. All participants were aged 50 years and over, this age restriction was seen as important and valuable in terms of exploring an under-represented community within the research arena of psychiatric services. Other factors with regards to researching older service users were also of interest such as generational differences (between current younger service users) whereby younger service users during the 1970s and 1980s did not have nationwide access to specialist services such as child and adolescent mental health services (Black & Gowers, 2005). In addition, 'community care' programmes were not well established, particularly in the 1970s, so many older service users may have been resident in psychiatric institutions prior to the introduction of the 'community care' programme (Parr, 1999). For some participants in my research project, there were intimations that some participants would still be residing in psychiatric institutions if the 'care in the community' programme had not been introduced.

One-to-one, semi-structured interviews were conducted in the day centre and were recorded using a digital recorder and transcribed *ad verbatim*. In practical terms, all participants within this research were in receipt of various state benefits and subsequently did not have access to funds to pay for their own car to enable wider socialisation outside of the immediate neighbourhood. Consequently, narratives emerged within the research data collection when discussing daily life of time spent at home or in a space of residential care.

For the purposes of this chapter, the experiential narratives of service users will be drawn upon to offer divergent accounts of the relational and emotional aspects of home spaces. These participants' extracts were selected for analysis to provide accounts of independent, single-occupancy living in council accommodation and the experiences of living in supported accommodation with other service users. All participants have very different experiences of the ways in which mental health and home spaces are embodied and the importance that this particular space has on their daily lives.

Analysis

Following transcription, all interviews were analysed using a thematic approach, following the six procedures of analysis as outlined by Braun and Clarke (2006). The emergent dominant themes discussed in this work are (a) Independent living in the community and (b) living in supported accommodation. While other themes are evident in the research data, such as the immediate neighbourhood, gendered practices and differing mental states and functionality in the home, these two main themes offer an insight into two key areas of daily service user life within home spaces. These data examples illustrate (via interpretation) the ways in which service users assemble and move within home spaces by drawing out the features of the data.

Independent living

Consider the following extract from Caroline, a 50-year-old service user, who has a psychiatric diagnosis of Borderline Personality Disorder and has spent some periods of time within psychiatric institutions, due to behaviours linked with drug and alcohol consumption coupled with self-harming practices and suicide attempts. Caroline lives alone in a council-owned, one-bedroomed flat with a small garden. Here she is discussing events when she went into hospital under 'voluntary' section as a consequence of her excessive drinking and smoking of cannabis (and in the following event her overt self-harming behaviours by cutting herself and taking a medicinal overdose) in the view of her immediate neighbours.

Caroline: I did go into town in (names town) bought a load of tablets and a bottle of wine and I went in the garden took the tablets and drank (sighs) and yeah, some cutting, self-harming and um you know

LAS: So it was actually somebody else phoning up (Caroline = yeah) for you?

Caroline: Yeah it was people and yeah the ambulance people and the police came as I did threaten somebody with a knife but she give me all that (imitates talking with hands) so I threatened her with a knife (LAS = yeah) yeah you know so (3)

LAS: So when the police came, they took you to (names local psychiatric institution) did they?

Caroline: No they got an ambulance as well (LAS = right) because the ambulance were called and because of the situation I was in and doing they have to have police escorts

LAS: Oh right . . . was that because they considered you dangerous at that time?

Caroline: Yes, yeah, yeah (sighs) . . .

LAS: And did you consider yourself dangerous at the time?

Caroline: I didn't give a shit at the time, I didn't give a shit (LAS = mmm) anyone got in my way then they would have got it (LAS = yeah) (clenches one fist) you know anyone but you know"

In this excerpt, Caroline frames her performance of drinking alcohol, taking an overdose of tablets and self-harming as manifesting in a confrontation with her neighbours within her garden. Rather than playing out her sequence of actions within her home 'behind closed doors', in a space away from prying eyes, Caroline opted to perform this elaboration of behaviours with an audience comprising of her immediate neighbours. What is interesting here is the spatial use of the garden where the visibility of her behaviour becomes more public (Brickell, 2012). Caroline is using the garden space to play out her heightened levels of distress – her garden is where her experience is spatially distributed (Tucker & Smith, 2014).

This is no spontaneous act as Caroline describes how she previously went into town to buy wine and tablets. Interestingly, she does allude to cutting herself at this point but does not mention the acquisition of a knife. On reading this further, the knife is not explicitly linked to her cutting behaviours but rather, the knife is central to the ways in which she expresses her distress by threatening somebody who was talking to her. She accentuates this threat of violence by clenching her fist. By setting the scene using these items act as a catalyst of an unfolding event, Caroline is marking out how her distress manifested at that time (Urry, 2005). Due to the circumstances of cutting and threatening another person, Caroline offers factual information of the legal and necessary involvement of others in the event (the police and ambulance services). Thereby, Caroline frames this intense period of crisis with a selection of objects (particularly the knife), her aggressive behaviours and the visibility of the garden to her neighbours are pivotal in how she expresses her experience but this is grounded within a psychiatric domain with a police escort for her being necessary to curtail her behaviours. Caroline is more than aware of the consequences. Here the cartographical markers within the garden space (both human and non-human) serve to stabilise her account of what undoubtedly would have been a volatile and erratic series of events (Wise, 2000).

Jackie is a 52-year-old service user who has a psychiatric diagnosis of bipolar affective disorder. She describes herself as a 'recovering' alcoholic and drug addict. Her addiction to substances began when she was a teenager where she was able to gain access by stealing prescribed medication such as Mandrax and amphetamines from her father who was a general practitioner. After finishing school, Jackie was employed as a catering assistant for a variety of touring rock musicians (e.g. Whitesnake, David Bowie).[2] This employment gave her the opportunity to indulge her alcohol and drug addiction further without any cost to herself as she readily admits that 'lines of cocaine', for instance, were freely available at any time of the day. She subsequently gave birth to a daughter who was granted full custody with her father due to Jackie's addictions and periods spent within psychiatric institutions. This maternal severing seemed to have the greatest impact on Jackie's psychological and physical well-being as she now is a regular attendee at Alcoholics Anonymous and attends a Christian church (although she is an atheist) to go some way to prove to her daughter that she is now a reformed and respectable person.

In the following excerpt, Jackie describes the ways in which her home space reflected her emotional and physical experiences at the time:

> I've got this picture of where I come from and I ended up hiding away for three years after I was sectioned, three years I lived on my settee just in darkness drinking and drinking and drinking and I'd go out to the shop at 5.30 in the morning, get my drink, come back and lie on the sofa all day and I would detach myself from reality (LAS = mmm) and my flat just became (5) (sighs) I can't tell you how degrading the state I got into . . . I had two sack fulls, bin bags black sack fulls of unopened post (LAS = mmm) (2) can you imagine the state I got into um (LAS = mmm) I hadn't been in the bedroom cos that was the last room my daughter went into and I just used to live in the lounge and I don't think I even washed my hair and I lost all my teeth (1) so I've got dentures now (3) . . . Sometimes I had the telly on um (2) I didn't really watch television though (4) I'd um run out of electric because I drank the money (LAS = yeah) . . . I smoked as well and my money went on cheap cider and um (4) fags and that was it and a can of cold baked beans now and again. Oh I didn't even go in the kitchen um (1) I didn't wash up for three years and I didn't have any knives left cos they were all in the sink (LAS = yeah) (2) the state I got in you would even believe (2) (LAS = mmm) I should have taken some photos you know (LAS = yeah) but I did get that low and I'd, I'd have sworn it was impossible for anybody to get that low to pull themselves back to the quality of life that I've got now.

In this extract, Jackie sets a psychopathological landscape when describing her home space. Here we are presented with an account that draws together the social, material and the spatialised body; "three years I lived on my settee just in darkness drinking and drinking and drinking". Spatially, the lounge is represented as the space where her experiences manifested, which is punctuated by the descriptor 'darkness' to possibly metaphorically reflect the emotional and physical desolation she felt at that time. These narratives of living in a world devoid of the cultural assumptions attached to normative constructions of home life and lack of self-hygiene is punctuated by the focus on the limited movement in her account (Blunt & Dowling, 2006; Cox, 2012). Here, the settee provides an anchor in that this particular piece of furniture is where her daily life at the time was played out – it is the space where she spent most of her day drinking and smoking. There is limited engagement with other areas of the home and Jackie maintains a concealment of her connections to the outside world by putting unopened post in a bin bag but she does leave the confines of her flat on a daily basis to purchase alcohol. What is interesting to note is how she frames this event by drawing attention to the time she emerges from her home at "5.30 in the morning". It would be reasonable to suggest that shopping at this time in morning does not fit in with 'normal' day-to-day life. Here Jackie may be highlighting that at this period of time in her life, her own social identity resided at the boundaries of what would be considered normative at this time. As a result, Jackie's spatial production of her home space is wrapped up in alcoholism together with personal and physical neglect – these narratives constitute a bleak time in Jackie's life and the home space is central to experience (Blunt & Dowling, 2006; Tucker, 2010a).

Living in supported accommodation

Jim is a 57-year-old service user who has a psychiatric diagnosis of paranoid schizophrenia. Jim lives in supported accommodation with other service users – this set up was a cul-de-sac of houses (it is worth noting that all research participants residing in supported accommodation called these 'units' as opposed to home/house) with a resident care worker. Service users have their own bedroom and share a living room – meals and liquid refreshments are provided centrally by a care worker. The following extract is by Jim, who is describing the structural and practical (in terms of social functioning) components of the supported accommodation he currently resides in:

Jim: Um three bedrooms in each little um made in a line all in a line and there was an office and respite room and um you got three bedrooms in each (LAS = mmm) one and that's about 12, 15 accommodation for 15 people suffering with mental illness . . . (LAS = oh right) . . . and I don't understand (why he lives in supported accommodation) probably because I need a bit more caring (2) I pay for me bath and I pay for me food, me rent and

I pay for me milk all me meals and what else do I pay for? (2) Water when I have a bath what else and um I think they pay for me clothes and I get it and this is what they gave me ages ago (shows jumper) (3) it's alright ain't it? . . . Um see my bedroom's small (LAS = yeah) and I couldn't get a telly or a record player or a disco in there or a big table as it's too small and I trip up all the time and my bedroom's like a cell the smallest room in (names location)

LAS: Does it feel like a cell to you?
Jim: It does . . . and lived in a cell all me life mmm

Jim provides details of the geometric framework of his accommodation by discussing the linear way in which these units are situated and for what purpose they serve. Drawing from the language embedded within mental distress (the respite room, an office), serves to anchor his narrative of the production of his spatialised surroundings as emanating from his distress (Tucker, 2010a). This crystallisation can go some way to counter his sense of uncertainty as to why he is living there by elaborating the material and practical services this space provides: "I don't understand (why he lives in supported accommodation) probably because I need a bit more caring." Here he is making the abstract characteristics of supported accommodation more concrete by providing a series of different territorialities and including the goods and services that are 'actively entwined', and therefore embodied within his own ordering of living arrangements (Rubinstein, 1989; Urry, 2005). His way of organising services and goods as pertinent characteristics from the broader (paying for the rent) to the more minutiae (paying for milk) are important elements encompassed within his sense of place. Jim's narratives here focus on the functional needs of this day-to-day life in line with local authority directives, but omitted here is any sense of this spatiality providing him with a place of sanctuary or indeed, he does not discuss any psychological attachment: "and my bedroom's like a cell". Fogel (1992) argues that this position is due in some part to practitioners underestimating the emotional needs of those within supported care by placing more emphasis on the bureaucratic components of providing definitive elements of practical care.

What we are presented with here is a catalogue of transactions that take place within the confined space of this accommodation. These are fairly significant as they are linked to his own embodied assumptions of what is appropriate for service users in supported housing to require: "and I get it and this is what they gave me ages ago (shows jumper) (3) it's alright ain't it". For Jim, this is what being bound within psychiatric services entails – no choice and no responsibility. Jim does not have the social functioning skills to even buy a pint of milk or an item of clothing.

In the following excerpt, Daisy discusses her home space, which she shares with another service user within a supported accommodation setting and describes the spatial production of her shared home space. Daisy is a 50-year-old service user with a diagnosis of Bi-Polar Affective Disorder. She used to live in an annex with Jim who was discussed earlier but has since moved to another section within the same collection of units.

LAS: So what is your favourite bit of the house where you live, your sort of favourite room?
Daisy: Um (1) I would say the living room (2) . . . um I've got pictures of Manchester United up and uh em I've got like my little pot dog on top of the telly (2) you know sort of homely things (LAS = yeah)
LAS: And do they mean something to you?
Daisy: Yes because I love dogs um and I've got a pot dog and I love Manchester United so I've got things I love around me
LAS: Do you have any photographs of family or friends?
Daisy: I don't cos it'd probably upset me too much so I don't um (LAS = yeah)

In this extract, Daisy sketches out some objects that she has acquired and has placed around the shared living room. Within this particular space she has a vested interest and staked out certain pockets within this space displaying her own desires. What is interesting is the way in which she talks about an emotional attachment she feels to objects not usually associated with home-making and strong expressions of love: "I love dogs um and I've got a pot dog and I love Manchester United so I've got things I love around me". Within the dominant cultural assumptions of adorning home spaces and indeed, in much research, objects such as pictures of a football team and a singular dog made of pottery, perched on top of the television are not generally equated with meaningful emotional and economical investments within home spaces. For example, focal points such as the top of a television are normally reserved for personal memorabilia such as photographs or family objects (Hurdley, 2007).

This is not the case for Daisy who does not place any photographs of family or friends in the space at all:

LAS: Do you have any photographs of family or friends?
Daisy: I don't cos it'd probably upset me too much so I don't um.

Daisy's explains her disengagement with placing photographic artefacts of family and friends as too upsetting to have around this particular room. Here we have some kind of trade off in creating Daisy's landscape, the items she loves that cannot possibly love her back, the football team who are most probably unaware of her existence and the pot dog she possibly purchased from the local discount shop. It is the negation of displaying cultural objects such as photographs that can create a topographical site from which the outside and interior world can map different times within one's life course that is interesting. Photographs can tell a story, and Daisy does not want to tell hers in this space.

In this way, her human and non-human (objects) relationships within the living room can be seen as a creative arena to display the transactions of consumption and exchange. Such processes can both form personal connections and conversely, blur other areas of experience (Smith, 2004). Daisy's sense of disenfranchisement, whether economical (Daisy is on benefits so would be unable to afford to purchase an abundance of objects) and more pertinently, the emotional (the hurt she expresses when discussing her family and friends) are creatively masked and visually eradicated, albeit temporarily, by drawing on objects she has access to that do not require such intense levels of engagement (Parkin, 1999).

I would like to continue with Daisy's narratives of living within shared accommodation because she has interesting ways of creating and producing space. In the following excerpt, Daisy discusses her bedroom, her private space within the supported accommodation she lives in:

> I'm quite an eclectic [sic] collect things you know that are mine and posters of dogs and um I've got an awful lot of um (2) um a lot of sort of personal things all in bags which are full of stuff and it needs clearing out to be honest but the more the better to more because they're all memories and I feel like (1) I've got you know more well too many things it's strange you know possessional [sic] things . . . Well (names member of staff) came in once and um she said Good God (laughs) you know and she complained about it and I said I'd actually tidied it up but I hadn't done and I only got rid of one bag or something but luckily she's um eh she's not said since you know which is a miracle.

Here Daisy talks about the ways in which she collects objects that belong to her "that are mine . . . a lot of sort of personal things". These items that she highlights belong to her and are personal (there is a social interaction here) may be a way of Daisy creating meaningful ownership within a shared space. These are her things, they only belong to her and by the very way she conceals these objects in bags: "all in bags which are full of stuff". There is a suggestion here that this is how Daisy intends her relationship with these objects to remain. She does not want her possessions open to the 'gaze' of others – they are not artefacts for general display to provide a visual mapping of her memorial experiences. These objects are important to her "because they're all memories", but only to Daisy. In this way, by concealing her collection of objects in bags, Daisy is both bulking out and controlling her 'private' bedroom space. Daisy may be packing out her space to make her feel safer and more secure as she discusses that the more bags she has in her bedroom the better, this is how she may have created her own 'haven of private' space.

By continuously filling her space with her own desires there is an acknowledgement that her packing out of space needs some rectification; "it needs clearing out to be honest but the more the better". Daisy is aware that she has too many things and her production of space may be visually messy and untidy and may alert the 'gaze' of unwanted eyes. She punctuates this point by drawing attention to her socially unusual behaviour by reverting back to the dominant codings when spatialising objects in home spaces: "I've got you know more well too many things it's strange you know possessional [sic] things". Daisy acknowledges here that how she hoards and packs many objects in one space is "strange". Her creativity here does not conform to the wider notions of mapping out home space whereby her

Spaces of 'sanctuary' **175**

practices and arrangements of decorations do align to the aspirational endeavours within television programmes such as *Escape to the Country* (Clarke, 2001).

This unconventional behaviour does not go unnoticed; "Well, (names member of staff) came in once and um she said good God (laughs) you know and she complained about it". This is where Daisy struggles to anchor her bedroom space. For Daisy, this 'private' space is not so private after all. Her interactions, both human and non-human, are continuously under potential scrutiny by more dominant others in her day-to-day life. Nevertheless, Daisy goes some way in temporally stabilising her sense of space by pretending to tidy her space: "I said I'd actually tidied it up but I hadn't done and I only got rid of one bag or something but luckily she's um eh she's not said since you know which is a miracle". There is no suggestion of stability here though – Daisy's 'private' space is always fleeting, it is always awaiting a destabilised act as dictated by others to curb her own creative use of producing space.

Discussion

In this chapter I have sought to explore the divergent ways in which mental health service users produce the spaces of home. What was of particular interest to explore further was the ways in which the social performance of behaviours was articulated within the garden and the home (Blunt & Dowling, 2006; Brickell, 2012). Rather than positioning these areas as a series of spaces merely consisting of square footage, a lawn and the structural separation of rooms, attention was given to how psychological phenomena and the organisation of space can become socially visible as joint and interactional entities (Smith, 2012; Tucker, 2010b; Tucker & Smith, 2014). Drawing from the data analysis, we were presented with a divergence of ways in which service users can either produce space or can be impeded by their own sense of lacking a spatial identity within independent and supported home spaces.

Here we are given familiar, everyday spatial backdrops from which to untangle unusual events relating to distress – we are able to make some sense of accounts we may not have or indeed, ever will experience. In this way, space can be shaped and experienced by using recognisable cartographical markers or objects, which in turn may create expressions of a fairly stable spatial territory from which to explore fluid identities further (Thrift, 2003; Wise, 2000). For example, Caroline's way of exerting a sense of temporal agentic power of controlling her own garden space as she drinks the wine, ingests the tablets, cuts herself and threatens others with no authoritative, outside control for a short period of time. The garden has become her stage and Caroline has the starring role, however, it does not last long before other actors become part of the performance. In this account, we have a concoction of the wine, tablets, the knife, aggression, the immediate neighbours, the authorities, the garden and Caroline all playing a part within an actualised performance of a psychiatric episode where Caroline ends up being 'sectioned' and taken to a psychiatric institution. This is an extraordinary event, taking place in an everyday space.

Likewise, Jackie maps out her independent home space as one imbued with mental distress and emotional negativity (Tucker & Smith, 2014). Nonetheless, Jackie does not simply bracket off these experiences but instead she illuminates on the events and draws the reader in to the potentiality of Jackie, 'becoming a respectable person'. She does this by contrasting her feelings of climbing out of the depths of depravation to the higher quality of life she has now. This is not simply a forward going linear trajectory – it is constituted by a series of contractions and expansions – of back and forth (Thrift, 2004). In this account, Jackie frames the process of transforming her home space from the immoral deprivation it was in her adverse past to a future, culturally ordered potential life imbued with positivity and morality.

In terms of living within supported accommodation, Jim discusses his only private space, namely, his bedroom. Jim is unable to stake out his space using objects as cartographical markers to create a space that has content and meaning for him. Jim's narratives can impart feelings of being inextricably and irrevocably entwined within psychiatric confinement as he has become an indelible part of the wider societal assumptions of extreme mental distress. Conversely, Daisy has to some extent created compartments of personalised space within a shared living room area but, as alluded to above, her creations do not fall within the cultural and social assumptions of cultivating a space imbued with past experience (Dovey, 1985). With regard to her 'private' bedroom space, Daisy's spatialised production is based on historical events (being asked to clear her mess), the near past (tidying up one bag only) and the future (the potential that she will be asked to clear out again). In this way, Daisy's bedroom is bound up within a mesh of "temporal qualities . . . which involve change and stability, recurrence and rhythm" (Altman, Werner, & Oxley, 1985, p. 6).

Conclusion

The spaces of home were crucial milieus for all service users, from which expression and identity emerged, which were largely enveloped (although not always contained) within psychiatric dialogues. Therefore, rather than these events being subject to open, public scrutiny by occurring in community spaces they were spatially distributed and expressed in semi-private (for Caroline, Jim and Daisy) landscapes (Parr, 1997). In addition, the culturally preferable features of creating the moral home of decorative order, cleanliness and socially acceptable behaviours, based on the notions of one needing to have attributes relating to positive mental health to enable this, were not seen as pivotal in terms of connecting exterior social interactions with others (Cwerner & Metcalfe, 2003). Negotiating strategies to produce home spaces were in a state of constant flux and unrest based on their individual situations. To summarise, at that time, these spatially distributed accounts give a sense that experiences, in terms of physical movement and psychological states, were inextricably linked to the psychiatric identities for all service users whether they lived independently or in supported accommodation.

Notes

1 When discussing spaces of the home this will normally refer to the home and garden spaces as interlinked spaces.
2 These were some of the names of musicians Jackie discussed in her interview.

References

Altman, I., Werner, C., & Oxley, D. (1985). Temporal aspects of homes: A transactional perspective. In I. Altman & C. Werner (Eds.), *Home environments* (vol. 8). New York, NY: Springer.
Bijl, R. V., & Ravelli, A. (2000). Current and residual functional disability associated with psychopathology: Findings from the Netherlands Mental Health Survey and Incidence Study (NEMESIS). *Psychological Medicine*, *30*, 657–668.
Black, D., & Gowers, S. D. (2005). A brief history of child and adolescent psychiatry. In S. D. Gowers (Ed.), *Seminars in child and adolescent psychiatry* (2nd ed.). London: Royal College of Psychiatrists.
Blunt, A. (2005). Cultural geography: Cultural geographies of home. *Progress in Human Geography*, *29*(4), 505–515.
Blunt, A., & Dowling, R. (2006). *Home*. London: Routledge.
Blunt, A., & Varley, A. (2004). Geographies of home: Introduction. *Cultural Geographies*, 11, 3–6.
Braun, V., & Clarke, V. (2006). Using thematic analysis in psychology. *Qualitative Research in Psychology*, *3*(2), 77–101.
Brickell, K. (2012). 'Mapping' and 'doing' critical geographies of home. *Progress in Human Geography*, *36*(2), 225–244.
Brown, S. D. (2001). Psychology and the art of living. *Theory & Psychology*, *11*(2), 171–192.
Brown, S. D., & Tucker, I. M. (2010). Eff the ineffable: Affect, somatic management and mental health service users. In G. Seigworth & M. Gregg (Eds.), *The affect reader*. Durham, NC: Duke University Press.
Cieraad, I. (1999). Introduction: Anthropology at home. In I. Cieraad (Ed.), *At home: An anthropology of domestic space*. New York, NY: Syracuse University Press.
Clarke, A. (2001). The aesthetics of social aspiration. In D. Miller (Ed.), *Home possessions: Material culture behind closed doors*. Oxford: Berg.
Cloutier-Fisher, D., & Harvey, J. (2009). Home beyond the house: Experiences of place in an evolving retirement community. *Journal of Environmental Psychololgy*, *29*, 246–255
Cox, R. (2012). Home: Domestic dirt and cleaning. In B. Campkin & R. Cox (Eds.), *Dirt: New geographies of cleanliness and contamination*. London: I. B. Tauris & Co.
Curtis, S. (2010). *Space, place and mental health*. Farnham: Ashgate
Cwerner, S. B., & Metcalfe, A. (2003). Storage and clutter: Discourses and practices of order in the domestic world. *Journal of Design History*, *16*(3), 229–239.
Davidson, J. (2003). *Phobic geographies: The phenomenology and spatiality of identity*. Farnham, UK: Ashgate.
Dovey, K. (1985). Home homelessness. In I. Altman & C. Werner (Eds.), *Home environments* (vol. 8). New York, NY: Springer.
Doyle, K. O. (1992). The symbolic meaning of house and home. *American Behavioural Scientist*, *35*(6), 790–802.
Fogel, B. S. (1992). Psychological aspects of staying at home. *Generations*, *16*(2), 15–19.
Graves-Brown, P. (2000). Introduction. In P. Graves-Brown (Ed.), *Matter, materiality and modern culture*. London: Routledge.

Hurdley, R. (2006). Dismantling mantelpieces: Narrating identities and materializing culture in the home. *Sociology*, *40*(4), 717–733.
Hurdley, R. (2007). Focal points: Framing material culture and visual data. *Qualitative Research*, *7*(3), 355–374.
Imrie, R., & Edwards, C. (2007). The geographies of disability: Reflections on the development of a sub-discipline. *Geography Compass*, *1*(3), 623–640.
Knappett, C. (2002). Photographs, skeuomorphs and marionettes. *Journal of Material Culture*, *7*(1), 97–117.
Lefebvre, H. (1999). *The production of space* (D. Nicholson-Smith, Trans.). Oxford: Wiley-Blackwell.
Low, S. M., & Lawrence-Zuniga, D. (2003). Locating culture. In S. M. Low & D. Lawrence-Zuniga (Eds.), *The anthropology of space and place: Locating culture*. Oxford: Blackwell.
McGrath, L., & Reavey, P. (2015). Seeking fluid possibility and solid ground: Space and movement in mental health service users' experiences of 'crisis'. *Social Science & Medicine*, *128*, 115–125
Massey, D. (2004). Space-time, 'science' and the relationship between physical geography and human geography. *Transactions of the Institute of British Geographers*, *24*(3), 261–276.
Miller, D. D. (2001). Behind closed doors. In D. Miller (Ed.), *Home possessions: Material culture behind closed doors*. Oxford: Berg.
Miller, D. D. (2004). Atypical antipsychotics: Sleep, sedation and efficacy. *Primary Care Companion to the Journal of Clinical Psychiatry*, *6*(2), 3–7.
Milligan, C., Gatrell, A., & Bingley, A. (2004). 'Cultivating health': Therapeutic landscapes and older people in Northern England. *Social Science & Medicine*, *58*, 1781–1793.
Mind. (2015). *Making sense of ecotherapy*. Retrieved from www.mind.org.uk/information-support/drugs-and-treatments/ecotherapy/#.V6hCJ7grLIU.
Parkin, D. (1999). Mementoes as transitional objects in human displacement. *Journal of Material Culture*, *4*(3), 303–320.
Parr, H. (1997). Mental health, public space and the city: Questions of individual and collective access. *Environment and Planning*, *15*, 435–454.
Parr, H. (1999). Bodies and psychiatric medicine: Interpreting different geographies of mental health. In R. Butler & H. Parr (Eds.), *Mind and body spaces*. London: Routledge.
Parr, H. (2007). Mental health, nature work, and social inclusion. *Environment and Planning D: Society and Space*, *25*, 537–561.
Pinfold, V. (2000). 'Building up safe havens . . . all around the world': Users' experiences of living in the community with mental health problems. *Health & Place*, *6*(3), 201–212.
Putnam, T. (1999). 'Postmodern' home life. In I. Cieraad (Ed.), *At home: An anthropology of domestic space*. New York, NY: Syracuse University Press.
Reynolds, R., Thornicroft, G., Abas, M., Woods, R., Hoe, R., & Leese, M. (2000). Camberwell assessment of needs for the elderly (CANE): Development, validity and reliability. *British Journal of Psychiatry*, *176*, 444–452.
Rubinstein, R. L. (1989). The home environments of older people: A description of the psychosocial processes linking person to place. *Journal of Gerontology*, *44*(2), 545–553.
Slade, M., Phelan, M., Thornicroft, G., & Parkman, S. (1996). The Camberwell assessment of need (CAN): Comparison of assessments by staff and patients of the severely mentally ill. *Social Psychiatry and Psychiatric Epidemiology*, *31*(3–4), 109–113.
Smith, L. A. (2012). *'Mad, bad and dangerous to know': Exploring the everyday spaces of older, mental health service users* (Unpublished thesis). University of Northampton, UK.
Smith, S. J. (2004). Living room? *Urban Geography*, *25*(2), 89–91.
Somerville, P. (1997). The social construction of home. *Journal of Architectural and Planning Research*, *14*(3), 227–245.

Thrift, N. (2003). Space: The fundamental stuff of human geography. In N. J. Clifford, S. L. Holloway, S. P. Rice, & G. Valentine (Eds.), *Key concepts in geography*. London: Sage.

Thrift, N. (2004). Movement-space: The changing domain of thinking resulting from the development of new kinds of spatial awareness. *Economy and Society*, *33*(4), 582–604.

Tucker, I. (2006). Deterritorialising mental health: Unfolding service user experience (Unpublished thesis). Loughborough University, UK.

Tucker, I. (2010a). Space, process philosophy and mental distress. *International Journal of Interdisciplinary Social Sciences*, *4*, 1833–1882.

Tucker, I. (2010b). The potentiality of bodies. *Theory & Psychology*, *20*(4), 511–527.

Tucker, I., & Smith, L. A. (2014). Topology and mental distress: Self-care in the life spaces of home. *Journal of Health Psychology*, *19*(1), 176–183.

Urry, J. (2005). The place of emotions within place. In J. Davidson, L. Bondi, & M. Smith (Eds.), *Emotional geographies*. Farnham, UK: Ashgate.

Williams, A. (2002). Changing geographies of care: Employing the concept of therapeutic landscapes as a framework in examining home space. *Social Science and Medicine*, *55*, 141–154.

Wise, M. J. (2000). Home: territory and identity. *Cultural Studies*, *14*(2), 295–310.

11
SPATIAL AND SOCIAL FACTORS ASSOCIATED WITH COMMUNITY INTEGRATION OF INDIVIDUALS WITH PSYCHIATRIC DISABILITIES RESIDING IN SUPPORTED AND NON-SUPPORTED HOUSING

Greg Townley

Introduction

Community integration refers to the notion that individuals with disabilities should have opportunities to live, work, engage with others, and enjoy recreational activities in the same manner as peers without disabilities (Wong & Solomon, 2002). In the twenty-first century, the ideal of individuals with disabilities enjoying equal opportunities to live and participate in their communities remains an unrealized goal. To address this issue, community integration research has emerged as a high priority among researchers studying the experiences of individuals with psychiatric disabilities living and engaging in community spaces. For example, Yanos (2007) instructs that "first and foremost, it is important that community integration be placed on the agenda of researchers who study the effects of place on people with mental illness" (p. 673), and Davidson (2005, p. 243) suggests that "the relatively uncharted territory of how people with severe and persistent mental illness navigate their immediate social environments becomes both a timely and important focus for empirical study."

Factors influencing integration in community space

Research literature generally reports three primary determinants of community integration. First, individual characteristics have been identified as potential predictors. There is some evidence that psychiatric symptomatology may make it difficult for individuals to work and participate in community activities (Badger, McNiece, Bonham, Jacobson, & Gelenberg, 2003). Other research suggests that symptom distress may actually facilitate individuals' ability to obtain social support from others, thus potentially increasing levels of inclusion (Gulcur, Tsemberis, Stefancic, & Greenwood, 2007). There is also evidence that individuals with higher psychosocial functioning report greater participation in activities (Felce, Lowe, & Jones, 2002; Kruzich, 1985; Prince & Prince, 2002) and more community connections (Wieland, Rosenstock, Kelsey, Ganguli, & Wisniewski, 2007).

A second primary category of community integration determinants, and one that is particularly relevant to an examination of the role of space in understanding mental health distress, concerns the influence of housing and neighborhood environments. In a study of 425 individuals with psychiatric disabilities living in supported housing, Townley and Kloos (2011) found that positive neighbor relationships, perceptions of safety, and neighborhood satisfaction predicted community integration. Similarly, Silverman and Segal (1994) found that individuals' satisfaction with their dwellings and neighborhoods, as well as their length of residence, were related to their perceptions of "fitting-in." There is also evidence that individuals in scatter-site apartments have more diverse social relationships than individuals living in congregate housing (i.e., housing in which all residents have a psychiatric disability) (Gulcur et al., 2007), while individuals in congregate housing experience higher levels of belonging (Townley, Kloos, Green, & Franco, 2011).

Community attitudes about mental illness are a final commonly reported category of factors associated with community integration. Numerous studies have found that increased acceptance by neighbors and lower levels of societal rejection are associated with increased community integration (e.g., Townley & Kloos, 2011; Sherman, Frenkel, & Newman, 1986). Prince and Prince (2002) examined the relationship between perceived stigma and community integration among 95 clients of assertive community treatment (ACT) teams and found that clients' perceptions of stigmatization were inversely related to their perceptions of community inclusion. Finally, in a qualitative study of 80 individuals with psychiatric disabilities, one-third of participants reported difficulties fitting in to their neighborhoods due to low tolerance for "different" types of behaviors (Yanos, Barrow, & Tsemberis, 2004).

Housing models for individuals with psychiatric disabilities

Given the history of institutionalization and the traditional model of taking individuals out of communities for care in hospital or residential treatment settings, a common focus of research examining the relationship between space and distress has been on the housing situations of individuals with psychiatric disabilities. This is particularly true among community psychologists in the United States, who have been instrumental in developing and evaluating a variety of housing approaches since deinstitutionalization in the 1960s. These models can be divided into two broad categories: *housing without rehabilitation* and *housing with rehabilitation* (Nelson, Aubry, & Hutchison, 2011).

Housing without rehabilitation

The vast majority of individuals who experience mental health challenges continue to live in housing in which no rehabilitative services are available (Newman &

Goldman, 2009). Two types of housing options that fit into this category are living with family members and utilizing the rental housing market (Nelson et al., 2011). Tsai, Stroup, and Rosenheck (2011) analyzed data regarding the living arrangements of 1,446 clients with schizophrenia and found that 46 percent of clients lived with family members. While families are often good intentioned and can provide emotional and material support, the lack of formal rehabilitative support can negatively impact both the caregivers and the family member experiencing mental health challenges (Chen, 2010; Solomon & Draine, 1995).

Little is known about the number of individuals with psychiatric disabilities who live independently in market-rate housing, but what is known is that affordability is the foremost determinant of their housing options (Newman & Goldman, 2009). Poverty is high among individuals with psychiatric disabilities. This often results in individuals living in substandard housing in disadvantaged neighborhoods that may jeopardize health and put them at increased risk of being victimized (Hiday, Swartz, Swanson, Borum, & Wagner, 1997)

Housing with rehabilitation

In the early 1970s, mental health systems began to develop housing focused on rehabilitation (Sylvestre, Nelson, Sabloff, & Peddle, 2007). Group homes, halfway houses, and supervised apartments were among the earliest settings used to house individuals with psychiatric disabilities (Leff et al., 2009). They were typically segregated from the community, professionally staffed, and congregate in nature. The programs were often based on a residential continuum theory in which clients follow a continuum of most-restrictive to least-restrictive settings as they reintegrate into the community (Ridgeway & Zipple, 1990).

In response to the criticisms of the residential continuum model, Priscilla Ridgeway, Paul Carling, and their colleagues called for the development of *supported housing*, marked by principles of choice, rent supports, holding a lease to community-based housing, and availability of flexible, individualized services (Carling, 1993; Ridgeway & Zipple, 1990). A major distinguishing feature of supported housing is an emphasis on community integration, in which clients have opportunities to become citizens who are engaged in all facets of community life.

The current study

There has been significant theoretical and empirical work conducted regarding factors that encourage and inhibit integration of individuals with psychiatric disabilities in community space. However, the vast majority of research been conducted among individuals living in supported housing, which is surprising given that the majority of individuals with psychiatric disabilities reside in housing without any services attached to it (Newman & Goldman, 2009). In addition to examining spatial and social features of housing environments for individuals with psychiatric disabilities, the current study intends to fill a gap in the literature by comparing facilitators and barriers to community integration between individuals residing in supported and non-supported housing (i.e., housing that is not attached to rehabilitative services). It is expected that findings will call attention to the role of physical and social space in understanding the community experiences of individuals with psychiatric disabilities and inform interventions aimed at promoting community integration.

Study context and procedures

This study reports findings from the *Networks of Community Support* (NoCS) study, a mixed-methods project funded by the Fahs-Beck Fund for Research and Experimentation (established with the New York Community Trust) aimed at examining differences in community living and community integration between individuals with psychiatric disabilities residing in supported and non-supported housing. For the study, a total of 100 individuals with psychiatric disabilities living in the southeastern United States (50 in supported housing and 50 in non-supported housing) completed a survey about their housing, neighborhood, and community environments. In addition to survey data, secondary data analyses utilizing Geographic Information Systems (GIS) were conducted to provide a broader understanding of the impact of physical and social spaces on participants' experiences. Finally, a subset of participants were invited to take part in a qualitative interview to further contextualize their community integration experiences and ensure that the perspectives of individuals with lived experience were adequately represented. The geospatial and qualitative components of this work will be the focus of the remainder of the chapter.

Sample description

Participants in the supported housing group were recruited from MIRCI (Mental Illness Recovery Center), a nonprofit mental health service organization in Columbia, South Carolina, USA. Services attached to housing include transportation, counseling, medication management, and rental assistance. The non-supported housing sample was comprised of individuals with psychiatric disabilities who live independently in housing with no support services and participate in services at a community mental health center affiliated with the South Carolina Department of Mental Health. On average, participants were 47 years of age. Some 52 percent of participants identified as female, 48 percent were Black, and 52 percent were White. At the time of the study, 68 percent of participants had graduated from high school, 4 percent were married, and 20 percent were working. Finally, 47 percent of participants reported a schizophrenia-spectrum diagnosis, while 53 percent reported depression or bipolar disorder.

Geospatial analyses

Geographic Information Systems (GIS) analyses provided one method of examining aspects of the spaces in which individuals with psychiatric disabilities reside that may impact their community integration. Participants were asked to provide their current addresses, which were then geocoded (i.e., converted to longitude and latitude coordinates) and plotted using ESRI ArcMap 10. This allowed for linkages of participant addresses to datasets of community indicators obtained through Dun & Bradstreet and the 2010 U.S. Census American Factfinder database. Two variables were computed using GIS analyses: (1) proximity to stores and services, and (2) the Community Integration Census Index (CICI). In order to protect the confidentiality of the study participants, addresses in the maps presented below were edited by adding random numbers ranging from 0 to 1,000 feet to their latitude and longitude coordinates. Thus, reverse geocoding could no longer be used to identify the participant but the overall pattern of addresses remained visually similar (Brusilovskiy & Salzer, 2012).

Proximity to stores and services

Living in close proximity to stores and services provides greater opportunities for activity involvement and engagement with community members. For this study, this variable was calculated by first obtaining coordinates of stores and services in Richland County, South Carolina from Dun & Bradstreet, which provides the location and sales information of U.S. and Canadian public and private businesses. Store and service coordinates were plotted in ArcMap along with participant addresses, and half-mile proximity buffers were created around each participant's home. These buffers were then joined to the store layers to obtain a count of the total number of stores and services within half a mile of each participant's home. Maps were generated to illustrate proximity of housing to stores and services (see Figure 11.1). The number of stores and services within a half mile of participants' residences ranged from 0 to 63, ($M = 10.70$, $SD = 9.28$). There were significantly more stores and services within a half mile of supported housing residences compared to non-supported housing ($M = 12.36$, $SD = 7.88$ and $M = 8.28$, $SD = 10.25$, respectively), $t(98) = -2.23$, $p < .05$). As was expected, proximity to stores and services was found to be significantly related to participants' involvement in activities ($r = .25$, $p < .05$) and their sense of community belonging ($r = .22$, $p < .05$).

Community integration census index

Variables obtained from the U.S. Census conducted every ten years can provide important information about the demographic and socioeconomic composition of the spaces in which individuals with psychiatric disabilities live. For this study, an index was created that combines seven census variables theoretically expected

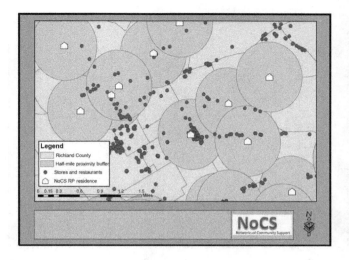

FIGURE 11.1 Proximity of NoCS participants to stores and services.

to promote community integration. The seven census variables selected for inclusion in this index (each measured at the block group level) were as follows: (1) *median household income* (with middle-range median household income expected to be more promotive of integration than lower-income or high-income blocks); (2) *median age* (with higher concentration of middle-aged individuals expected to be more conducive to integration); (3) *percent occupied housing*; (4) *percent owner-occupied housing* (with higher percentages of both occupancy variables expected to promote integration); (5) *percent single-person households* (with lower percentage of single-person households expected to promote greater integration); (6) *average household size* (with larger household size expected to be related to integration); and (7) *census block racial diversity* (with more diverse blocks hypothesized to be more conducive to integration). A quartile split was conducted on each variable whereby participants received a score of 1 to 4 depending on where their score on the particular census variable fell in the quartile split. For instance, scores ranging from 0 to .26 on the racial diversity index received a 1; scores ranging from .27 to .45 received a 2; scores ranging from .46 to .53 received a 3; and scores ranging from .54 to .66 received a 4. The individual variable scores (each ranging from 1 to 4) were then summed to create an overall composite index of community integration, referred to as the *Community Integration Census Index (CICI)*.

CICI Scores ranged from 10 to 25, ($M = 17.85$, $SD = 2.94$) (see Figure 11.2). CICI scores were higher among residents of supported housing than non-supported housing ($M = 18.56$, $SD = 2.56$ and $M = 16.84$, $SD = 3.88$, respectively, t (98 = -2.61, $p < .01$. That is, participants in supported housing were significantly more likely to live in neighborhoods whose social composition may be more conducive to community integration experiences than participants in

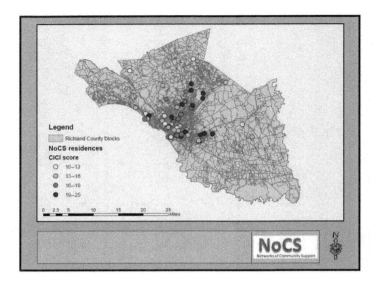

FIGURE 11.2 Participant residences with Community Integration Census Index (CICI) scores.

non-supported housing. Participants in neighborhoods with higher CICI scores also reported increased levels of belonging to their communities ($r = .33$, $p < .001$).

Qualitative analysis

As discussed previously, 30 individuals (15 from each housing type) were selected from the broader study to participate in a qualitative interview aimed at examining barriers and facilitators of community integration. After asking participants questions about their daily activities and neighborhoods, the author asked semi-structured questions focusing on barriers to and facilitators of activity participation and engagement in the community. In a few cases, and with consent, photographs of participants were taken to highlight their housing and community experiences. Modified grounded theory was used to analyze data. That is, theory informed but did not constrain the coding process. Participants are identified by housing type (SH for supported housing, NSH for non-supported housing), race, and gender (WF for white females, BF for black females, WM for white males, and BM for black males). For example, "SHWF" would be used to identify a white female participant residing in supported housing.

What are potential facilitators of community integration?

Participants discussed numerous factors that facilitate their involvement in community life. These factors are summarized in Table 11.1 and discussed in detail below.

TABLE 11.1 Facilitators of community integration identified by participants

Facilitator	Supported housing (n = 15)	Non-supported housing (n = 15)
Social support	12 (80%)	10 (67%)
Housing/neighborhood	11 (73%)	8 (53%)
Transportation	6 (40%)	7 (47%)
Mental health services	6 (30%)	5 (33%)
Finances	2 (13%)	4 (27%)

Social support

Social resources were the most frequently reported facilitators of community integration (n = 22, 73 percent). This support was described as being emotional (e.g., receiving encouragement from staff or friends to start new activities); informational (e.g., receiving suggestions from others about community engagement opportunities); and material (e.g., individuals receiving money or transportation that facilitates their involvement in activities). The latter type of support was described as particularly helpful for one participant:

> Well, my sister is very supportive. She signed for me to get my lease here because they didn't take Social Security. She always loans me money if I'm in a pinch, and she never holds it over my head. I really don't know where I'd be without her.
>
> *(NSHBF)*

Participants in supported housing were particularly vocal about the supportive role they can play for each other when performing activities of daily living, such as shopping or eating in restaurants: "We go shopping together, we eat together, we sit outdoors at night together and talk. We're a team out here" (SHBM).

The importance of social experiences was not limited to close relationships. Participants also spoke of the important role that casual conversations in community settings can have in feeling part of the broader community:

> I will socialize with people at those coffee houses. I will sit down, and I will have conversations with people. It's very important for me to be able to talk to people . . . All I got to do is walk. As long as I can walk, I can go somewhere and talk to somebody.
>
> *(NSHWM: see Figure 11.3)*

Housing/neighborhood

A large group of participants in both housing types (n = 19, 63 percent) discussed the role of their housing and neighborhood environments in their community

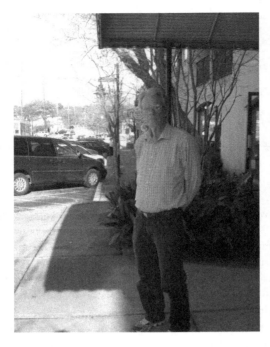

FIGURE 11.3 Gary enjoys meeting new people on his regular walks to coffee shops and stores in his neighborhood.

integration experiences. Most typically, this facilitator was described in terms of the location of housing. In line with the geospatial findings presented above, participants reported enjoying accessibility to stores, services, and transportation. A few participants also reported that the socio-demographic characteristics of their neighborhoods encourage them to participate in the local community: "It's pretty diverse racially, and I enjoy people from the university. A lot of professors and college kids live in the area. I like seeing them at Publix, Dano's, Pizza Man" (NSHWM). Six of the 11 supported housing participants who discussed housing/neighborhood environments as a facilitator of community integration also reported appreciating the availability of on-site support services from mental health staff and peers: "It's easier for us to talk to each other—your neighbors—when you have a mental illness also. It also makes me feel safer walking to the store with them than by myself" (SHWF).

Transportation

Participants who had access to transportation described it as a major facilitator of community participation (n = 13, 43 percent). Transportation access ranged from owning cars, to living close to bus lines, to utilizing transportation tied to mental

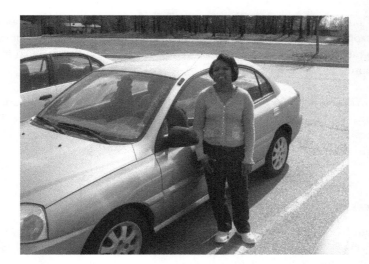

FIGURE 11.4 Pauline values her car because it provides her with the freedom and flexibility to engage in activities in her community.

health services: "I've become eligible for DART, which will take you where you want to go on the—it's for people with disabilities—a bus" (NSHWF).

> It helps me to go places where I can relieve my stress. Having a car is an advantage because you can just go in the car to go ride. Like, I do, when I get so bored and just need to get out. I get in my car and just go to the mall, or I just go to McDonald's and sit down and eat.
> *(SHBF: see Figure 11.4)*

The latter quote highlights the importance of transportation as a resource that provides participants with freedom and flexibility to access community locations in the same manner as peers who do not have a psychiatric disability.

Mental health services

Over one-third of participants of both supported and non-supported housing discussed the role of mental health services in their community integration experiences. For example, one participant said: "If I do get depressed, or I do have a day where my mental illness won't let me get outta bed, I can pick up a phone knowing there is somebody staff-wise that I can talk to" (SHWF). Although participants of non-supported housing do not have the same level of access to staff support as participants in supported housing, five participants did report receiving assistance from mental health staff. One participant relayed a poignant story about feeling unable to interact in social settings for years because he talked to himself out loud—responding to auditory hallucinations that were a symptom of his schizophrenia. His psychiatrist worked with him to find a better combination of medications that would help quiet the hallucinations; he also coached him on social norms of communication:

> I had this problem of talking out loud to myself or thinking out loud. My psychologist said it was alright to do that at home but not outside, so I have been practicing that, and it seems to be working. He also taught me to ask a question, wait for an answer, and then ask another question.
>
> *(NSHWM)*

Finances

Although it was the least-reported facilitator of community integration, several participants (n = 6, 20 percent) discussed the positive role of financial factors. Receiving supplemental security income (SSI), housing assistance vouchers, employment income, and money from family allowed participants to be able to shop, eat at restaurants, and engage in hobbies: "I've been working, so I was able to afford to enter my painting into the contest. It was 15 bucks, and as a result, it's very important to me" (NSHWF) (see Figure 11.5).

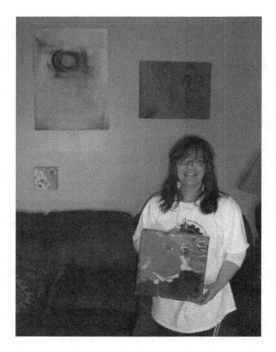

FIGURE 11.5 Cynthia poses with artwork she created and entered into a local community auction.

What are potential barriers to community integration?

Many of the factors identified as facilitators were also identified as potential barriers to engaging in community life (see Table 11.2). In addition, two new clusters of community integration factors were identified as barriers—*mental health stigma* and *health*.

Mental health stigma

Most participants (n = 24, 80 percent) discussed mental health stigma as a barrier to community integration. This barrier was more of a concern for participants in supported housing than participants in non-supported housing. This appears to be primarily due to the recognizability of supported housing and transportation as being tied to the mental health center, as well as the high number of community activities done with other service users. Ten supported housing participants spoke about the van that picks them up from their housing sites to go to activity locations in the community: "Man, it's like riding the short bus. All the people in the neighborhood ask us why we're getting on that van, and what's wrong with us, and all that" (SHBM). Participants were even more vocal about the fact that their checks clearly identify them as mental health service users, which causes fears of being recognized and treated differently in community settings:

> The thing that bothers me the most is, I get my check, and it says "Mental illness Recovery Center." There's a level of embarrassment when I go to Wal-Mart and have to pay with a check that's made out to Wal-Mart from "Mental Illness Recovery Center." And stamped on the check, it'll say, "Cash back not to exceed $5.00." That kind of makes me feel like a child or like I can't maintain my own finances.
>
> *(SHWM)*

Similarly, engaging in community activities with other service users increases the likelihood that community members will treat them differently: "Oh yeah, they see all of us coming in together and know who we are—there's those crazy people again" (SHBF).

TABLE 11.2 Barriers to community integration identified by participants

Facilitator	Supported housing (n = 15)	Non-supported housing (n = 15)
Mental health stigma	15 (100%)	9 (60%)
Health	9 (60%)	10 (66%)
Transportation	8 (53%)	7 (47%)
Mental health services	7 (47%)	6 (40%)
Finances	6 (40%)	4 (27%)
Housing/neighborhood	5 (33%)	4 (27%)

Although not as frequently discussed, nine participants in non-supported housing expressed concerns about stigma limiting their ability to be involved in community life. For example, one participant who lives in a large apartment complex made careful decisions about disclosure based on such concerns: "There's a lot of stigma here. I'm sure there is. It's stigma about mental illness—so I keep my mental illness a secret here" (NSHWF).

Health

The majority of participants reported health-related experiences as barriers to community engagement (n = 19, 63 percent). In over two-thirds of these cases, health was discussed in terms of the impact of psychiatric symptomatology on participants' ability to participate in activities and engage with community members. One participant spoke poignantly about feeling out-of-step with other parents when he goes to watch his daughter play soccer:

> I mean, you work through all the crap in life that I have worked through, and I still deal with a lot of crap inside because of a mental illness. It's just a daily fight to be functional, you know? Sometimes I'm weird and sometimes I'm not. I'd like to be more friendly and outgoing with people. But, I just sit back.
>
> *(NSHWM)*

Numerous participants reported that symptoms of mental health distress can make it difficult to be motivated to leave the house and engage with others in the community:

> The main obstacle to me doing stuff is my mental illness because when I go through a period of depression, it's all about isolation. It's locking myself in my cave, cutting off contact with friends and family, and just losing interest in all the things that interest me. I'll stare at walls all day or sleep all day, that kind of thing.
>
> *(SHWM)*

Symptoms of some types of schizophrenia, including paranoia and disorganized speech, may make it particularly difficult for individuals to interact with community members:

> I used to be more paranoid. I was scared of people—thinking they weren't thinking well of me. When I would get sick, I used to yell at people a lot—in grocery stores, the mall, restaurants. It got really bad—so bad that I would then isolate out of shame and being nervous that they would recognize me if I went back.
>
> *(NSHWF)*

Although not discussed as frequently as mental health challenges, five participants discussed the impact of physical health on community integration. Difficulties walking, being overweight, and having cardiovascular disease were all described as barriers to participating in the community.

Transportation

Just as having access to transportation was described as a facilitator of community integration, not having access was discussed by half of the participants as a barrier to participation in activities. Participants discussed not having cars, not being able to walk to bus lines, and being scared to walk or drive to activity locations. Even when participants could access bus lines, the schedule was described as not being conducive to certain types of activities:

> The issue I have is the bus line because it only runs every hour to hour and a half out here, and then it stops at 6:00. So, if you have a job that you work over, then you ain't got no way home. You gotta pay a cab, which is $40.00 or $50.00 at least.
>
> *(SHBM)*

Transportation difficulties were particularly salient for participants who had once owned vehicles and were used to the independence provided by mobility:

> I'm thankful for the MIRCI van coming to pick me up, but I'd rather be driving and be completely independent . . . When I did drive, I used to be a member of a group called Meetup.com. That was real important to me. I enjoyed doing things with them. People would spontaneously just decide on, "Hey, I want to go to a movie, and I think I'll invite whoever wants to go with me to a movie." And then 30 or 40 people would show up and go to a movie together . . . There were a lot of things that I used to do that I can't do now because I don't drive.
>
> *(SHWM: see Figure 11.6)*

Mental health services

Although participants discussed ways in which mental health services facilitated community integration, almost half of participants (n = 13) also discussed the negative impact that service providers and lack of activity programming have on their ability to engage in activities. First, participants noted that service providers seldom discuss the importance of community integration in the recovery process: "They encourage us to go to doctor's appointments on our own, but that's it. They never give us ideas of other things to do" (SHWF). In some cases, they may even discourage engaging in activities:

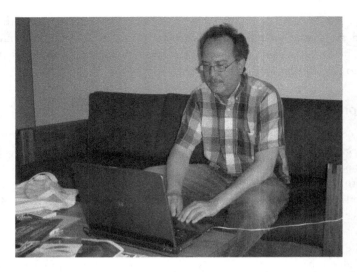

FIGURE 11.6 Roger keeps in touch with friends online, but he misses being able to drive to attend events he learns about on meetup.com.

> You know, I think they encourage them to be more isolated—or else just to interact with other people who have mental illness. My recent experiences with the mental health center has been a lot more negative than in the past—they even told me to stop doing my work with the NAMI walk.
>
> *(NSHWF)*

Second, participants in both housing types discussed the impact of mental health activity programming (or lack thereof) on their ability to fully enjoy community life. Several participants reported feeling that more could be done to help residents "combat boredom":

> People sit around here all day, all the time, and there's nothing to do. There's nowhere for us to go to conversate and be around friends and stuff. The boredom makes people get sick—their mental illness, it climbs because there's nothing to do. I know they're short on staff and money, but there has to be something they can do.
>
> *(SHBF)*

Finances

Ten participants (33 percent) discussed the negative impact that their financial difficulties have on their ability to participate in community activities. This was particularly true for participants who are not working and who do not receive a monthly SSI check: "Money right now is a huge barrier for me because I'm not getting an SSI check. I'm barely treading water" (SHBM). However, even clients who receive SSI noted the difficulties of meeting basic needs, let alone having money left over for leisure and recreational activities: "And then when you get your Social Security Income, it's like—it's not enough money to support yourself with. When you only get $550 a month, and you gotta pay bills, buy groceries, child support. There's nothing left. Nothing" (SHBM). Financial difficulties were also cited as reasons for individuals having to stop regular activities at gyms, pools, and social clubs:

> I was also involved a lot with Capital Senior Center and Shepherd Center, which are places for retired adults to go and take different classes and stuff. It draws from the professional people who were in professional fields, and they have different kinds of educational classes and stuff like that. The thing is, it got to be too expensive. The membership cost too much, and I had to stop going. I really miss it though
>
> *(NSHWF)*

Housing/neighborhood

Finally, nearly a third of participants discussed the negative impact that physical and social components of housing and neighborhood environments have on community integration. First, as has already been discussed, the location of housing plays a large role in participants' ability to access stores, services, and activity locations. Second, perceptions of safety impact whether or not participants feel comfortable talking with neighbors or walking in their neighborhoods: "It's been nothing but trouble since I've had this place. My door was broken into, my wall was smashed. I don't like walking in the neighborhood—even up to the store—because I think I'll get jumped or something" (NSHWF). Participants also discussed the role that negative relationships with neighbors can play in their perceptions of belonging to the neighborhood:

> People go around calling me crazy all the time, and I just don't like it here. I do not fit in here because I'm like totally different from other people. Usually, I don't go outside because I don't want to hear all the gossip and people talking about me.
>
> *(SHWF)*

Discussion

This study represents one of the first attempts to compare the spatial and social environments and community integration experiences of individuals with psychiatric disabilities living in supported and non-supported housing. Results suggest numerous factors that may facilitate or impede the ability of individuals with psychiatric disabilities to engage in activities, socialize with community members, and perceive a sense of belonging with the broader community. Although there are some notable differences in the spatial and social environments of individuals residing in supported and non-supported housing, qualitative results highlight more similarities in community integration experiences between the two groups than differences.

Summary of major findings

Geospatial analyses revealed that individuals in supported housing live in closer proximity to stores and services and reside in neighborhoods whose demographic and social composition may be more conducive to community inclusion (e.g., higher percentage of occupied than vacant housing, larger household size, and residents who are more racially diverse). This may reflect strategic planning and locating of housing sites on the part of the supported housing provider. It may also reflect the increased variability of neighborhood types among non-supported housing participants. For example, some individuals in non-supported housing lived in rural neighborhoods characterized as being less proximal to stores and services and having lower scores on the Community Integration Census Index (CICI). For individuals in both types of housing, spatial and social features of their housing and neighborhood environments were significantly related to important community integration experiences, including activity participation and sense of belonging.

In qualitative interviews conducted with participants, social support was the most commonly reported facilitator of community integration, with participants discussing the importance of various types of support as they engage in community activities. Other facilitators included features of the housing/neighborhood environment, transportation, and mental health services. Mental health stigma was the most frequently discussed barrier to community integration, with participants expressing fears of or actual experiences with negative treatment from community members. Physical and mental health issues were also commonly discussed as barriers to community engagement, as were transportation and finances.

Qualitative analyses suggest more similarities in community integration experiences between individuals in supported and non-supported housing than differences. Areas of discrepancy primarily related to specific components of the supported housing environment. For example, more participants of supported housing listed mental health stigma as a barrier to community integration, due primarily to the fact that transportation, housing sites, and more frequent participation in activities with other mental health service users make them more identifiable (and thus more likely to be discriminated against) by community members.

Community and clinical implications

Several of the findings synthesized above have the potential to impact mental health practice related to housing and community integration. First, it is important to uncover practical mechanisms through which service providers, community supports, and service users themselves can promote community involvement of individuals with psychiatric disabilities. Community integration should be a priority when formulating treatment plans. Individualized treatment plans can include goals for number of activities to perform on a weekly or monthly basis, number of job or housing applications to complete, timelines for enrolling in college classes, and so forth. Additionally, rehabilitative services tied to mental health settings may encourage individuals to integrate into the community through provision of skills that help individuals socialize with others, fulfill activities of daily living, and obtain education and employment.

Besides relationships tied to mental health settings, evidence from this study suggests the importance of working with individuals to bolster networks of relationships in broader community spaces. These may include friends and family, relationships tied to housing (e.g., neighbors and landlords), relationships at activity settings (e.g., co-workers, congregation members, and members of hobby groups), and even casual community relationships developed via regular contact with individuals who live and work in the community.

Findings also inform suggestions for developing and locating supported housing sites to allow maximum potential for residents to be integrated into the community. This includes designing housing so that it blends into the neighborhood; locating housing in residential areas that are within walking distance to stores and services; and providing opportunities for independent and group activities that encourage community involvement.

Given evidence that negative community attitudes may discourage community integration, interventions aimed at changing attitudes may be helpful. Mass-media campaigns that include facts about mental illness, personal narratives from service users, and information intended to dispel common stereotypes have been successful in achieving population-level change (Clement, Jarrett, Henderson, & Thornicroft, 2010). Similarly, more targeted interventions intended to educate family members, friends, and neighbors about the realities of mental illness have also been effective in reducing stigma (Rusch, Angermeyer, & Corrigan, 2005). Finally, neighborhood block parties can help individuals meet and discuss important neighborhood issues. Communication opens doors to interactions, thus reducing stigma and fear in the neighborhood and facilitating social integration.

Conclusions

It is important to understand community integration from the perspectives of individuals with lived experience of mental health challenges in order to make recommendations for interventions and service delivery. This study points to numerous types of support, including people (e.g., friends, family, and mental health staff); places (e.g., activity settings, homes, and neighborhoods); and things (e.g., transportation, finances, and hobbies) that may encourage participation in activities, utilization of diverse social networks, and perceptions of belonging in a wide variety of community spaces.

References

Badger, T. A., McNiece, C., Bonham, E., Jacobson, J., & Gelenberg, A. J. (2003). Health outcomes for people with serious mental illness: A case study. *Perspectives in Psychiatric Care, 39*(1), 23–32.

Brusilovskiy, E., & Salzer, M. S. (2012). A study of environmental influences on the well-being of individuals with psychiatric disabilities in Philadelphia, PA. *Social Science Medicine, 74*(10), 1591–1601.

Carling, P. J. (1993). Housing and supports for persons with mental illness: Emerging approaches to research and practice. *Psychiatric Services, 44*(5), 439–449.

Chen, F.-P. (2010). Assisting adults with severe mental illness in transitioning from parental homes to independent living. *Community Mental Health Journal, 46*(4), 372–280.

Clement, S., Jarrett, M., Henderson, C., & Thornicroft, G. (2010). Messages to use in population-level campaigns to reduce mental health-related stigma: Consensus development study. *Epidemiologia E Psichiatria Sociale, 19*(1), 72–79.

Davidson, L. (2005). More fundamentally human than otherwise. *Psychiatry, 63*(3), 243–249.

Felce, D., Lowe, K., & Jones, E. (2002). Association between the provision characteristics and operation of supported housing services and resident outcome. *Journal of Applied Research in Intellectual Disabilities, 15*(4), 404–418.

Gulcur, L., Tsemberis, S., Stefancic, A., & Greenwood, R. M. (2007). Community integration of adults with psychiatric disabilities and histories of homelessness. *Community Mental Health Journal, 43*(3), 211–228.

Hiday, V. A., Swartz, M. S., Swanson, J. W., Borum, R., & Wagner, H. R. (1997). Criminal victimization of persons with severe mental illness. *Psychiatric Services 50*(1), 62–68.

Kruzich, J. M. (1985). Community integration of the mentally ill in residential facilities. *American Journal of Community Psychology, 13*(5), 553–564.

Leff, H. S., Chow, C. M., Pepin, R., Conley, J., Allen, I. E., & Seaman, C. A. (2009). Does one size fit all? What we can and can't learn from a meta-analysis of housing models for persons with mental illness. *Psychiatric Services, 60*(4), 473–482.

Nelson, G., Aubry, T., & Hutchison, J. (2011). Housing and mental health. In J. H. Stone & M. Blouin (Eds.), *International encyclopedia of rehabilitation*. Retrieved from http://cirrie.buffalo.edu/encyclopedia/en/article/132/.

Newman, S., & Goldman, H. (2009). Housing policy for persons with severe mental illness. *Policy Studies Journal, 37*(2), 299–324.

Prince, P. N., & Prince, C. R. (2002). Perceived stigma and community integration among clients of assertive community treatment. *Psychiatric Rehabilitation Journal, 25*(4), 323–331.

Ridgeway, P., & Zipple, A. (1990). Challenges and strategies for implementing supported housing. *Psychosocial Rehabilitation Journal, 13*(4), 115–120.

Rusch, N., Angermeyer, M. C., & Corrigan, P. W. (2005). Mental illness stigma: Concepts, consequences, and initiatives to reduce stigma. *European Psychiatry, 20*(8), 529–539.

Sherman, S. R., Frenkel, E. R., & Newman, E. S. (1986). Community participation of mentally ill adults in foster family care. *Journal of Community Psychology, 14*, 120–133.

Silverman, C. J., & Segal, S. P. (1994). Who belongs? An analysis of ex-mental patients' subjective involvement in the neighborhood. *Adult Residential Care Journal, 8*(2), 103–113.

Solomon, P., & Draine, J. (1995). Subjective burden among family members of mentally ill adults: Relation to stress, coping, and adaptation *American Journal of Orthopsychiatry 65*(3), 419–427.

Sylvestre, J., Nelson, G., Sabloff, A., & Peddle, S. (2007). Housing for people with serious mental illness: A comparison of values and research. *American Journal of Community Psychology 40*(1–2), 125–137.

Townley, G., & Kloos, B. (2011). Examining the psychological sense of community for individuals with serious mental illness residing in supported housing environments. *Community Mental Health Journal, 47*(4), 436–446.

Townley, G., Kloos, B., Green, E. P., & Franco, M. (2011). Reconcilable Differences? Human diversity, cultural relativity, and sense of community. *American Journal of Community Psychology, 47*(1–2), 69–85.

Tsai, J., Stroup, T. S., & Rosenheck, R. A. (2011). Housing arrangements among a national sample of adults with chronic schizophrenia living in the United States: A descriptive study. *Journal of Community Psychology, 39*(1), 76–88.

Wieland, M. E., Rosenstock, J., Kelsey, S. F., Ganguli, M., & Wisniewski, S. R. (2007). Distal support and community living among individuals diagnosed with schizophrenia and schizoaffective disorder. *Psychiatry, 70*(1), 1–11.

Wong, Y.-L. I., & Solomon, P. (2002). Community integration of persons with psychiatric disabilities in supportive independent housing: Conceptual model and methodological issues. *Mental Health Services Research, 4*(1), 13–28.

Yanos, P. T. (2007). Beyond "landscapes of despair": The need for new research on the urban environment, sprawl, and the community integration of persons with serious mental illness. *Health and Place, 13,* 672–676.

Yanos, P. T., Barrow, S. M., & Tsemberis, S. (2004). Community integration in the early phase of housing among homeless persons diagnosed with severe mental illness: Success and challenges. *Community Mental Health Journal, 40*(2), 133–150.

12
SOCIAL MEDIA AND MENTAL HEALTH
A topological approach

Lewis Goodings and Ian Tucker

Introduction

The use of social media in mental health provision is increasing in the UK. Social media offer new ways for people who are suffering with ongoing mental health problems to seek support and care. The Internet provides almost endless possibilities to seek information about one's mental distress, and social media broaden this in providing digital tools to communicate with others. Social media refers to a range of digital technologies that emphasise the importance of connecting across a network, including technologies such as Twitter, Social Network Sites (SNSs), LinkedIn and YouTube. This chapter focuses on Elefriends, which is a relatively new SNS that is dedicated to mental health issues. Elefriends is specifically designed for people experiencing mental distress and has been operating since 2012. The main strength of this site is the ability to connect with other people with similar experiences in a peer support environment. In this chapter we draw on concepts from topology to analyse the communication in Elefriends. Our aim is to develop knowledge regarding the impact of social media on practices of care and support for those users suffering with ongoing distress, and then to highlight the possibilities for the development of future care practices in mental health.

Digital spaces and mental health

Bauman and Rivers (2015) recognise how tools for supporting people with mental distress now take on a number of digital forms, ranging from digital versions of existing therapeutic practices (e.g. computerised CBT) to a growing number of social network sites (and other digital media e.g. mental health apps) that can provide people with support alongside formal care practices. Social media are an attractive tool for connecting people who are in need of support (Mental Health

Foundation, 2013) and the use of social media in mental health services has increased significantly in recent years. This will impact on the overall experience of mental distress as digital technologies contain their own set of practices, meanings, discourses and ideas. Lupton (2012) argues that these technologies have the power to reflect back on the users and embed a form of subjectivity and meaning that is derived from the technology. These practices are then incorporated into the everyday experiences of the users. The introduction of digital technologies in mental health results in bodies becoming characterised by the movements of both human and non-human actors.

The process of entering an atmosphere (any kind of space or place, be it digital or otherwise) involves a process of feeling the space – the sense of others, how they relate and our position in that particular space. Atmospheres are also felt through the body in terms of the smells, tastes, sounds and other sensory information that contribute to the feelings associated with a space. This experience of digital spaces is also felt through the body. Goodings and Tucker (2017) recognise that users' experiences of distress is shaped by the mediation of their bodies in digital spaces in which both body and technology are co-emergent in the process of distress. In this chapter we will develop an approach that conceptualises technologies as agents in the operation and organisation of communication within networks of users. This will develop an argument for topological psychology as a profitable way of further conceptualising digital spaces.

Topological psychology

> If you take a handkerchief and spread it out in order to iron it, you can see in it certain fixed distances and proximities. If you sketch a circle in one area, you can mark out nearby points and measure for of distances. Then take the same handkerchief and crumple it, by putting it in your pocket. Two distance points suddenly are close, even superimposed. If, further, you tear it in certain places, two points at the close can become very distant. The science of nearness and rifts is called topology, while the science of stable and well-defined distances is called metrical geometry.
>
> *(Serres & Latour, 1995, p. 60)*

The above quote comes from an extensive set of interviews between Michel Serres and Bruno Latour. Serres is detailing his theory of topology through the act of folding a handkerchief. He argues that, while laid flat, the handkerchief presents a metric space with clearly defined distances between certain points. For Serres, this represents the common experience of space as defined by extensive properties of Euclidean geometry. It is when the handkerchief is 'crumpled-up' that we can see a topological sense of space as the distances are transformed, what was far is now close, what was close is now distant. Serres' point is that the analogy of a handkerchief folding is much closer to capturing our experience of space and time than the idea of a flat handkerchief with clear metric dimensions.

The handkerchief example differentiates between topology and geometry. The traditional model of space is focused on the idea of spaces as containers, with fixed metrical properties. Topology offers an alternative view, with space seen as relational and formed through processes of connection. Topology emerged from the mathematical theories of Reimann in the late nineteenth century and has been a theoretical resource for the social sciences to understand the operation of social worlds. In social psychology topological ideas have been drawn upon in theories of the relations between psychological experience and the environmental context of such activity. This work builds on the earlier theories put forward by Kurt Lewin (see Brown, 2012; Brown & Reavey, 2015; Tucker & Smith, 2014).

In *Principles of Topological Psychology* (1936), Kurt Lewin explores the interaction between our experiences and the spaces that we inhabit, mind and body together in action. Lewin looks closely at the content of spaces (or 'environments') and how physical spaces contribute to our potential for movement. Bringing together the role of the environment and the individual aspects of the person in a way that gave equal importance to the impact of both these dimensions, unrivalled in psychology at the time and perhaps even still today. Lewin describes the coming together of the person and the environment as the 'life-space'. This, however, not only depends on an 'immediate' physical relation, e.g. between an individual and their immediate environmental context, but can involve the 'connecting' of many different spaces (including those in the past and future). In defining the principles of psychological life-space, Lewin illustrates how the potential for a person to act is bound up with the arrangement of physical life-space: the two forms of experience are intertwined in movement through a field. This is fundamentally a *dynamic* framing of space in which any given situation is analysed in terms of possibilities for action. Lewin argues that

> if one approaches the description of a situation from a dynamic point of view (that is, from a point of view that should finally allow prediction), one has to understand the situation as a totality of possible events and actions.
> *(Lewin, 1936/2013, p. 16)*

Life-space aims to identify the *totality* of a set of events that that might determine behaviour in any given moment. Lewin extended this argument to pose that anything has the potential to impact on behaviour ('what is real has effects'). Anything that *feels* real has the ability to impact on the way that a person thinks about a given situation; so much so, that our fantasies are even deemed to be real because they have the capacity to affect behaviour.

Lewin argues that psychological life-space is defined by relations, which can involve people, places, spaces, things and ourselves. All relations can be expressed mathematically. For example, at its most simple, behaviour (B) is the function of person and environment, expressed as $B = f(PE)$. This approach develops a vocabulary for the multiplicity of sources that impact on how we might act and feel in any given situation. Psychological events can be mapped topologically by identifying the variety of sources that present at a given moment and Lewin suggests that identifying the forces at play in the psychological life-space requires understanding the different forces at play. This involves moving outwards from a single act in order to recognise how that action is embedded in a network of relations. As one of the key works to illustrate the power of Lewin's work in relation to psychology, Brown and Reavey (2015) demonstrate the potential for the topological approach to provide a way out of the some of the mathematical assumptions that typically dominate psychology (see Brown, 2012; Brown & Reavey, 2015). As they argue:

> Psychologists often implicitly rely upon Euclidean or Cartesian procedures of applying external measures and scales. This is why human perception is conceptualised in terms of stimuli that are 'near' to us rather than 'far' away . . . However, near and far, along with recent and old (or present and absent), are relations that are relative to the to the topological properties of the space under construction.
>
> *(Brown & Reavey, 2015, p. 60)*

Near and far, recent and old, are all topologically equal in a life-space. It is for this reason that we must avoid applying external points of reference on the experience and how all forms or properties of a life-space have the potential to impact on experience. This means that focus is not on the digital architecture of digital 'spaces', but rather what kinds of relation are made possible through them. Space as a metric property becomes redundant in such analysis. Time also becomes a psychological process as part of the life-space. As Lewin notes, life-spaces do not rely on a concept of time as a linear process. Instead, past, present and future can all feature as part of experience. This resonates with a Bergsonian reading of time, in which present experience is always-already a relation between past and present, but not in a chronological sense of the past being a 'stored resource', accessible for retrieval as per present need. Instead, for Bergson (1911/1988, p. 78), the present is driven by the presence of an ever growing past pushing into the future: '[B]ut already we may speak of the body as an ever advancing boundary between the future and the past, as a pointed end, which our past is continually driving forward into our future'. There is no disconnect between past and present, rather experience is constituted through the continuous flow of past into future, through the present.

Our argument in this chapter is that social media provide new experiences of space and time in which notions of distance and nearness are replaced by those of connection and relation (see also Tucker & Goodings, 2014b). We argue that topology is a useful theoretical device to explore the impact of social media on mental distress as it avoids falling into the trap of labelling digital space as virtual (not real). Instead the focus on connections and relations speaks precisely to the operation of social media, and its power to connect people, largely irrespective of geography. Topology additionally provides a challenge to the so-called 'primacy of technology' (Marres, 2012), in which agency is predominantly located with technology, rather than the social and psychological practices with which it intersects.

We develop a topological approach that sees agency as mobile, unfolding as part of ongoing socio-technological processes, rather than as operating between two ontologically distinct entities (humans–technologies). This framing helps as a way of theoretically mapping what is at stake with increased social media use in mental health. Doing so involves understanding what kinds of connections are made possible, not only between people, but also with the technologies through which social media activity operate. Both these relational layers have affective power, and interweave in the unfolding of experience. For example, a post in an online social network site may be tied to an earlier conversation with a family member, or part of an ongoing dissatisfaction with one's mental health care team or linked to ongoing austerity measures and the changing landscape of mental health care in the UK. A topological approach also recognises how we also have capacity to act into these networks of relations. Whereby we actively engage with these networks in order to create meaning in the world. Brown and Reavey (2015, p. 176) state: 'Life-space expands when we work together to construct "common notions". It is on the basis of this commonness that we are able to make connections and to expand our joint capacities to feel and act, to build futures together'. Here there is particular concern with the way that life-space can be expanded through the ongoing process of folding the past into the present in the everyday practices of remembering. Clearly, this is a process that is not without its challenges; but, for the people involved the rewards of connecting with a sense of commonness of memory affords movement into another way of thinking and feeling about a particular experience. Topological psychology offers a way of identifying how people act into the world to create meaning. For example, if a person is told to try a new medication in response to their mental health they may feel anxious or unsure about how the new drug will affect them. However, if this person was to talk to someone who already had experience of the drug, who reports a positive experience, this may allow the person to feel confident about their own future experiences of the medication. This is describing the collective capacity to establish meaning and how alternative ways of feeling and being can be the result our embodied relations with other bodies.

Elefriends and mental health in the UK

In this chapter we are concerned with identifying how the life-spaces of people suffering with ongoing mental distress are shaped through use of the social media site Elefriends. This involves considering in what ways people expand their experience in order to create new opportunities for constructing 'common notions' about mental health? How is that space narrowed or expanded through the use of the site? As mentioned earlier, Lewin focuses on the totality of life-space, where thought and action come together in the precise assemblage of any given moment. Therefore, in looking at Elefriends we cannot contend that a certain action is directly related to the actions in a social media site; alternatively, we are proposing that Elefriends offers a *potential* opportunity for a different affective direction.

In making this distinction the aim is to avoid treating 'online' and 'offline' as separate entities that do not collide. Instead, in thinking of the total life-space, the relations become of most importance and the movement that is made possible or restricted via these relations.

Elefriends is SNS for people who experience mental distress (www.elefriends.org.uk, see Figure 12.1). The site is similar to other SNSs in style, layout and forms of communication. Elefriends was designed and developed by Mind, the mental health charity. Members of Elefriends can see recent activity from other users via a newsfeed and can post to the wall for everyone to see or can choose to message other members individually. The site also includes the use of specifically designed buttons that signal a reaction to some content e.g. Elefriends has a button in the shape of an ear that stands for 'I hear you'. Communication in Elefriends centres around members discussing recent incidents relating to mental health and other members providing support or advice. Elefriends is a supportive community that harnesses the power of peer support and provides a space outside of formal health care practices for accessing help. Elefriends is designed around the image of the kind and helpful elephant (hence 'Ele' friends) and as of August 2016, Elefriends has approximately 45,000 users.

Elefriends is a safe space to speak about mental health issues and is moderated by a team of people at Mind. They are happy for people to talk about whatever they wish, but they may remove posts that could be considered to be harmful or dangerous to others (in line with their 'house rules'). Mind use an image of elephant (called the 'Ele') to deliver their messages to the community. Elefriends is one of a number of SNS that are designed to focus on mental health issues (for another example see *The Big White Wall*). Conversations in Elefriends frequently involve speaking about a recent experience of medical intervention, a difficult period of

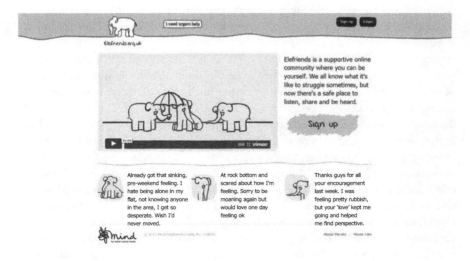

FIGURE 12.1 Elefriends website.

distress or more general conversations about a range of mental health issues. Users are encouraged to respond to posts and many conversations have input from lots of different members. Mind has designed Elefriends to be a supported community that aims to deliver a high quality of peer support. Elefriends is indicative of the way that mental health services are no longer tied to institutional settings. Elefriends is moderated by a dedicated team of staff (although not overnight) and Mind have designed Elefriends to be a safe and supported community that aims to deliver a high quality of peer support.

It is very important to understand what kind of connections and relations are formed in and through social media in communities suffering from ongoing mental distress. The value of peer support is well known, and yet underexplored in relation to the digital. The increase of mental health-related social media makes this a live issue in current mental health care and support. Our focus on Elefriends provides an important example through which to examine these issues.

The study

Fifteen interviews were conducted with members of the Elefriends community. This was part of a larger project that looked at the role of peer support in mental health social media. The interviews were conducted in July 2014 via Skype. The participants responded to a post from the Ele that asked people to take part in the interviews. A high proportion of the interviewees were female, and ranged in age from 22–55. The participants were spread across England, Wales and Scotland. They also ranged in terms of time spent on the site with some have been members of Elefriends for less than one month and others having joined the site nearly two years ago (which would have been close to the launch of Elefriends).

Interview questions covered areas including time spent using Elefriends, experience of seeking and providing support, comparison with offline services and perceptions of using digital technologies for mental health care. The interviews were transcribed verbatim, without minor non-textual expressive features (e.g. ums, ers, etc). Transcripts were analysed using Thematic Decomposition (Stenner, 1993), which encourages a close reading of the text in order to identify meaningful units of text in terms of patterns, themes or stories in the data. This approach shares an interest with Discursive Psychology (see Edwards & Potter, 1992) in the way that discourse is considered to be constructed in the process of social interactions. The analysis focused on developing thematic patterns in the data relating to the experience of connecting with others through Elefriends. This relates to the theoretical orientation and experience of using Elefriends for support relying on the kinds of relation and connection made possible by the site. Additionally, analysis needs to be able to capture the ways that connections and relations can transcend the material conditions of an environment. So, analysis did not only focus on the technological connections made possible by the design of Elefriends, but also the life-spaces emerging and operating in relation to Elefriends. Thematic decomposition has featured recently in topological studies in psychology as a way of capturing the relation and process orientation of experience (Reavey, Poole, & Ougrin, 2017). The study received ethical approval from the University of East London Research Ethics Committee. Standard ethical procedures for qualitative research were put in place to ensure the protection of the participants during the transcription phase (i.e. all participant information was anonymised in the written transcripts).

Life-spaces in Elefriends

The analysis that follows aims to provide topological understanding of the kinds of life-space that develop in and through use of Elefriends. This involves 'mapping' some of the relations and connections formed in terms of covering a range of different 'stages' of people's experiences with Elefriends. We will see that using Elefriends involves becoming attuned to operating in what feels like a space occupied by many other people, but that actually operates on the specific relations that constitute individuals' life-spaces, which themselves are subject to movement over time. In the first extract we see an example of the experience of starting to use Elefriends:

> **Extract 1**
>
> *Int.:* What were your first impressions of Elefriends?
> *Janet:* A bit wary to start with because I wasn't sure how anonymous it was. I suffer with a lot of paranoia, so that doesn't help when you're on a website with other people that you think might be NHS staff masquerading as patients and getting information about you and stuff like that. But I've come, over time, to realise that it's not like that and it is a very supportive community that helps you through good times as well as the tough times.

When service users first start using Elefriends they do so from a context largely shaped by offline services. Seeking care and support through social media is no straightforward task, as it is often shaped by a concern about the potential for social media activity to be seen by others. Janet's use of Elefriends comes at a time when she was feeling particularly vulnerable due to experiencing paranoia. As such, she was already concerned about expressing her feelings, for fear of what that might mean for her relationships with other services (e.g. NHS). What if someone recognised her, and gained information that Janet did not want to be shared? What if this was happening surreptitiously (e.g. NHS staff masquerading as service users)? For Janet, the initial dynamics at play were not easy to manage. It was not as if she was entering a space that afforded immediate peer support (Elefriends' main objective). Janet's initial use of Elefriends was a new relation through which she tried to manage her ongoing distress.

The question of anonymity shaped Janet's initial feeling about using Elefriends. This does not just refer to the specifics of Janet's activity through Elefriends, but rather about the process by which it became part of her life at the time. Social media have considerable power to connect, and yet Janet did not feel able to harness this power initially. They are not, by definition, fixed and stable. This means they are not tools in a traditional sense (as in having one fixed function), but technologies that facilitate, although not determine, new experiences. Indeed, we follow the idea that to understand the impact of digital technologies on social and cultural practices, we should adopt a techno-genetic approach, premised on the idea that people and technologies are co-evolving actors in the ongoing production of our social worlds (Hayles, 2012). Technologies are not just tools, and humans are not the sole agents. Extract 2 shows another participant discussing their experience of learning to trust other members of Elefriends, through which meaningful practices of support can emerge:

Extract 2

Int.: Cool. So when you say that you began to realise that it wasn't like that, was there anything that helped you to realise that?

Daniel: Just the things that the other Elefriends were saying. Like, if you put down 'Is there any Elefriend suffering from the same diagnosis that I've got?' they were coming out with the same symptoms and with the same thoughts on how they were treated at A&E and the same sort of drug reactions and the – you knew that they were real people and that other people were suffering the same as you are.

The status of Elefriends as a medium designed to facilitate peer support is clear in this extract. Daniel comments on how members of Elefriends share details of distress and associated contact with health services. This resonates as an attempt to form 'common notions' (Brown & Reavey, 2015) as a way of expanding life-space to afford different ways of feeling. This talk of treatment could be considered as part of the conversational work that allows common notions to develop, which has the potential to expand Daniel's life-space. This expansion is not just about an increase in the number of relations Daniel has (e.g. connecting with more people), but the sharing of experiences creates a collective pool of shared knowledge, which can in turn, expand the life-spaces of those involved. Crucially, this particular expansion is only made possible through the relations formed through Elefriends. It does not emerge from each individual user, as if they are sharing a part of themselves, but unfolds as a relational form. This in turn 'acts back' on users by enhancing their powers to act. Sharing stories and the subsequent understanding that one is not alone in the experience of being distressed, creates an affirming affective experience. Common notions can be seen to develop through a set of embodied and social practices unfolding 'outside' of the digital environment of Elefriends. Daniel talks about the role that physical symptoms and experiences of medication play in the development of common notions. In Extract 3, we can see how Elefriends can expand life-space at a time when connections are limited in formal care services:

Extract 3

Peter: I'm on Elefriends to a lot of professional help because I've often thought, in my experience, when I've gone to seek, or I've had visits – well, you know, whether it's hospitals or psychs or anything like that – then they couldn't really understand. They may have been qualified and they might know about which meds to prescribe and they may have seen people all the time, who have mental health concerns, but they don't live it day to day, every day, every day, so talking to people on Elefriends, a lot of them do. I've had conversations with other Elefriends on the site and we agree that, yeah, we're the only ones who can understand each other because we go through it all the time. We're living this and it's not impersonal because you talk about your own experiences and you can trade ideas or helping, coping mechanisms. So this is a really useful tool for support.

Peter describes how the members of Elefriends are the 'only ones' who can understand what he is going through and further illustrates how the 'common notions' function works to connect users with alternative ways of feeling. This extract also shows that Elefriends users are known to explicitly discuss this connection and commonality. As Peter states, 'I've had conversations with other Elefriends on the site and we agree that we're the only ones that can understand'. This conceptualisation resonates with what Brown and Reavey (2015) describe as the 'feelings of affordance'. Peter can sense the way that Elefriends (and the relations therein) offer a range of actions that could offer up alternative possibilities for thinking and feeling. The outcome of such a large number of people being present in Elefriends means that individual experiences quickly become entangled with the experiences of others, becoming reconstructed in light of those relations. It is almost impossible to tell where one experience begins and another one ends.

Key here is the way that Elefriends facilitates possibilities to develop common notions through connecting service users with similar experiences of distress and associated challenges. For example, while a doctor may have expertise regarding possible side effects of a psychiatric medication, she cannot empathise through having experienced the medication. Only other service users have similar embodied experience, and it is the ability to connect with other similar bodies that Peter reports as beneficial. This distinguishes Elefriends from the care and support Peter has received from formal mental health services. A clear distinction between offline and online experience is not a universal part of experiences of using Elefriends. Indeed, the idea of a life-space constituted as simultaneously on- and offline is highlighted in Extract 4 in which feelings of distress do not 'stop' at a perceived boundary of physical-digital, but very much shape the experience of using Elefriends:

Extract 4

Tracy: The very first time I started using it, I thought it was brilliant – like Facebook but without – you could say what you wanted to say rather than – Facebook is very – it's more difficult to say how you feel on there. Then after a while, I started to feel really lost, like everyone else knew what they were doing and I didn't and I got really – also I was quite suspicious of people being nice to me. I thought I didn't know anything, that it wasn't real, I thought they were all being fake. I went through quite a wobbly patch and didn't really trust anyone, and didn't feel like I fitted in. That actually lasted quite a while, like, coming and going. I think I'm kind of into it now and – yeah and with the aftermath this depression (laughs) . . . I suppose the reasons I had problems trusting people is much the same as in real life, so I think Elefriends is like this, it's the miniature version of the world and all the problems I have in real life come out in Elefriends as well. But because it's online and it's remote, it makes it just slightly easier to deal with than in real life. So there were a few trust issues with a few people and I've become friends with them, which I think might have been harder in real life, but – I think that's what's helped me to feel safer, to be honest, is to connect with a few people who I know quite well. So I know that when the say that they care, that it's like it means something.

Tracy's extract demonstrates how feelings of trust and support can fluctuate over time. Her initial positivity regarding Elefriends waned through becoming suspicious of the motives of the sheer number of people being nice to her (something she may not have experienced before). This speaks to a common part of using social media, namely acknowledging the potential high-level visibility of one's activity online, to multiple unknown others. As there are many people in this space who want to communicate and share their experiences, this can lead to being overwhelmed with support and make it difficult to identify if people are being genuine. As a response to this, Tracy has extended practices from her offline network of relations that helps her to avoid these issues. She maintains a close group of friends in Elefriends that she speaks with regularly. As she states, 'when they say that they care, that it's like it means something'. These are not challenges that people are unfamiliar with, as Tracy states, Elefriends is a 'miniature version of the world', in which existing problems in life are played out and worked through. The simultaneity of experience moving in and through digital and physical worlds is seen in Tracy's extract when she discusses how it took a while of 'coming and going' before she was able to build a network of friends, through which Tracy developed feelings of trust. This gives a sense of how life-spaces are not static, but formed through process of movement, and that it's not just physical spaces that are moved through, but also digital ones. The topological principles of connection, relation and movement are the same. Elefriends can also give rise to complex or ambivalent experiences that are afforded by the ever-changing assemblage of relations. For instance, Extract 5 we can see how the use of Elefriends leads to new experiences of distress, in which users can feel over reliant on the site:

Extract 5

Int.: Cool. You've been there for a while, so has the way you used it, do you think it's changed over the time you've been there?

Allison: Well, I used to be on it sort of all the time and I didn't want to leave it at one time, but then I thought, well, this is silly; I can't be on it all day and all night. So I probably – the way I use it probably has changed. It's probably only when only when I'm triggered and really stressed out and upset that I go on it.

In Extract 5, the initial expansion of life-space enacted through Elefriends can, over time, take a form that limits the connections with other parts of life. For Allison, a concern developed that she was using Elefriends too much, as her life was becoming predominantly constituted through the relations developed through Elefriends. The dominance of the expanded life-space threatens a narrowing of other parts of her life-space, those typically associated with offline relations outside of Elefriends. Although the overall life-space stays connected, its shape becomes too narrowed in terms of relations operating through Elefriends. This acts to limit movement in other areas of Allison's life, and shows how relations can transform over time.

Life-spaces are not rigid, but shift according to the relations present at a given time. For Allison, Elefriends created an expanded feeling of support initially, which was a positive experience. Over time though, Allison has found herself spending a significant proportion of her time on Elefriends, which threatens to dominate the life-space. Allison has recognised this, and reports attempting to re-configure the life-space by reducing time spent with Elefriends. There is an element of unpredictability about Allison's use of Elefriends though, as it is not possible to organise precisely when she will use it. Her distress comes to structure usage, as Allison will engage with Elefriends when she is feeling particularly distressed ('when I'm triggered'). Its always-on presence here services as a positive and a negative. It can lead to Allison over using, and neglecting other parts of her life. And yet, when her distress is triggered, it is a source of immediate support. Consequently, there exists a tension in her relationship with the site.

Conclusion

The increased presence of social media in mental health presents a need for understanding the challenges and benefits they bring to those they are designed to help (Tucker & Goodings, 2018). This involves expanding the existing focus on ecologies of distress from the bricks and mortar of physical spaces of care to digital environments with significant powers to connect (McGrath, Reavey, & Brown, 2008). The value of topology for understanding of multiple ways that service users' experiences of distress are inter-connected with the spaces and places in and through which they unfold has been demonstrated in a number of contexts (e.g. Brown & Reavey, 2015; McGrath & Reavey, 2015; Tucker, 2018; Tucker & Goodings, 2014a, 2014b; Tucker & Smith, 2014). In the present chapter we have sought to develop these understandings through expanding the topological lens to include 'digital environments', which are underpinned by principles of connection and relation.

The topological approach moves us away from the idea that spaces are static, towards a perspective that emphasises movement and inter-connectedness. A person's experience of Elefriends, as a 'space', is interconnected with multiple other spaces (past, present and future), and as such, their activity always emerges through an inter-relational context. Using Elefriends adds new layers to these experiences, e.g. the value of being able to connect with other people with similar diagnoses and experiences. This though involves exposing oneself to an increased visibility to unknown others, which can be particularly challenging when it involves posting information about one's mental distress. Consequently, using Elefriends can at first feel very strange. Talking about one's distress commonly occurs in spaces perceived to be safe and secure (whether part of formal care services or not). Moving this activity into a digital realm can be anxiety provoking in itself, as people do not necessarily feel safe and secure online. We can see how this involves an additional affective layer that can develop just through connecting with Elefriends as a technology (Hansen, 2015). Using Elefriends is not just about connecting with other people, but about doing so through social media. The technology is an active agent in the activity, not just a passive tool facilitating communication between users.

The value of expanding life-space through common notions can, over time, develop into a concern about the extent of use. Allison's extract demonstrated a concern that Elefriends can become an obstacle to everyday life, in terms of taking up too much time, and shifting focus away from other important parts of life. The value of life-space as a concept is how it helps avoid the common spatial binary between real–virtual, offline–online, which can de-value the nature of the experience of social media. Life-space situates and contextualises social media activity within the broader ecology of distress (i.e. everyday life environment) of people suffering with ongoing mental health problems. This means not analysing what happens online in isolation, but rather widening the analytic lens to capture the entire environmental context from which social media activity emerges. This is important given the increased digitisation of mental health care and support, in which focus can become dominated by the perceived benefits of the digital, to the exclusion of wider life-spaces.

References

Bauman, S., & Rivers, I. (2015). *Mental health in the digital age*. Basingstoke: Palgrave Macmillan.
Bergson, H. (1911/1988). *Matter and memory*. London: George Allen.

Brown, S. D. (2012). Memory and mathesis: For a topological approach to psychology. *Theory, Culture & Society*, *29*(4–5), 137–164.
Brown, S. D., & Reavey, P. (2015). *Vital memory and affect: Living with a difficult past*. London: Routledge.
Edwards, D., & Potter, J. (1992). *Discursive psychology*. London: Sage.
Goodings, L., & Tucker, I. (2017). Digitizing care and support for mental distress: Bodies, affect and Elefriends. *Sociology of Health & Illness*, *39*(4), 629–642.
Hansen, M. N. B. (2015). *Feed-forward: On the future of 21st century media*. Chicago, IL: University of Chicago Press.
Hayles, N. K. (2012). *How we think: Digital media and contemporary technogenesis*. Chicago, IL: University of Chicago Press.
Lewin, K. (1936/2013). *Principles of topological psychology*. New York, NY: McGraw-Hill.
Lewin, K. (1948). Resolving social conflicts: Selected papers on group dynamics. *Resolving social conflicts field theory in social science*, 422 ST.
Lupton, D. (2012). *Medicine as culture: Illness, disease and the body*. London: Sage.
McGrath, L., & Reavey, P. (2015). Seeking fluid possibility and solid ground: Space and movement in mental health service users' experiences of crisis, *Social Science and Medicine*. *128*, 115–125.
McGrath, L., Reavey, P., & Brown, S. D. (2008). Spaces and scenes of anxiety: Embodied expressions of distress in public and private. *Emotion, Space & Society*, *1*(1), 56–64
Marres, N. (2012). On some uses and abuses of topology in the social analysis of technology (or the problem with smart meters). *Theory, Culture & Society*, *29*(4–5), 288–310.
Mental Health Foundation. (2013). *Starting today: The future of mental health services*. London: Mental Health Foundation.
Reavey, P., Poole, J., & Ougrin, D. (2017). The ward as emotional ecology: Adolescent experiences of managing emotional distress in inpatient settings. *Health & Place*, *46*, 210–218.
Serres, M., & Latour, B. (1995). *Conversations on science, culture, and time, studies in literature and science*. Ann Arbor, MI: University of Michigan Press.
Stenner, P. (1993). Discoursing jealousy. In E. Burman & I. Parker (Eds.), *Discourse analytic research: Repertoires and readings of texts in action* (pp. 94–132). London: Routledge.
Tucker, I. M. (2018). Shifting landscapes of care and distress: A topological understanding of rurality. In K. Soldatic & K. Johnson (Eds.), *Disability and rurality: Identity, gender and belonging*. Farnham, UK: Ashgate.
Tucker, I. M., & Goodings, L. (2014a). Mediation and digital intensities: Topology, psychology and social media. *Social Science Information*, *53*(3), 277–292.
Tucker, I. M., & Goodings, L. (2014b). Sensing bodies and digitally mediated distress. *Senses & Society*, *9*(1), 55–71.
Tucker, I. M., & Goodings, L. (2018). Medicated bodies: Mental distress, social media and affect. *New Media & Society*.
Tucker, I. M., & Smith, L.-A. (2014). Topology and mental distress: Self-care in the *life spaces* of home. *Journal of Health Psychology*, *19*(1), 176–183.

13
WALKING THROUGH AND BEING WITH NATURE

Meaning-making and the impact of being in UK wild places

Elizabeth Freeman and Jacqueline Akhurst

The developing field of eco-therapy directly focuses on the interactions of people and natural spaces, and meaning-making is core to the relationship between people and their environments. This chapter explores the social and material contexts of people in natural settings and how these shape and structure experiences and influence well-being, providing an insight into meaning related to artefacts in the landscape, cultural influences and dynamic transitional experiences within and between space and place. A custom-designed walking and solo experience (WSE), suited to UK conditions, is discussed in relation to underlying processes and as a potential well-being intervention. Perspectives were gathered from pre- and post-experience interviews, journal writing, group discussions and a nine-month follow-up interview that considered what endured for participants after their experiences. Findings highlighted important elements for programme design related to group and individual benefits and overall, the work suggests that interactions between people and natural landscapes are intricate and bound by cultural influences, with dynamic transitions and interactions happening within place, space and time. These findings provide an insight into the meanings associated with being in the outdoors and the processes that unfold. Implications for research, practice and policy are proposed, with recommendations for potential applications.

Nature experiences and well-being

The breadth and number of studies and literature on the relationship between humans and nature in relation to health and mental health is driven by the widespread assumption that the natural environment is essential to human fulfilment and meaning, at both the individual and the societal level (Pretty et al., 2007). The benefits of nature experiences are now more widely accepted by organisations such as DEFRA and Natural England and they are more concerned with understanding how best to harness the benefits of and protect nature. With the reported growth in mental health problems, particularly anxiety, stress and depression, in the UK being 1 in 4 people (Mental Health Foundation, 2014) it is essential for people's mental health and well-being to understand and harness the potential benefits of nature experiences and nature-based interventions. Indeed, in a recent report by Natural England (2016) nature-based interventions were found to reduce stress-, anxiety- and depression-related symptoms. Contact with nature is not enough to foster meaningful and long-lasting benefits though – it is the type and quality of the experience that makes a difference and requires further examination.

Eco-therapy capitalises on the human–nature relationship and, based on ideas in eco-psychology that involve the integration of psychology and ecology, utilises a broad range of nature-based methods of psychological healing grounded in the idea that people are nurtured by healthy interaction with the earth (McCallum, 2007) and that disconnection with nature is damaging to mental health (Kelly, 1996). Eco-therapy consequently aims to restore the natural balance between the inner and outer person through physical connections with nature and restoring mental and emotional balance (Capra, 1982): feeling better for having a better connection with nature and moving away from the ego to the eco (McGeeney, 2016). Wilderness and adventure based therapy, survival training, gardening, meditation in nature, rites of passage and rituals, shamanic counselling and walking outdoors can all be employed as part of an eco-therapy programme (Kelly, 1996; McCallum, 2007).

Jungian approaches to eco-therapy involve archetypal landscapes to evoke the history of human nature (Chirot, 1993), where physical terrain provides the challenges and obstacles required to face danger and confront fear. Set within an empathic environment, challenges are seen as natural obstacles within a journey, rather than contrived ones, and encourage a group to persevere and rely on each other. Eco-therapy views symptoms as signals of distress in a larger social context; an individual's symptoms reflect what is going on in the world as a whole (Conn, 2006). The emphasis is therefore on healing people within their environments and at the same time healing communities and building trust (Kelly, 1996). This is counter to traditional Western psychological approaches that tend to identify pain as a pathology, disorder or illness in an individual or family.

Nature and landscape is therefore central to eco-therapy and natural environments have, for a long time, been viewed as therapeutic landscapes – as 'healing places' (Baer & Gesler, 2004). The therapeutic landscape concept is a useful way for social scientists to frame both real and imagined connections between place and human health (Gesler, 1992) and draws from humanism and the philosophy of holistic health, resisting and criticising what is seen as the positivist hegemony of the biomedical model. For example, Akhurst (2010) explores similarities between walking in wild places and therapeutic experiences but also highlights that potential difficulties inherent in experiences have not been consistently considered by some of the studies in the eco-psychology literature. There is also little research in this area that is process orientated rather than outcome orientated (Revell, Duncan, &

Copper, 2013) and that also focuses on meaning, place and well-being (Freeman, Akhurst, Bannigan, & James, 2016). An examination of the nuanced and complex ways that people make meaning from their experiences in nature could be beneficial, particularly due to the impact on well-being, the affordability and potential to engage 'hard to reach' groups, including males experiencing mental distress. Below, we provide an examination of eco-therapy utlising a walking and solo experience (WSE).

The walking and solo experience

The WSE aimed to provide a safe, enjoyable and challenging experience 'in' and 'with' nature. This involved a five-day experience *walking through* nature (the exploration and journey phase) and *sitting within* nature (the solo phase) and was influenced by many outdoor experience and therapy approaches, but particularly Jungian approaches, using the landscape as a provider of challenge and instigator of change. During the more physically challenging aspects of the WSE, participants are more likely to be experiencing being 'in' nature, with the predominance of psychological and personal sensations encouraging the awareness of physical and social selves (Russell & Farnum, 2004). These aspects of the WSE were apparent during the 'journey' phase of the WSE that involved walking from one place to another, with all that they needed being carried in a rucksack. During the less physically demanding aspects of the WSE, the 'exploration' and 'solo' phases, participants are more likely to experience being 'with' nature; having time to listen to, be aware of and connect with nature on a sensory and more emotional level.

The phases (exploration, journey and solo) were used to describe the structure of, and identify transitions in, the WSE; from landscape to landscape (between urban and natural) and between activities ('walking through' and 'sitting within'); these facilitated the experiences of nature and the emotional, social and physical journeys of the participants. The purpose of the exploration phase was to gradually and safely ease participants physically and psychologically into the unfamiliar wild place; walking was relatively short in distance and duration. The journey phase provided an opportunity for participants to move through the landscape over larger distances, involving greater challenge. Challenge also occurred during the solo phase, providing a more intensely psychological experience including reflection and introspection, while also being an opportunity for relaxation, mindfulness and extrospection.

Despite its Jungian influences, the WSE does not identify symptoms or involve any direct form of therapy. Instead, the WSE provides an environment and space for individuals and the group to explore their feelings and experiences in a novel non-judgemental space/place 'held' by the walking guide. The WSE is therefore not 'therapy' but rather 'therapeutic' in its effects (Davis-Berman & Berman, 1993).

In study 1, the WSE was in Northumberland during September and comprised a consecutive five-day experience (from Sunday to Friday). In study 2,

North Nidderdale provided the location during August/September, also a five-day experience but over two weekends with a two-week interval, so as to explore whether the WSE would be effective in a potentially more accessible and affordable form that may be more appropriate for mental health services. The distributed structure of study 2 was also an opportunity to examine the differences between the two WSE models, to further investigate the transitions between space and place (e.g. wild place and everyday life), and understand the role of meaning-making more clearly. In both studies there was stable weather with very little rain, but cold evenings. Participants wild camped, carried all their equipment and food and experienced a 34–36-hour solo phase (no people within 100 metres, no movement beyond 30 metres of their tents, no electronic equipment or books allowed, but a journal could be kept). The leadership structure for both studies involved a summer mountain leader (who was also the researcher) and another facilitator (who was there to help in any emergency).

Space, place and meaning-making

Identifying and understanding meaning-making within space and place is important when examining experiences (Tuan, 1977) and the impact on a person's sense of well-being. People come to know and construct their realities through direct (passive and active), and indirect ways of experiencing: using symbols is indirect, visually perceiving is active and the senses of touch, taste and smell are passive. Knowing is mediated and limited by the direct and indirect nature of experiencing, with direct experience allowing one to know something intimately (like a home) whereas indirect experience is conceptual, allowing one only to know about something (like a country). Tuan (1977) aptly highlights, however, that a person may be able to articulate ideas but may have difficulty expressing what they perceive through their senses, which may lead to some people suppressing that which they cannot communicate. For this reason some people deem these more subtle experiences and meaning-making as private, thus difficult to access and capture during data collection.

Illustrating the ambivalences and nuanced nature of experiences in nature with many shades of meaning is therefore important, despite the challenges in doing so (Freeman & Akhurst, 2015). Meanings are acquired through activity – the sharing and interchange of personal opinions, knowledge claims and experiential understanding/reflection – so this work focuses on individual and social meaning-making activities. It is acknowledged that social and individual meanings are rarely separable, thus no attempt will be made to do so.

Capturing experiences

To capture this complexity, a multi-method approach to data collection was taken. Pre- and post-interviews were employed so that a comparison could be made before and after the WSE, and journals and group discussions were used to capture more 'in-the-moment' experiences during the WSE. The nine-month follow-up assessed the temporal effects of the experience and any changes in perspectives. This approach hoped to capture the 'whole' experience of preparing for and doing a WSE, avoiding 'partial' data collection and exploration, resulting in a rich dataset. Audio recordings of interviews and group discussions were transcribed and analysed using Thematic Analysis (TA; Braun & Clarke, 2006), coding and highlighting parts of text and labelling them with 'tags' in NVivo data management system.

Data was generated by students from counselling degree programmes, who volunteered to participate in the two studies. Four participants volunteered for study 1 (by pseudonym with age in brackets): three females, Kit (22), Sam (37) and Alex (42) and one male, Joe (39); Kit and Joe knew each other socially. Five participants volunteered for study 2: two males, Dannie (23) and Leslie (36); three females, Nina (20), Sarah (23) and Alex (43), and Joe from study 1 acted as a facilitator (helping the researcher with group safety). Ethical approval was granted by the university Ethics Committee and informed consent was gained from all participants, ensuring knowledge about the right to withdraw, confidentiality and proper assurances of anonymity in communications.

Findings

The therapeutic quality of the WSE was shown as changeable over time, person, space and experience. Half of the participants reported that at the time of the study they were experiencing anxiety and depression. One participant was recovering from drug addiction and was particularly fearful about the solo experience, worried about relapsing and how she was perceived by others. Common distress experienced across all participants was worrying about day-to-day responsibilities like bills and deadlines. The findings will illustrate participants' experiences and how wild spaces alleviated and sometimes transformed participants' distress. Facets of the WSE that fostered relief from stress, anxiety and depression will be explored and two themes "Time to chill out" and "I don't have to wear a mask" will be explained.

"Time to chill out": stresses of everyday life, responsibilities and time pressure

All participants reported how distressing they found everyday life, responsibilities and time pressures. Relinquishing responsibilities and escaping everyday life and pressures was pervasive in participant reports and thoughts of responsibilities were an unwelcome and a distraction from experiencing the wild place and connecting to nature (n = 8), interrupting the calmness they felt.

Alex, Sarah and Dannie report the pressures and pace of society and everyday life and how wild places can provide an escape from those stresses, with Alex describing everyday life like being "trapped in our own little prisons because of the rules we have to abide by", and Sarah, stating she gained perspectives on life:

SARAH, FOLLOW-UP INTERVIEW, STUDY 2

S: [. . .] I think the memory is more linked to like a really nice feeling of (.) everything being really peaceful and open (.)I think it's the space that really like made it very relaxing and really different from just being in a green (.) part of York (.) cos (.) there is something (2) really whatever the opposite of pressurising is (.) pressure relieving (.) about erm it's about being in this massive open space and kind of all my (.) daily life agenda crap bags goes out the window and that was nice: cos I (.) I don't get much perspective in the city and I get really obsessed about (.) daily living and concerns and even though like we've done existential philosophy and counselling it's still hard to get hold of unless you've got like a (.) prompt. (.) I think that's what it kind of (.) so like: oh yeah see how you were worried about all this crap that's going on at uni and the (.) finer points of this essay well: it doesn't really matter because here are some birds (.) and isn't that the point really like (.) all this stuff is just constructs and that is real so it makes me feel better (.) so I guess that's what stuck just the feeling of being like (.) when I need peace then that's when I need to go somewhere (.) green: and open (.) yeah (.) I go in the forest when I need a hug [. . .] being reminded of like (.) well this is (.) it's the ultimate point of life and the ultimate point of all this crap that we do to ourselves like making ourselves do stupid degrees is it because we are supposed to enjoy it at some point (.) and we're supposed to feel happy at some point and just (.) be alive and experience being alive and so it takes like it literally takes my seeing ducklings to be like (.) oh: yeah (.) like you don't have to do anything to be happy (.) you just have to notice what's already there.

Sarah mentions the pressures of everyday life several times and describes the wild place as a "massive open space", unlike greenspaces in York, where she can have relief from the stress, be happy, experience vitality and gain perspective. Green open space fosters peace and perspective and forests are a comfort. Knowing she has the option to go to nature to *feel better* is meaningful to her and empowering, providing her with a choice, control and confidence to deal with life and her experiences of anxiety and depression.

Dannie similarly finds wild places relaxing and pressure relieving:

DANNIE, POST-EXPERIENCE INTERVIEW, STUDY 2

D: it's just escaping somewhere just (.) stepping out of normal like
    [. . .] it's just like stepping off that conveyer belt (.) so you're like not getting pushed along (.) just a place where basically time doesn't matter to me just a

(continued)

> *(continued)*
>
> place where you're not being rushed but time's not an issue (.) that's (.) that's basically it doesn't matter how long you're there for you're just there for until you feel like coming back that's that the main thing about it (.) just there's no rush (.) cos it's like every day you (.) you usually rushed by something even if it's down to just (.) even if you've got a day off (2) or something like (.) for me anyway (.) there's still (.) there's still a bit of pressure (2) even if it's self-applied to do something with your day cos otherwise you feel like you've wasted your day [. . .] just being able to relax and not feel (2.5) I feel quite free I suppose you know just (.) feel free to just be a human being and sat in a place (.) rather than (.) be (2) this person who is a (.) who does (.) who has to do (.) you know and all these other terms (.) that society places on us sort of [. . .] I suppose it's getting closer to actually being wild you know like [. . .] existing rather than (.) having to earn money (.) get a grade and (.) please somebody and do something (.) you know (.) just the mundane things that everybody has to do in society to get along in society.

Dannie talks about feelings of everyday pressures as being on a conveyer belt resonating with Alex's comments about feeling trapped in a prison and, like her, his aspiration for escape from the everyday is strong. Dannie's enjoyment of and desire to have a simpler, freer life is clear, making a distinction between being a *person* and being a *human being*. Being a 'person' is associated with normal conformity, routines and responsibilities, whereas being a 'human being' is associated with being wild and free. Restorative places are characterised by Dannie as wilder and freer than everyday places, where time has less relevance.

Nina also captures the essence of feeling free, reporting:

> **NINA, JOURNAL, STUDY 2**
>
> It's weird I've left all the stress and worry at home and I'm enjoying myself and feeling a hell of a lot better already! I'm just having fun and being myself which is great I can finally breathe, I'm free!

Feeling a sense of freedom for Alex was similarly strong and was one of the main motivations for her own personal walking and wild camping trips to the Scottish Highlands after the studies. Here she explains how multi-faceted the experience of freedom was:

> **ALEX, POST-EXPERIENCE INTERVIEW, STUDY 1**
>
> I: would you partake in the wilderness programme again?
> A: oh yeah now yeah come on [laughter] [. . .] because it was fantastic it was just that freeing that (.) that freedom I felt and that peace of mind (2)

> just everything [. . .] it's like when I was there and it's totally given me a different light (.) and I've been reading a few spiritual books (.) especially just recently (.) and (2) it's like when (.) when I was there I didn't actually feel like I was in a body if you (.) it wasn't an out-of-body experience or anything (.) it was just more like this is nature you know (.) and we are one basically [. . .] it is a really (.) really freeing really freeing you know and you get a real awareness of you [. . .] so (3) personal growth [. . .] and gaining confidence.

A sense of freedom here is associated with having a sense of tranquillity within and a spiritual/eco-centric perspective. Alex's passion about the feeling of freedom is clear from her emphasis on and repetition of *freeing* and *freedom*. Alex also explains that the wild place also promoted growth in self-awareness and confidence.

A sense of freedom and escape was not always easily attained during the WSE as Nina (journal, study 2) reports: "I found a nice spot in the middle of the stream to sit down. I tried to clear my mind but I was still thinking about things that needed to be done or what time it is." Trying to recreate the feeling of freedom at home was also hard as Alex explains, suggesting that wilder places have particular facilitative qualities:

ALEX, JOURNAL, STUDY 2

I've been trying to capture the feeling I get when out in the 'wild place', I've tried laying on the couch, with my windows open, in silence I've tried having a relaxing bath. But nothing is the same, nothing gives me that same feeling of freedom – which I believe comes from within, but out in the wild place I feel truly free.

Overall, wild places offer respite from responsibilities and foster calmness and happiness among participants. After the WSE Sam (post-experience interview, study 1) states how invigorating the experience was for her: "I was just so chilled out to a point I've never been before really (.) yeah I really felt quite invigorated from the experience" – an experience of de-stressing and recuperation that she remembers strongly nine months later:

SAM, FOLLOW-UP INTERVIEW, STUDY 1

E: is there anything in particular during the time of being alone (.) that seemed to make it important for you?
S: I think it was just time to chill for me and not (.) being sort of (.) being both a student and a mum and running a house I think it was really just

(continued)

> *(continued)*
>
> total time out for me when sometimes you can do something for yourself at home but it's probably an hour (.) you know if you go do something like tai-chi or go out on your bike it's a little snap shot and then you're back into that (2) whereas that (the WSE) was a longer period so it was really time to totally chill out.

Sam reports the pressures of family life and being a mother and how the solo experience offered her time out. Complete relaxation seemed to be afforded by the long duration of the solo, highlighted when Sam compared the solo experience to an hour of leisure activity.

As well as open space and slower sense of time, noticing nature, being still in nature and being by water helped foster participant experiences of calmness and sense of freedom within wild places. Participants (n = 9) became more aware of their surroundings and took greater interest in nature as time went on during the WSE which provided fascination and affected some participants' moods:

> **DANNIE, POST-EXPERIENCE INTERVIEW, STUDY 2**
>
> D: I started seeing little insects and weird things like I saw a big massive dragonfly that went under this big (.) fallen tree that looked like it were sort of man-made archway [. . .] definitely the surroundings and the different parts where we were affected my mood I think (2) it made me feel better.

> **SARAH, FOLLOW-UP INTERVIEW, STUDY 2**
>
> S: [. . .] it takes like it literally takes my seeing ducklings to be like (.) oh: yeah (.) like you don't have to do anything to be happy (.) you just have to notice what's already there.

During the WSE Dannie experienced back pain and his reflections about his change in mood when noticing nature illustrates natures influence on the way people feel. Noticing nature can also have more profound effects as Sarah highlights when she reports how it changed the way she thinks about life and happiness is more easily attainable than she thought, realising that valuing what you have can bring happiness. This appreciation occurred after the WSE in her home city, suggesting that the benefits of the WSE have the potential to be fostered in semi-natural or urban areas.

Participants (n = 7) predominantly noticed nature during the solo experience while being still, which also provided space and time to reflect and relax. Joe reports how he wanted to hold on to that experience of stillness in mind and in time, while also revealing the challenges of doing this with a competing sense of daily routine:

JOE, POST-EXPERIENCE INTERVIEW, STUDY 1

J: [. . .] there was a particular moment for me when I woke up in the morning on the 24-hour period and I just sat for ten mins in the tent just at the door of the tent eh just it was just sitting (2) I did this before everything that I (had) to engage in so just as I knew that this was going to last for maybe five or ten minutes and then once I had to move then everything else would have to start (.) the day would just unfold in its way [. . .] so it's that experience of that kind of stillness both in myself and in nature that kinda comes to mind.

The experience of *just sitting* was precious to Joe, alluded to by his reference to it as being a *particular moment*. Joe's certainty that being still in mind can only be short in duration implies a norm of routine and habit, and he regards movement as something that will disrupt or change the fragile 'moment' of calm.

For Sarah, it was not just the experience of being still that was profound for her but the realisation that she could experience stillness as she normally finds stillness very difficult to deal with. Sarah transforms this realisation into an empowering coping mechanism:

SARAH, POST-EXPERIENCE INTERVIEW, STUDY 2

S: I think what I'll really keep which is really lovely (.) is that that realisation that like (.) I have the potential to stand still (.) because I honestly don't do that ever [. . .] it's really a nice realisation (.) that like oh it is possible for me (.) because I just assumed it wasn't (.) [. . .] so it's nice that there's an outlet that I do feel dead calm (.) really good (.) because I think it's something to try and incorporate into my life (.) that will be really healthy (.) and that's really positive (.) I don't have that much (3) apart from friends and stuff in my life that (.) I enjoy (.) like pleasure activities and that's the hardest part like (.) if you are having a period of like mental ill health (.) is that that's the significant thing that everyone always asks like what can you do to make yourself feel better (.) and that's what I'm lacking (.) the thing that (2) that therapeutic thing that just makes you feel better (.) I don't really have one (.) so (2) yeah that's like (.) a massive thing for me (.) wee hee [laughs]

The profoundness of her realisation is accentuated by the level of detail in this extract. Being still in nature seemed to be a way in which Sarah could relax and be calm in mind as well as body, providing relief from mental ill health. Nature becomes her *outlet*, her *therapeutic thing* that she felt she was *lacking* in her life and as such is especially significant to her. The use of words like *potential, it is possible for me* and *I just assumed it wasn't* shows changes in her perspective, emphasising the transformative characteristic of this account.

For some participants (N = 4) being near water was a sensual and calming experience. Joe found that water provided an escape from troubling thoughts: "My day now draws to evening after spending the afternoon at the waterfall I feel refreshed and less troubled with thoughts" (Joe, journal, study 1). For Sarah, the memories of her experiences near water alleviate depressive thoughts:

SARAH, FOLLOW-UP INTERVIEW, STUDY 2

S: I think when you get used to functioning every day without being particularly happy like the (.) the most I expect out of life is just to not to be chronically unhappy and when those times (.) when you actually have real happiness and not just okay-ness that you really notice it (.) and I think that's when I almost got a bit like euphoric when I was in that stream and the same thing happened again when we found another stream (3) something about streams.

The feeling of happiness and euphoria she describes when she found streams during the WSE seemed to trigger a realisation in her that she could be a happy person rather than just a *functioning* person that only felt, and could feel, *okay-ness*. The realisation that she does not have to be content with 'not' feeling *chronically unhappy* is freeing and important to her, recollecting nine months after the WSE.

Finally, returning back home was not always easy (N = 7) and reports often also highlighted how much of an impact the WSE had on people's behaviour, thinking and sense of well-being. Joe reports attempts to try and maintain his sense of well-being in his journal, reflecting about the day he left the wild place, the first full day back in everyday life and then nine days after the end of his WSE:

JOE, JOURNAL, STUDY 1

18th/19th [. . .] Coming back I noticed smells more strongly such as perfume from passers-by and sense of well-being, it also struck me I had not even thought about what was happening in the news and when I did begin to watch it I just turn it off (not like me) I felt a bit more sensitive to the negative reports on it. I had some wine with my dinner but felt I did not really want it! (another not like me) Later I switched the TV off as I found the noise distracting and just sat in the silence and by candlelight. I still have a feeling of being connected to the outdoors for the moment . . .

20th Really feeling like getting back out there by myself, usual distractions alcohol, shops and TV seem little hollow at the moment! Feeling really chilled still and a little removed to my usual concerns [. . .] Did not have any alcohol last night, usually I would but felt my mind was still out doors, thinking of lying out on the heather star gazing, went to bed earlier as well, about the same time I had been over the past week whilst outdoors.

28th Still have a strong urge to head outdoors, it feels more comforting than ever before! I know that when I do go trekking again I will find it a cathartic experience. This was something I had forgotten from when I was younger and have now re-experienced as an adult.

Joe's journal entry builds up to his realisation about a *forgotten, cathartic* emotion that he had only experienced when he was *younger* describing going outdoors as *comforting*. Joe's connection to nature persists over a number of days after the study, demonstrated by his heightened senses and contributing to his *sense of well-being*; relinquishing everyday routines and habits seems to be an attempt to try and maintain the well-being and calm.

Maintaining a sense of calm and well-being after leaving the wild place was a challenge however, as Alex explains:

ALEX, JOURNAL, STUDY 2

Just walked into town and it felt really full – the atmosphere people everywhere – really annoying – and money – I don't need money in the wild place, but here everything stems from money. I think the whole wild experience – such as bills, money, food, even the toilet reminds me of why I used drugs in the first place. Trying to understand what's normal to people – I'd rather run away from it all – the busyness of towns [. . .] I just don't like the fullness, the hustle and bustle of this life – I felt a kind of freeness on drugs and no responsibilities, here today I feel responsibilities weighing me down and to experience the wild place was like feeling from the past – in a strange way.

Returning back to everyday life was an intense experience for Alex, alluded to by her lists and fragmented writing. The town reminded her of all the things she dislikes about society, particularly the weight of responsibilities and norms, and about how being a drug addict allowed her to relinquish herself of responsibilities and exist somewhat outside of society, which she finds freeing.

"I don't have to wear a mask": ruminating and worrying about what others think

Open space, lack of distractions and increased sense of time for some participants (N = 5) both facilitated and relieved them of unwanted ruminations and worrying thoughts. For most participants (n = 7) they were doing the WSE not to prove anything to anyone else but rather prove to themselves they can do it as Sam illustrates:

SAM, FOLLOW-UP INTERVIEW, STUDY 1

S: I was just doing it for me (.) not to prove (.) anything to anybody else (.) I think it was my own doing (.) and I think that was what was good for me cos it's just when you're always doing things for other people at home and putting other people first then it was kind of (.) that, it was good for me.

The WSE provided an opportunity for Sam to put herself first, which was a welcome change for Sam who has many responsibilities at home as a mother and a student. Participants, including Sam, could not always prevent their worrying and ruminating though.

Joe finds the start of the solo experience difficult to start with:

JOE, JOURNAL, STUDY ONE

18th/19th September
I found the morning of the 24hr difficult in the sense I had unwanted thoughts come up, and negative feelings from past and current stuff. This seemed to be tied in with my expectation of it being therapy it felt I put myself on road to experience these feelings and thought but what to do with them was the difficult thing, being out in the wilderness seemed to intensify the feelings as there seemed no distractions.

However, when I explored around my tent I came across a small waterfall, there I spent the rest of the day and as I did I let go of the idea of it all being therapy and tried to be just present in my surroundings, in the 'here and now'. When I did this the intensity of feelings lessened and I became more peaceful within myself.

Initially experiencing unwanted thoughts and feelings, Joe blames the lack of distractions and his preconceptions that the solo should be like *therapy* for this and looks to nature for consolation. He soon realises that focusing on the 'here and now' would be more beneficial for him. His ruminations impeded being in the present moment but shifting towards thinking about himself in nature rather than just himself, helped finally bring about peace within.

For Kit, the wild place helped her gain confidence, clarity and stop ruminating about what to do about her relationship with her family:

> **KIT, JOURNAL, STUDY 1**
>
> When I got back I was so happy and eager to do as much as I could in a day. I've not had such a positive mentality for so long to this extreme [. . .] Since the time away I've known exactly what I've wanted and needed to do with my current relationships, family and work, when before I was a little stuck. It's been absolutely amazing.

Kit reports her motivation and positivity after the WSE, finding that she is more confident about dealing with some issues that previously had been difficult for her. In other parts of her diary she discloses how much she cares and worries about what her family think of her. Kit is surprised about the intensity and duration of her feelings suggesting that it was perhaps an unexpected but special outcome to her.

Alex also explains the perspective, confidence and insights into herself that she gained as a consequence of time away in the wild place:

> **ALEX, POST-EXPERIENCE INTERVIEW, STUDY 1**
>
> A: it just really opened my mind you know (2) I can be on my own (2) can survive on my own [. . .] not one thought about using drugs which really really surprised me because in that situation at home you know I 'used' but since I've come back I haven't done anything I've been quite content being on my own at home [. . .] I just know that I want to reach the goals I want to reach (.) yeah (.) yeah more determined than ever [. . .] my confidence as well has gone up definitely erm mainly around doing things that I don't know (2) usually I like to change [. . .] I feel different I feel like I don't need others to help me strive for what I want usually I fix myself from other people [. . .] I'm aware of erm (2) what goes on around me influences me (.) you know (2.5) I was before but not to the extent that I am now (.) like the way people look at me (2) I think they can see me the way I used to be (.) and stuff like that [. . .] I'm more aware (.) cos I've never had that feeling before (.) never had that feeling that I'm not an addict (.) and I looked at that I thought oh my [laughter] you know (.) [laughter] why didn't I?

The WSE provided Alex with a realisation that she can *survive*, providing determination, motivation and *confidence* to reach her goals and do novel things. Though she knew how other people influenced her, the wild place – devoid mostly of everyday people that worried her – allowed her to relinquish her label as *addict*. The newness of this feeling made Alex question why she had not felt it before in other situations, making her consider how much people influenced the way she feels about and defines herself, also reiterated in her journal during second WSE (study 2):

ALEX, JOURNAL, STUDY 2

In the wild place I don't have to wear a mask – in the solo phase I can just be me – and I am so looking forward to it. [. . .] Oh it will be so good to get away from what's going on in the world, (pretend) it's not happening. I am so looking forward to not having to spend time making sure my hair's ok and not worrying about what my clothes look like, or what I look like. [. . .] Here there were no distractions, I won't get hurt from another person, I am safe in this place. I don't have to put on an act – a mask I can just be me with no distractions.

Alex conveys a desire to have distance from the world and escape to the wild place where she feels empowered and free, with the notable comments *I don't have to wear a mask* and *I can just be me*, evading worries about her appearance. In doing so, Alex describes the solo experience like a safe haven, explaining that it allows her to get away from *distractions* and pain other people cause her.

Discussion

It is clear that the findings support the large body of research that claims the benefits of being out in nature (e.g. Gladwell, Brown, Wood, Sandercock, & Barton, 2013; Keniger, Gaston, Irvine, & Fuller, 2013) and of Jungian approaches to eco-therapy (with landscape as a provider of challenge and instigator of change). The WSE, particularly open space, noticing nature, being still in nature and being by water, provided opportunities to reflect, de-stress and recuperate. Feelings of escaping life, pressures and responsibilities, heightened awareness and noticing nature contributed to the restorative benefits noted in several other recent studies. Being away from everyday pressures (Heintzman, 2006, 2009; Hinds, 2011), being somewhere with a sense of remoteness (Glaspell, Watson, Kneeshaw, & Pendergrast, 2003) and being in conditions of solitude and simplicity (Hinds, 2011; Nicholls, 2009) were similarly found to be important for restoration. Solo experiences were also reflective (Brookes, Wallace, & Williams, 2006; Hinds, 2011) promoted self-awareness (Kaplan, 1995) and led personal growth (Sklar, 2005). Participants' preferences for the length of solo varied, thus it is important to negotiate an appropriate time length with the participants, while also balancing it with the aim of the programme or experience.

Participants also benefitted from time away from everyday contexts with increased reports of embodied experiences. For example, two participants described their experiences of relinquishing their social 'masks' to just *be*, supporting findings that connection to nature fosters a positive body image (Hennigan, 2010). Recognising everyday influences and relinquishing these can lead to positive experiences during and after the WSE. This suggests that the transferability of benefits is possible (although not predictable or assured) since participants sought to re-experience aspects of the WSE in order to reduce anxiety (supported by Pearson & Smith, 1986), increase self-esteem (Barton & Pretty, 2010; Pretty et al., 2007) and enhance their well-being (Alcock, White, Wheeler, Fleming, & Depledge, 2014; Bragg, 2014).

Strengths and limitations

The findings provide insight into the ways certain aspects of the natural environment might impact upon the therapeutic relationship (e.g. the effect of the interaction with the landscape on emotion, perception and meaning-making) in outdoor therapies. Using multiple sources of information we created a rich and extensive dataset that enabled us to examine personal and socially reflective processes, nuance and complexity. Photos were also shared at the end of each WSE (a process greatly enjoyed by participants), which encouraged further recollection and reflection, showing that such a method may also enhance debriefing in other outdoor experiences, helping people share their experiences and potentially prolonging the benefits.

A more developmental and longitudinal approach, with exposure to more than one WSE, is needed however. Alex's data (participant in study 1 and 2) suggests that repeated supported experiences might enhance the positive effects of being in nature (e.g. increased confidence and sense of gaining competence) and a collaborative inquiry would be suitable to explore this further (Reason, 1995), including how different contexts and groups influence benefits. Further research could also lead to the development of guidelines and resources for effective reflection, application of phases (e.g. how best to transition between exploration, journey and solo phases, as well as entering and exiting the WSE landscape), and overall design that would be useful to training leaders or practitioners and inform services and service users.

Implications

Practical implications

There is a need for more creative and affordable ways to meet the needs of people experiencing mental health problems. The built environment is expanding and mental illness is increasing leading to strains on health provision. In the UK, only a quarter of people with a mental health problem receive ongoing treatment (Health and Social Care Information Centre, 2009). The total cost to the UK society is £70 to £100 billion each year in lost earnings, productivity and reduced quality of life (OECD, 2014) and therefore services need to be able to address the needs of many including 'hard to reach' groups like men, who may enjoy this more indirect and active approach to improving well-being and mental health.

For practitioners and 'decision makers', the current research highlights that this relatively simple approach to WSE is viable, affordable and beneficial to implement. Employing an unhurried approach to leadership with two main features – walking through and being with nature (i.e. the solo experience) – provided an enjoyable and enriching experience and opportunities to reflect, as found in other studies (Nicholls, 2009). Before embarking on using a similar design, practitioners or service staff need to be trained in outdoor leading or employ outdoor leaders who can be guided by staff expertise in working with specific groups of people. Generally though, due to its structural simplicity with no talking therapy per se, it is a feasible approach to implement in various contexts but also has the flexibility to be enhanced by complimentary therapeutic approaches.

Present findings also suggest a greater focus on the solo phase in structured outdoor experiences is beneficial and might be implemented on its own, without lengthy exploration and journey phases, in more accessible local greenspaces. Nicholls (2008) reports the benefit of self-initiated time alone, providing some support for this idea. Indeed, shorter solos in local greenspaces have been shown to be beneficial to people and foster a sense of well-being (Freeman, Robinson, & Harland, 2016). Having a place nearby that is more accessible to participants may mean more autonomy and control over when and length of time spent alone.

Establishing a good balance between group and solo elements is also important and an aspect to consider further due to the lack of consensus about the benefits of group approaches (Heintzman, 2008). The present study showed participants' fluxing attitudes towards being part of a group. Appropriate framing, group bonding and forming working agreements before a trip are advisable. Additionally, asking participants whether they prefer walking with the group or alone may reduce any unpleasant experiences. This may, however, compromise the positive aspects of challenge related to being part of a group. Indeed, there are studies that have found participants valued group elements highly, despite apprehensions (Revell et al., 2013).

Participants could also have more say in location, route choice and duration of experiences, giving them greater levels of control, which can be empowering and lead to greater and longer-lasting benefits (e.g. increased knowledge, confidence and competence may lead to greater accessing of natural environments and increased well-being), making structured experiences in nature more beneficial and sustainable. However, it needs to be remembered that people with little previous experience may feel overwhelmed by the choices and responsibilities. Also, the weekend study (2) was regarded as a less 'powerful' experience than the five-day consecutive study (1). Nevertheless, providing more training and shorter experiences before and after a WSE may be effective in making the benefits more sustainable and transferable.

Political and policy implications

In the UK there have been policy developments that could support nature-based initiatives, particularly around service-led and personalisation agendas. However, more evidence is needed rather than more policy; some policy exists but examples of implementing it in practice are needed. More established structured outdoor experiences, e.g. NHS walking schemes and green exercise programmes, still remain on the margins of environmental policy and public health (Barton, Bragg, Wood, & Pretty, 2016); and further evidence is needed about people's associations with aesthetic features of natural environments or their benefits (Cavill & Roberts, 2011). It is also important to safeguard these environments and make sure that outdoor programmes do not jeopardise these, since many of the benefits associated with them are likely to disappear if they are degraded. In order for natural environments to be protected, a more ecological or holistic approach in public health and environment policy is therefore required (Pretty, Griffin, Sellens, & Pretty, 2003). Furthermore, how the outdoor space is perceived, concerns for personal safety and ease of access to natural environments all influence usage (Gladwell et al., 2013).

Conclusion

These findings highlight that an eco-therapy approach (including modest activities of walking through and being within nature), in a programme designed to incorporate evidence collection, can alleviate stress, anxiety and symptoms of depression. Interactions between people and natural landscapes have been demonstrated to involve dynamic transitions and interactions happening within place, space and time and are intricately bound by cultural influences, providing useful insights into the processes that unfold during nature-based interventions and their meanings for participants. As a result, ways of using WSEs and applying the designs more widely within different communities and through services are suggested, with proposals for further research, practice and policy.

References

Akhurst, J. E. (2010). Exploring the nexus between wilderness and therapeutic experiences. *Implicit Religion*, *13*(3), 295–305.
Alcock, I., White, M., Wheeler, B., Fleming, L., & Depledge, M. (2014) Longitudinal effects on mental health of moving to greener and less green urban areas. *Environmental Science and Technology*, *48*(2), 1247–1255.
Baer, L. D., & Gesler, W. M. (2004). Reconsidering the concept of therapeutic landscapes in J. D. Salinger's *The Catcher in the Rye*. *Area*, *36*(4), 404–413.
Barton, J., Bragg, R., Wood, C., & Pretty, J. (2016). *Green exercise: Linking nature, health and wellbeing*. London: Earthscan.

Barton, J., & Pretty, J. (2010). What is the best dose of nature and green exercise for improving mental health? A multi-study analysis. *Environmental Science & Technology, 44*(10), 3947–3955.

Bragg, R. (2014). Nature-based interventions for mental wellbeing and sustainable behaviour: The potential for green care in the UK (Thesis submitted for the degree of Doctor of Philosophy in Environmental Sciences). University of Essex.

Braun, V., & Clarke, V. (2006). Using thematic analysis in psychology. *Qualitative Research in Psychology, 3*(2), 77–101.

Brooks, J. J., Wallace, G. N., & Williams, D. R. (2006). Place as relationship partner: An alternative metaphor for understanding the quality of visitor experience in a backcountry setting. *Leisure Sciences, 28*(4), 331–349.

Capra, F. (1982). *The turning point.* New York, NY: Simon & Schuster.

Cavill, N., & Roberts, K. (2011). *Sources of data for investigating the influence of the environment on physical activity and diet.* Oxford: National Obesity Observatory.

Chirot, D. (1993). *Social change in a peripheral society: The creation of a Balkan colony.* New York, NY: Academic Press.

Conn, S. (2006). *Ecotherapy and development.* New York, NY: McDonald Press.

Davis-Berman, J., & Berman, D. S. (1993). Therapeutic wilderness programs: Issues of professionalization in an emerging field. *Journal of Contemporary Psychotherapy, 23*(2), 127–134.

Freeman, E., & Akhurst, J. (2015). Rethinking notions of therapeutic landscapes: A case study exploring perceptions of a wild place experience (WPE). In C. L. Norton, H. Carpenter, & A. Pryor (Eds.), *Explorations: Adventure therapy around the globe, international perspectives and diverse approaches* (pp. 210–234). Champaign, IL: Common Ground Publishing.

Freeman, E., Akhurst, J., Bannigan, K., & James, H. (2016). Benefits of walking and solo experiences in UK wild places. *Health Promotion International, 32*(6), 1048–1105.

Freeman, E., Robinson, E., & Harland, K. (2016). Understanding the power of the 'solo'. In *Well-Being 2016: Third International Conference Exploring the Multi-Dimensions of Well-Being*, Birmingham City University, 5–6 September 2016.

Gesler, W. M. (1992). Therapeutic landscapes: Medical issues in light of the new cultural geography. *Social Science & Medicine, 34*(7), 735–746.

Gladwell, V. F., Brown, D. K., Wood, C., Sandercock, G. R., & Barton, J. L. (2013). The great outdoors: How a green exercise environment can benefit all. *Extreme Physiology & Medicine, 2*(3) Retrieved from www.extremephysiolmed.com/content/2/1/3.

Glaspell, B., Watson, A., Kneeshaw, K., & Pendergrast, D. (2003). Selecting indicators and understanding their role in wilderness experience stewardship at Gates of the Arctic National Park and Preserve. *George Wright Forum, 20*(3), 59–71.

The Health and Social Care Information Centre (2009). *Adult psychiatric morbidity in England.* Results of a household survey. London: Health and Social Care Information Centre.

Heintzman, P. (2006, April). Men's wilderness experience and spirituality: A qualitative study. In R. Burns & K. Robinson (Eds.), *Northeastern recreation research symposium* (pp. 216–225). Newtown Square, PA: US Department of Agriculture, Forest Service, Northern Research Station.

Heintzman, P. (2008). Men's wilderness experience and spirituality: Further explorations. In *Proceedings of the 2007 Northeastern Recreation Research Symposium* (pp. 55–59). Newtown Square, PA: US Department of Agriculture, Forest Service, Northern Research Station.

Hennigan, K. (2010). Therapeutic potential of time in nature: Implications for body image in women. *Ecopsychology, 2*(3), 135–140.

Hinds, J. (2011). Exploring the psychological rewards of a wilderness experience: An interpretive phenomenological analysis. *The Humanistic Psychologist, 39*, 189–205

Kaplan, S. (1995). The restorative benefits of nature: toward an integrative framework. *Journal of Environmental Psychology, 16*, 169–182.

Kelly, J. G. (1996). *Ecology constraints on mental health services*. Basingstoke: Palgrave Macmillan.

Keniger, L., Gaston, K. J., Irvine, K. N., & Fuller, R. A. (2013). What are the benefits of interacting with nature? *International Journal of Environmental Research and Public Health, 10*, 913–935.

McCallum, I. (2007). *Ecological intelligence: Rediscovering ourselves in nature*. Cape Town: Africa Geographic.

McGeeney, A. (2016). *With nature in mind: The ecotherapy manual for mental health professionals*. London: Jessica Kingsley.

Mental Health Foundation. (2014). Retrieved from www.mentalhealth.org.uk/help-information/mental-health-statistics/.

Natural England. (2016). A review of nature-based interventions for mental health care (NECR204). Retrieved from http://publications.naturalengland.org.uk/publication/4513819616346112.

Nicholls, V. E. (2008). Busy doing nothing: research the phenomenon of 'quiet time' in a challenge-based Wilderness Therapy (Unpublished thesis). Faculty of Education, University of Wollongong, New South Wales, Australia.

Nicholls, V. E. (2009). Quiet time: A sense of solitude. Outdoor education research and theory: Critical reflections, new directions. *Fourth International Outdoor Education Research Conference*, Beechworth, Victoria AU. Retrieved from www.latrobe.edu.au/education/downloads/2009_conference_nicholls.pdf.

OECD. (2014). Retrieved from www.oecd.org/els/emp/MentalHealthWork-United Kingdom-AssessmentRecommendations.pdf.

Pearson, M., & Smith, D. (1986). Debriefing in experience-based learning. *Simulation/Games For Learning, 16*(4), 155–172.

Pretty, J. N., Griffin, M., Sellens, M., & Pretty, C. (2003). *Green exercise: Complementary roles of nature exercise and diet in physical and emotional well-being and implications for public health policy* (CES Occasional Paper 2003-1). University of Essex, UK.

Pretty, J. N., Peacock, J., Hine, R., Sellens, M., South, N., & Griffin, M. (2007). Green exercise in the UK countryside: Effects on health and psychological well-being, and implications for policy and planning. *Journal of Environmental Planning and Management, 50*(2), 211–231.

Reason, P. (1995). *Participation in human inquiry*. London: Sage.

Revell, S., Duncan, E., & Copper, M. (2013). Helpful aspects of outdoor therapy experiences: An online preliminary investigation. *Counselling and Psychotherapy Research*. Retrieved from: http://dx.doi.org/10.1080/14733145.2013.818159.

Russell, K. C., & Farnum, J. (2004). A concurrent model of the wilderness therapy process. *Journal of Adventure Education and Outdoor Learning, 4*(1), 39–55.

Sklar, S. L. (2005). Positive youth development: The case of a wilderness challenge intervention (Doctoral dissertation). University of Florida.

Tuan, Y. F. (1977). *Space and place: The perspective of experience*. Minneapolis, MN: University of Minnesota Press.

PART III
Interventions in space and place

14

GEEDKA SHIRKA (UNDER THE TREE)

Cultural, migratory and community spaces for preventative interventions with Somali men and their families

Amira Hassan, Iyabo Fatimilehin and Carolyn Kagan

Introduction

In this chapter we will report on the use of cultural, migratory and community spaces in working on a long-term, community-based, preventative action research mental health project, undertaken with Somali men of different generations, living in Liverpool, UK.

We take a complex and multi-layered approach to the concepts of space and place, moving beyond the physical features of a location to the meaning it has and the way this meaning is represented. In this, we are drawing on interdisciplinary space-place studies, in particular, critical geography, cultural studies and post-colonial studies (see Giesling, Mangold, Katz, Low, & Saegert, 2014), most specifically derived from the works of Harvey and Lefebvre. Our chapter concerns different generations of migrants to the UK and embraces the ways in which local and translocal spaces are understood and negotiated. Indeed, the core of the intergenerational tensions and their resolution that we discuss below can be understood in terms of both the spatial imagination of both generations (the meanings attached to space and place here and now) and the spatial imaginaries they hold (the values, institutions, laws and symbols of the place called Somalia, both held in the imagination and transposed to the new location, Liverpool). The spaces and places that permeate the project we discuss are inextricably bound to identity: we take the view that people are both shaped by and shape the places they inhabit and move through. Harvey (2005) argues that spaces are socially produced: whereas absolute space refers to bounded territories with a strong degree of permanency, relational space-time refers to the ways in which spatial meaning comes through the memories and attachments we forge through relationships.

We will outline the different action research cycles and will highlight the central place held in the project of intergenerational storytelling sessions, essentially exploring different spatial imaginations, accompanied by a meal in locations not normally frequented. These facilitated storytelling sessions drew on narrative and community psychological approaches. Both storytelling and the sharing of food resonated with the traditions of Somali culture that had translocated from Somalia to Liverpool. We discuss the project in terms of the role of participation, the creation of 'third places' and new social settings.

Somali culture

The Somali community is, of course, not homogenous. Nevertheless, across class, clan, predicament and geography, some commonalities generally hold in what we can call the spatial imaginary, reproduced strongly by the older generation and felt by the younger generation. In Somali culture, the family is the most important unit of society and collectively takes precedence over its individual members. The traditional Somali family is characterised by a sense of unity based on shared language, traditional values and Islamic teachings that provide the moral framework governing behaviour and rules within the family. In Somalia, family roles are well defined with the father being at the top of the hierarchy and responsible for providing financial security. Mothers are responsible for all work in the home including cooking, cleaning and raising the children. These responsibilities are often undertaken communally and this is reflected in the pooling of resources. Many children are expected to show unquestioning respect to their elders and a certain degree of corporal punishment is an acceptable form of discipline. The communal aspect of Somali culture also means that children will be regarded as the responsibility of the whole community with any adult having the right to speak to any child about their behaviour (Harris, 2004). In Liverpool 8, the Somali families we worked with reproduced a translocated Somali way of life – fulfilling their everyday needs and activities in the local area, interacting by and large only with other Somali migrants. The older generation had created a boundaried space in which their identities were inextricably tied up with the place in which they lived and the spatial imaginary of 'Somalia'. Younger family members crossed the boundaries of space and identity.

Migration, space and place

Migration is one of the most radical transition and life-changing experiences that a family can face. As Watters (2011) says, migration is marked by both fixity and continuities in space, as well as being a transformative process. Liebscher and Dailey-O'Cain (2013, p. 17) stated that:

> In migration, there is always a change of location from one place to another, so the concept of place is always imminent. When migrants move from one place to another, they bring concepts; ideas and habitual practices associated with their *place of origin* . . . with them, and then proceed to work with these concepts, ideas and practices in some way in the new *place of living* . . . Some

may try to repress this place of origin and some may try to recreate it, while still others may do both at different times, but it is present either way. The ways in which immigrants 'work with' their place of origin have consequences for them individually, of course, but these also have consequences for the social spaces they construct in the new place of living. Through the use of grammatical and interactional linguistic resources in the practice known as *positioning*, people describe themselves as being either inside or outside of spaces, or in the middle or at the edges of them. They can do this because positioning makes use of *indexical meanings*, or semiotic links to linguistic forms. But since the indexicality between a space and a place is much more remote in a situation of migration, and because spaces do not have the same sort of solidity of material form that places do, immigrant groups need to constantly continue to construct their group's space in the new place of living in order to maintain it. (Emphasis in original)

Migration and mental health

Migration is an inherently stressful process with specific risk factors that can lead to increased vulnerability to mental health difficulties. Once uprooted from their culture, migrants may suffer a sense of loss, particularly in the case of forced migration: loss of home; separation from family and community; loss of a job, position in society and the resulting identity loss; loss of support networks; and an uncertain future for the individual or the family. When settled in host communities, a variety of factors may increase psychosocial vulnerability, such as cultural differences, racism and unemployment. Language barriers further hinder communication and can lead to isolation and feelings of helplessness (Greeff & Holtzcamp, 2007).

One of the major psychosocial changes experienced by immigrants is acculturation, which is the process of cultural change and psychological change that results following meeting between cultures. Within immigrant families there are different speeds of acculturation. Parents and adults have reached maturity in their culture of origin, may have difficulty learning a new language and be slow to adapt. They typically have less contact with the larger society than do their children, and tend to maintain traditional collectivist values. As a result, an acculturation gap develops between the generations, particularly notable in those families whose heritage-culture holds collectivist values as opposed to the individualistic ones of the receiver-culture.

The acculturation gap may intensify the common parent–child conflicts that occur in families with adolescents and heighten intergenerational conflict. As immigrant children in the UK acculturate and English becomes their preferred language, protective family ties and effective parental communication and monitoring can erode. In families where the parents rely on the youth for communication in English dependency roles may be reversed. This role reversal could jeopardise the parent–child relationship.

Living with these tensions can affect family functioning and the mental health of family members. Maintaining communications within the family is one way of strengthening family resilience, and it is in this arena that the importance of the project can be understood.

The Fathers and Sons Project

This was a community psychological, action research project, which can be described in three stages or cycles, each building on and learning from the other: (a) consultation and strengths-needs assessment; (b) narrative meal-based events and follow-up initiatives; (c) cross-generational learning and activities.

We were each positioned differently in relation to the project. Amira and Iyabo worked in Building Bridges, a specialist child and adolescent mental health service within Alder Hey Children's NHS Foundation Trust, with an ethos of prevention, working in partnership and with the strengths of communities using community psychology approaches and principles (Fatimilehin, 2007). Amira designed and carried out the project and Iyabo contributed to the interventions, managed and supervised the work and supported Amira. Carolyn acted as critical friend from a university base and supervised a linked research student.

Cycle 1: consultation and strengths-needs assessment

In 2002 a community counselling and mental health promotion framework was used by Amira to work with adults in the Somali community. Because the older Somali generation lived out most of their lives in Liverpool 8 it is important to note that Amira went to the families, to their spaces, rather than asking them to come to the Building Bridges offices. Discussions with the women in the Somali community suggested a breakdown in family relationships, which was having an impact on psychological well-being in some sections of the community. The women were particularly concerned about intergenerational conflict between fathers and sons and asked us if we could address the difficulties. These issues were also evident in our therapeutic work with individual families.

In 2003, Building Bridges developed a meal-based consultative event in collaboration with women from the Somali community and with local agencies. Both fathers and sons were involved in its planning and implementation. The aims of this event were to raise awareness of the impact of living between two cultures and promote dialogue between fathers and sons in the Somali community. Participants indicated that the event had met its aims, and proposed a number of other ideas for initiatives that would further communication between younger and older generations. A video of this event was produced as a resource for promoting dialogue in the Somali community.

Cycle 2: narrative meal-based events and follow-up initiatives

In 2006 we built on this consultation and continued the work with the Somali community, with funding from the Parenting Fund.

We used a narrative and participative approach (Denborough, 2010; Denborough et al., 2006). We chose this because it is a respectful, non-blaming approach, which positions people as the experts in their own lives. It views concerns as separate from people and assumes people have many strengths – skills, competencies, beliefs, values, commitments and abilities – that will assist them to change their relationship with concerns in their lives. This mirrored the values and ethos of Building Bridges and is to be contrasted with the more usual pathology-based approach, which highlights people's and communities' deficiencies thereby making it harder for people to bring about positive change. Furthermore, storytelling is a traditional art in Somalia, and people gather around the fire at night to share anecdotes about values, fears, beliefs and heroism that have been passed from one generation to the next.

The aims and objectives of this cycle were to:

- help fathers and sons understand the impact of living between two cultures on their relationship and appreciate the situation from each other's perspective;
- provide opportunities for fathers and sons to come together and promote dialogue between them;
- maximise family functioning.

The project was underpinned by strong partnerships. The Liverpool Arabic Centre (LAC) was the major partner in making the application. A consortium of a wide range of local voluntary, statutory and community stakeholders formed an advisory group from the start. The partnership with the Research Institute for Health and Social Change (Manchester Metropolitan University) enabled us to appoint a research student to undertake a participative action research evaluation, and we employed an assistant psychologist to deliver a quantitative evaluation.

This cycle of the project had three phases: consultations and development of narratives; the meal event; and development and delivery of initiatives.

Consultation and development of narratives

A total of 12 Somali fathers and 12 sons were recruited through the Somali umbrella group or via our links with the Somali community. Weekly consultations took place in separate groups over a period of three months. The groups were co-facilitated by Building Bridges staff and a middle-generation Somali, who was a father and a son and had good relationships with the older and the younger generations. This co-facilitator also acted as interpreter for the fathers' group as many fathers did not speak English. The sons' groups was run in English.

Each consultation group was asked about (a) their worries and concerns about living in this country and how this affects their relationships with each other as well as their parenting skills and status; and (b) how they thought the situation could be improved in terms of help to retain parenting skills, bridging the gap between fathers and sons and what it would take for both fathers and sons to make the situation better.

Project workers worked in collaboration with members of the community to identify places, outside the usual community or professional places, in which to hold the workshops. They then worked collaboratively with the fathers and sons to develop composite narratives. They drew on the group discussions and their own experiences to produce 'concern' and 'solution' narratives. In total, four fictional narratives were developed: two contained themes regarding the worries of fathers and of sons; and two contained ideas from fathers and from sons about how to improve the relationship between them. The fathers and sons were not aware of each other's stories, and the narratives were developed and written in both English and Somali.

Somali fathers' 'concerns' narrative (abridged)

Al salamu alaykum, my name is Mohammed and I am 45 years old. I came to Britain in 1993 after the civil war broke out in Somalia. I have a brother already in Liverpool so I came to him. I brought my wife Anab and my five young children with me . . . I used to be a skilled carpenter in my village back home, which enabled me to support my immediate family – my mother, my sister and her children. One of my sister's daughters got married last month and I have to support my sister by sending large amounts of money for the wedding and for clothes and presents – I am expected to do this because I live in England . . . Since we have been here, I have become frustrated because I can't find work – any kind of work at all . . . Some men feel that they are losing their status as fathers and as breadwinners because the family depends on government benefits and not them. This can cause fighting and then the family ends up splitting up or the husband wants to avoid the fighting and arguing and ends up staying out and chewing khat all night . . . I also worry about my children and how they are going to grow up here. Whether they will get a good education and find jobs or whether they'll follow the ways of other children in this country. Will they be good Muslims and will they respect their elders?

Somali fathers' 'solutions' narrative (abridged)

We love our sons, and we want to see them being successful, educated and happy living in this country. They are our future, and we want what is best for them without losing any of their heritage and culture. We would like the opportunity to talk with our sons, and listen to what they have to say too . . . We feel that social services sometimes come between us and our children because of their lack of knowledge about our traditions and culture. It would be helpful to us if social services knew more about our culture. This could be done by organising awareness days run by us and our sons . . . We think having parenting gatherings or groups will make us realise that we are all dealing with similar issues and hence unite the community and bridge the gap between fathers and sons . . . We think having a community centre where families can come together as one unit so it will promote closeness and family togetherness, rather than having only women or men centres.

Somali sons' 'concerns' narrative (abridged)

Salaam Alekum, my name is Ali, and I am 22 years old. I came to this country when I was 13 years old, with my mother, father, two brothers and two sisters . . . Liverpool was very strange to me. I went to school but I did not understand the lessons, and there was no one to help me. In the canteen, I always sat by myself. There were other Somali boys in the school but their English was better and they laughed at me when I tried to speak English . . . One of my brothers is now 14 years old and is doing well in school. But he has problems because he is always quarrelling with my father. He wants to go out to the youth club with his English friends but my father is worried about what they will be doing there.

Somali sons' 'solutions' narrative (abridged)

We know there is a big difference between the culture our fathers were raised in, and this culture we are growing up in. Therefore we understand our fathers' stresses and worries. We sometimes feel our fathers do not appreciate how difficult it is for us. It would be nice for our fathers to tell us traditional Somali stories that can also teach us about Somali morals. We think it would be a great idea to make a book of these Somali tales, and of life in Somalia. The stories can be told by our fathers and we could do the writing. We need to know about our history and heritage; it will give us a sense of belonging, pride and identity . . . We would like to tell them stories about life for us in Liverpool and our concerns for our parents' health and well-being. We worry about our fathers chewing khat and us not being able to spend time with them. We do not have many opportunities to share our ideas and feelings with our fathers. For this to happen we need to have more communication with our fathers, which means we both need to listen to and make time for each other.

The meal-based narrative event

After the narratives had been prepared, the meal event, designed in close collaboration with fathers and sons, took place. The event was centred on the telling and sharing of the narratives. It involved the use of facilitators and a team of reflective listeners. The facilitators were community members, professionals and community workers. All the community members were male and were fathers and sons who had attended the consultation groups. The professionals consisted of psychologists, social workers and community workers who were employed by Building Bridges and local services. In addition, there were workers from local Somali community organisations.

The team of reflective listeners consisted of a group of professionals as well as fathers and sons from the community. Their role was to note carefully the important knowledge and skills spoken about by the people at the event. Both the professionals and community members were trained in the Outsider Witness framework (White, 2000). The Outsider Witness is a process in which people who know about or have experience of a particular concern are invited first of all to listen and then to talk about what resonates for them when they hear about the concern. Following this, the people who brought the concern reflect on what they have just heard and what new perspectives it has given them. The key to the whole experience is resonance with the person's hopes, values, dreams, strengths, coping strategies, positive qualities and skills. The idea is to minimise the concern story yet respectfully draw attention to the alternative story (for example, how has the community got through this? What values have helped? Where did these values come from?).

Some 28 fathers and 18 sons attended the event. The mean age of fathers was 55 years and that of sons was 19 years. The two concern narratives were read by a father and a son to the whole group at the beginning of the day. This was followed by small group discussions in which groups of fathers discussed the sons' narrative and groups of sons discussed the fathers' narrative. Each group had a facilitator who acted as an interpreter and took notes, as well as being a reflective listener. The following questions were asked and discussed in each group:

1. As you heard the stories being read by the father/son, what caught your attention?
2. How is it to be a Somali son/father living in Liverpool?

Following this, a father and a son read the two solutions narratives and addressed the following questions in small group discussion in the same way as they did with the concerns narratives:

1. What caught your attention as you heard these second stories being read by the father and the son?
2. What did you discover as you were listening to these stories (the fathers' story and the sons' story)?
3. What solutions can our group come up with?

At the end of the discussions, the reflective listeners gave feedback, which focused on special knowledge and problem-solving skills that were heard from fathers and sons, and what resonated with them. Finally, the fathers and sons commented on what they thought were the most important messages that they had received from the reflective team.

'Concern' narratives and reactions

Sons responded to the fathers' concern narrative by highlighting fathers' loss of economic and family status, and the identification of cultural issues such as responsibilities for family members in Somalia and expectations of respectful behaviour towards fathers. There were negative comments about the fathers spending too much time playing cards or chewing khat. One significant theme related to discussions about the reasons for 'family breakdown', including different child-rearing practices such as the use of physical punishment, unemployment and excessive amounts of time spent out of the home chewing khat. The sons expressed a range of emotions regarding the fathers' narrative, from sympathy regarding the high expectations of fathers to sadness about the issues that fathers face.

The fathers responded to the sons' concern narrative by discussing and acknowledging the universality of generation gaps between fathers and sons and said that this is evident in all nationalities. However, they also talked about the importance of changing their expectations of their sons due to the different cultural context in which they are being raised. The fathers expressed an interest in gaining a better understanding of their sons' experiences but also wanted them to retain aspects of their religion and culture as Somalis and Muslims. Fathers also identified racial discrimination as a factor that affected their aspirations negatively and talked of cultural issues such as responsibilities for family members in Somalia and expectations of respectful behaviour towards fathers.

Solution narratives and reactions

The sons endorsed many of the ideas in the fathers' solutions narrative. They agreed with many of the suggestions put forward, including the development of a community centre for both men and women, the potential for community members to train social care service staff and the possibility of learning from fathers about their lives in Somalia. They felt that they could talk to their fathers about the effect of khat on the family and stories about how they experience life in England. The sons also suggested joint activities with fathers such as playing football. However, the sons expressed some reservations about parenting programmes for fathers and were concerned that this could lead to gossip and negative stories circulating in the community about individuals or families.

The fathers responded to the sons' solutions narrative by acknowledging the importance of spending time talking with their children and sons. They expressed sadness and remorse that chewing khat reduced the opportunity to spend time with the family. However, they were happy that their sons were concerned about the negative experiences that they had had, and that the sons want to know more about their history and culture. They liked the idea of producing a book and sharing their childhood games and memories.

Feedback from the reflective listeners

The points made by the reflective listeners included the difficulty of the journey (physically and psychologically) for fathers, the importance of hearing concerns in order to identify solutions, shared feelings of exclusion, the fundamental difference between being a father in Somalia and in the UK, fathers' pride in their sons' feelings, finding the balance between culture and relationship building and the ability to learn from each other in a culturally acceptable way.

Following the event, we met with the fathers' and sons' consultation groups for a review of the event and to identify some initiatives that would improve the relationship between fathers and sons. The consultation groups then became working groups to support and develop the initiatives. The initiatives they chose were (for fathers) a forum for talking about issues to do with parenting, and (for sons) the production of a magazine about Somali culture and heritage.

Again, through consultation, a broad range of parenting sessions were planned over a three-month period, and included the impact of life in Britain (including racism) on the psychological well-being of parents; knowledge of British customs and way of life and how this affects Somali teenagers, relationships between teenagers and parents and difficulties dealing with social services.

The Somali sons worked on both the content and technical aspects of producing a high-quality magazine, interviewing parents for stories of life in Somalia and Britain and including their own commentaries on life. Their final product was called *Geedka Shirka*, which means 'under the tree', a reference to the outdoor storytelling traditions in Somalia. For both these series of workshops professionals and other 'experts' were brought out of their institutional spaces into community spaces, thereby contributing to the changing meanings and understandings of those situations.

Dissemination event

An important part of the process of the project was its wider dissemination, enabling more people to benefit from the insights gained and lessons learnt from the initiatives. A large event, attended by families, community representatives and professionals took place. Fathers talked of their experiences in the parenting discussion groups and sons talked of their experiences making the film and producing the magazine. Both talked of how the activities had forged bridges between the two generations. The film was shown and the magazine circulated. By the end of the dissemination event a working group had been formed of different stakeholders (including men and women, young and older from the community) to develop ongoing activities and seek further funding for initiatives.

Cycle 3: cross-generational learning and activities

Further funding was obtained from the Parenting Fund by the Liverpool Arabic Centre in 2009, to build on the narrative- and action-oriented second stage of the project discussed above. The aims were the same as those described in Cycle 2.

Some sessions in the Mosque were set up for the fathers, enabling discussion with a prominent Imam on guidance on how to raise children in the West. Similar sessions were arranged for the sons. Both groups found the sessions useful and informative and thought there should be more sessions like these, possibly including mothers and daughters in the discussions. As a result of the feedback from the sessions a learning tool was developed in the form of a DVD, sharing advice to fathers and sons from the Imam on how to raise sons in a Western context, as well as guiding sons on how to respect fathers.

Three well-attended storytelling sessions took place where the khat sessions were held at the weekends. Further cultural sharing activities were introduced. Somali sons had said they wanted to learn a traditional game from the fathers. The sons and project workers collaboratively designed and produced Shax, a chess like game that is traditionally played in the sand, but produced here as a board game. These storytelling and games sessions all had the effect of enabling both fathers and sons to learn more about their cultures and to learn from each other. Fathers reported an increased sense of pride and of feeling valued again as they were able to share their knowledge. Sons expressed feeling more connected with their pasts and their culture. What in effect was happening through these activities was the emergence of cultural hybridity – something new arising from negotiation of spatial meaning and cultural representation. Homi Bhabha suggests that "the importance of hybridity is not to be able to trace two original moments from which the third emerges, rather hybridity is to me the 'third space' which enables other positions to emerge" (Rutherford, 1998, p. 211). These shared activities also helped improve communications within families, creating bonds, listening, respecting and valuing each others' experiences. Relationships were built through the shared activities.

A further dissemination event was held that enabled information and innovative practice to be shared across organisations. It was agreed that the learning tools and other products from the project would be available from the Liverpool Arabic Centre, for wider community and professional use.

Discussion

This project aimed to improve relationships between Somali fathers and sons. These relationships had been strained by migration and an acculturation gap, which meant that tensions had developed within families that were affecting family functioning and the well-being of family members. The project worked to normalise these experiences and externalise them, thus reducing any sense of blame or pathology. Furthermore, it encouraged fathers and sons to think about their concerns as collective rather than individual experiences. The project also highlighted the skills that fathers already possessed and enabled them to deploy them in a different cultural context. Evaluations of the parenting sessions with fathers showed an increase in the reported frequency and duration of talking to their sons, and described a wider range of topics (e.g. relationships, sports, local and world events) than they did previously (e.g. culture, religion, language, Islam, sons' behaviour). In addition, there were more reports of fathers attending the mosque with their sons. Fathers who contributed to storytelling sessions reported feeling valued by the younger generation and proud that they were interested in their history and heritage. Sons reported feeling closer to their fathers and being respected, which in turn increased their confidence to approach the older generation. Thus there were clear improvements in family functioning and an enhanced sense of well-being for both fathers and sons who participated in the project.

Participation in this kind of project is multi-layered and underpinned by the extensive relationship building, not only with members of the different communities, but also with relevant agencies, undertaken by Amira and Building Bridges. This groundwork enabled Amira to engage with families and to gain the trust and secure the involvement of men of different generations. Not everyone participated, and of those who did, not all participated in every stage of the project. This is the nature of participation: it is fuzzy and people move in and out of active involvement. However, the different activities, coupled with the dissemination events, enabled many more people to participate in one way or another throughout the project. Even though the work was directed at younger and older men, women took part in family discussions and dissemination events, which also functioned as learning events for professionals. Considerable effort was made in this project to support those participating. It was this active contact and support that enabled men of both generations to continue their involvement.

Building Bridges was based in the community and worked with people within their 'natural' settings (e.g. community centres, khat chewing sessions). Our location also meant that we could be flexible about timing and be available when community members were ready. The narrative meal events and subsequent activities, all enabled men from different generations, members of the wider communities and workers in relevant agencies to come together in new ways. Not only did they come together in community venues, but the structure of the work around narratives and activities building on these narratives enabled them to relate to each other in new ways. Through holding sessions in negotiated places, outside community and professional boundaries, the project facilitated the formation of 'third spaces' – locations used for new purposes, and the negotiation of different spatial imaginations. As Soja (2009) suggests, 'third space' is a transcendent concept that enables the contestation and re-negotiation of boundaries and cultural identities. Another way of thinking about how places were transposed to be sites of identity negotiation, is to see the project as creating *new social settings* (Kagan, Burton, Duckett, Lawthom, & Siddiquee, 2011), which facilitated the sharing of both strengths and concerns and built skills, knowledge and understanding. The creation of new social settings involves complex negotiations and collaborations with different groups, agencies and stakeholders. It is the creation of new social settings and the negotiation of spatialised identities (Fine & Sirin, 2008) that makes this work community psychological. Rather than working with individuals and families, the work is targeted at community level – at the links between individuals and families, families and agencies, the different groups and agencies with each other. These complex webs of relationships underpin community psychological place-based, preventive mental health work.

Acknowledgements

We would like to thank the Somali men and women, Liverpool Arabic Centre, members of the advisory group, Building Bridges staff and Joanne Hilton, without whom the project would not have been possible.

References

Denborough, D. (2010). *Kite of life: From Intergenerational conflict to intergenerational alliance.* Adelaide: Dulwich Centre.
Denborough, D., Koolmatrie, C., Mununggirritj, D., Marika, D., Dhurrkay, W., & Yunupingu, M. (2006). A narrative approach to working with the skills and knowledge of communities. *International Journal of Narrative Therapy and Community Work, 2*, 19–51.
Fatimilehin, I. A. (2007). Building bridges in Liverpool: Delivering CAMHS to Black and minority ethnic children and their families. *Journal of Integrated Care, 15*(3), 7–16.
Fine, M., & Sirin, S. (2008). Negotiating the Muslim American hyphen: Integrated, parallel and conflictual paths. In S. R. Sirin & M. Fine (Eds.), *Muslim American youth: Understanding hyphenated identities through multiple methods* (pp. 121–150). New York, NY: New York University Press.
Giesling, J., Mangold, W., Katz, C., Low, S., & Saegert, S. (Eds.). (2014). *The people, place and space reader*. London: Routledge.
Greeff, A. P., & Holtzkamp, J. (2007). The prevalence of resilience in migrant families. *Family & Community Health, 30*, 189–200.
Harris, H. (2004). *The Somali community in the UK: What we know and how we know it: The Information Centre about Asylum and Refugees in the UK (ICAR)* London. Retrieved from http://icar.livingrefugeearchive.org/somalicommunityreport.pdf.
Harvey, D. (2005). The sociological and geographical imaginations. *International Journal of Politics, Culture & Society, 18*(3/4), 211–255.
Kagan, C., Burton, M., Duckett, P., Lawthom, R., & Siddiquee, A. (2011). *Critical community psychology*. Chichester, UK: Wiley-Blackwell.
Liebscher, G., & Dailey-O'Cain, J. (2013). *Language, space and identity in migration*. Basingstoke: Palgrave Macmillan.
Rutherford, J. (1998). The third space: Interview with Homi Bhabha. In J. Rutherford (Ed.), *Identity, community, culture, difference* (pp. 207–221). London: Lawrence & Wishart.
Soja, E. W. (2009). The city and social justice. *Space and Justice, 1*, 1–5.
Watters, J. (2011). Migrant networkscapes: Spatialising accounts of migrants' social practices. *Translocations: Migrants and Social Change, 7*(2). E-journal. Retrieved from www.translocations.ie/docs/v07i01/Vol%207%20Issue%201%20-%20Peer%20Review%20-%20Migrant%20Networkscapes,%20Watters.pdf.
White, M. (2000). *Narrative means to therapeutic ends: Maps of narrative practice*. Adelaide: Dulwich Center.

15

TEA IN THE POT, 'THIRD PLACE' OR 'SOCIAL PRESCRIPTION'?

Exploring the positive impact on mental health of a voluntary women's group in Glasgow

Maria Feeney

Introduction

Tea in the Pot (hereafter TITP) voluntary women's group in Govan, Glasgow provides a safe place for women to meet in which they can enjoy the company of other women while developing new skills should they wish. Set within the context of place-based literature, place is here to be understood in terms provided to us by Creswell when he argues that 'places provides the conditions of possibility for creative social practice' (2004, p. 39). Related to this perspective on place, TITP can be regarded as what Oldenburg (1989) refers to as a 'third place'. Simply put, third places are places away from home (the 'first place') and work (the 'second place') where people can come together and socialise. More fully reflecting the key characteristics of third place, as identified by Oldenburg, members report that attending the group helps to alleviate feelings of isolation and loneliness, builds confidence and a sense of belonging, and connects them to their wider community. However, the growing use of the group by statutory services and the third sector to provide what some groups have referred to as a 'social prescription', particularly in the area of mental health, has raised concerns and particular challenges for all who benefit from the informal and safe environment that Tea in the Pot currently provides. In addition volunteers and referring bodies alike do not have any clear and agreed understanding of what social prescribing is and this has led to confusion and even contradiction in some instances. In the literature, an 'ideal type' of social prescription can be described as "a *formal* means of enabling primary care services to refer patients with social, emotional or practical needs to a range of non-clinical services, and provide a framework for developing alternative responses to meet needs" (Brandling & House, 2007, p. 3, my emphasis).

There is, however, no single definition of what constitutes a social prescription and in some cases the term is used interchangeably with 'social intervention'

(Kimberlee: 2015). For Friedli and Watson, (2004) social prescribing is beneficial in three key areas: improving the mental health outcomes of recipients, improving community well-being and reducing social exclusion. These potential benefits, however, may be dependent on the type of social prescription available to individuals. Drawing on empirical evidence collated from focus groups and individual interviews with group members and referring bodies, this chapter explores the role played by the group in the lives of members with a focus on the mental health benefits that attending the group has provided. It clearly shows that those who use and run the group very much identify with the view that TITP provides a third place experience for all who use it rather than a social prescription although elements of one can be seen in the other in some places.

TITP began after a local lone parent completed a six-month 'Regender' project run and funded by Oxfam. Following initial meetings in December 2004, TITP was formally constituted on 22 July 2005. In 2007 the group was granted charitable status. From its inception, TITP have been keen to emphasise that they are an informal group at which women can meet without being, or continuing to be, involved with statutory services. The group meets twice weekly and women of varying ages and backgrounds attend. Some women come because they feel lonely and isolated, many have or have had mental health problems, others have experienced abuse, but all come because TITP provides a safe space for women to meet and enjoy each other's company and build their skill set should they wish. Employing the concept of 'third place' (Oldenburg 1989), this chapter will first examine the role played by TITP and the impact it has had and continues to have on the lives of its members and the wider community. It will then go on to explore the way in which statutory and third sector organisations utilise the services provided by TITP and determine whether or not the group is providing a 'social prescription' or indeed whether it should go down that route.

In his thesis on place, Oldenburg (1989) argues that to lead a more fulfilled life, individuals should have access to places away from the 'first place' (home) and the 'second place' (work), in which they can interact with people other than family or colleagues. In his analysis, Oldenburg identifies eight key features that should be found in an ideal-type third place. They should be: (1) neutral; (2) non-hierarchical; (3) interactive; (4) accessible and accommodating; (5) welcoming; (6) ordinary; (7) sociable; and (8) comfortable. For Oldenburg, such places are particularly beneficial to the elderly and those on fixed incomes.

Oldenburg's argument is that the process of urban change in the post-war period (urban clearances, deindustrialisation, decline of high streets and rise of out of town shopping malls, etc.), meant a sharp decline in the number of accessible third places. Although Oldenburg was writing about the United States, these kind of processes were particularly marked in the city of Glasgow and especially in working-class communities like Govan, which was devastated by deindustrialisation and has never recovered either economically or socially. Therefore, Oldenburg's arguments can be seen as particularly relevant to the community served by TITP.

Utilising Oldenburg's concept to examine the use of third places more widely, it has been argued that, in the commercial setting, some restaurants and 'service places' can be considered to be third places especially for the elderly. Commentators have argued that such places can meet the needs of older patrons by providing socio-emotional support, encourage social interaction, combat feelings of isolation and loneliness, bring about a sense of empowerment, increase feelings of self-worth and can become like a 'home away from home' (Cheang, 2002; Meshram, & O' Cass, 2013; Rosenbaum, 2006, 2009). In the non-commercial setting, Oldenburg's concept has also been adapted to demonstrate that not-for-profit organisations dealing with individuals with cancer, can provide the 'third place experience', As with commercial third places, members have reported the benefits of social interaction, which helps to reduce loneliness and isolation induces a sense of belonging along with the overall therapeutic benefits of these 'restorative servicescapes' (Glover & Parry, 2009; Rosenbaum & Smallwood, 2011). Research carried out in six areas of deprivation in the UK (Hickman, 2013) found that particularly for the elderly, single mothers, the unemployed and those on fixed income, the recent recession has had a negative impact on the availability of places where these groups can engage in meaningful social interaction. He notes that although there has been a good deal of literature examining social interaction and community engagement, there has been limited engagement with third place literature. Hickman argues that these third places serve three key functions in areas of deprivation. First, they play an important *social* function because they are valued by the community. Second, they play an important functional role as service providers. Finally, they have a symbolic role as a marker of the 'health' and 'vibrancy' of the community. Hickman (2013) calls for further research to examine the effects of third place interaction on the attitudes and behaviours of those living in deprived areas and the significance of that social interaction to their lives. Drawing on the above discussion, the benefits of 'third place' interaction can be considered in four key areas:

- fostering social interaction;
- engendering a sense of belonging;
- reducing feelings of isolation and loneliness;
- helping participants to feel part of the community.

Employing this model as a basis of discussion, volunteers and women attending TITP were invited to take part in focus groups and individual interviews or to provide 'witness testimonies' to explore their views and feelings on what the group provides for them and its impact on the local community.

Methods

Original empirical research from two interrelated projects was undertaken. In the first instance and related to TITP as a 'third place' two focus groups were convened; the first in November 2013 had 11 participants and the second in

March 2014 had 6 participants. The group also provided 'witness testimonies' that they had gathered over a number of years attesting to the positive role the group had played in their lives. Finally, one member and one volunteer asked for their experiences to be recorded as individual interviews. The focus groups and interviews were held at the meeting place of TITP.

For the second part of this research and in relation to the concept of social prescribing, five interviews were carried out in March 2016. Those interviewed were the two volunteers from TITP, representatives from two statutory services, one dealing specifically with mental health and the other dealing with mental and physical health issues who either bring or refer women to TITP and a representative from a charitable mental health organisation who brings women to the group. This part of the research was to ascertain how respondents understood the concept of the social prescription and to determine whether TITP can or should be regarded as a social prescription service. As above, all interviews and focus groups took place in the meeting place of TITP.

All data was analysed using thematic analysis. Data was transcribed and archived in accordance with the 1998 Data Protection Act. To ensure anonymity the names of individuals and organisations represented are not provided.

Supporting positive social interaction

It is well known that positive social interaction plays a key role in an individual's sense of well-being. Rosenbaum (2006), for example, argues that social interaction in a 'third place' has key restorative benefits. At TITP, social interaction is a fundamental aspect of what the group provides for both volunteers and members alike. Social interaction is also linked to the alleviation, or at least lessening of isolation and loneliness, to the development of a sense of belonging and to the improvement in mental health problems. This is strongly evidenced by the women.

Catherine, who had been coming to the group for three years, had not long left an abusive and violent relationship where she had felt 'silenced and invisible'. She first came to the group through a referral from a mental health organisation and was suffering from severe depression and anxiety. She was accompanied by a support worker as she did not feel strong enough to come on her own. Initially she was unable to interact with members of the group and only able to sit for a short period before becoming anxious and having to leave. However, over time and with the help and support of the members and volunteers, she began to build trust and was eventually able to converse with them. Catherine puts this down to the sense of friendship and trust members have in each other. This is something that members stressed and highly valued. Coming to the group is a very important part of their lives. The women explained that coming to the group and sharing similar concerns (very often around issues of mental health) is very important to them. Linked to this trust is the non-judgemental attitude members have toward each other in relation to the private issues that are often discussed. Lee sums this up very clearly by saying, "I've seen me telling people in here that I wouldn't go and say to my sister or any of them.

In here people listen to you." Here, Lee is echoing a wider sentiment within and about the group. The fostering and building of relationships of trust allows for the sharing of personal stories in an open and frank way that would not otherwise be possible for group members. Moreover, such relationships provide the context in which the women feel they are listened to and not just heard, that what they have to say has value. Theresa reinforces this, saying: "You know that people are really interested [here] and they're concerned, that's quite important to me . . . it's another kind of lifeline." This use of the term 'lifeline', is more than a casual metaphor as it express a sentiment that is shared widely by group members. Being part of TITP has allowed for the kind of social interaction – both within the group and in the wider community – that has encouraged members to renew old hobbies and pursue new ones through the discovery of shared interests and the encouragement and support offered by group members.

An engendered sense of belonging

Literature on third place (Rosenbaum, 2006, 2009) demonstrates that such places engender a sense of belonging among those who attend. This is strongly evidenced at TITP, where women come to feel themselves as important and valued members of the group. For example, if any of the women have not attended for a while, a volunteer will get in touch to find out how they are. This is not seen as being intrusive but makes them feel as if they 'belong'. Theresa sums up the general views of the women in saying that:

> It's not just an exercise, it's not just like "ah well, she didn't turn up so she couldn't quite like it", ehm you're kind of hunted, they track you down to make sure you are still breathing. It's good, it sounds horrible, but it is a really, it's a good feeling, it's a kind of security blanket . . . it makes you feel kind of important.

Some members talked about going to other groups, where they had not felt this same sense of belonging and said that in comparison, TITP felt like 'a home away from home'.

The meeting room is set out like a large but cosy sitting room as opposed to the more 'formal' setting of some groups. Jean sums up the view of members in saying that TITP premises are like "something you would like to be your home. When you come in here . . . you feel comfortable." Other members likened coming to the group to "going to see your mammie [mother]".

The location of TITP has furthered this sense of belonging. Members who have used or been referred to services that deal specifically with issues of domestic violence or mental health issues said that, in some instances, they felt that they were going into an office where everyone knew why they were there, making them feel exposed and vulnerable. However, because TITP is located in a building that several community groups also use, this afford them a degree of privacy.

Reducing loneliness and isolation

Oldenburg (1989) argues that third places are particularly beneficial to the elderly or those on a low income. The vast majority of TITP members fall into at least one of these categories. When setting up TITP volunteers, perhaps serendipitously decided to hold the group on Mondays and Fridays. Tricia, a volunteer, explains that in hindsight opening on a Friday benefits those who attend by "[g]iving them a wee boost for whatever they have to cope with at the weekend, be that a violent partner or coping on their own because they have no family or friends around them". She adds that opening on a Monday provides members with a "place to offload". Several members say that they can cope better with evenings and weekends when they have been to TITP during the week and that TITP is an antidote to feelings of loneliness and isolation.

Given that the vast majority of those attend TITP are on a low income, their choices of places to socialise are extremely limited. TITP is a free service that provides women with the opportunity to meet and interact with others. This is viewed by members as a crucial factor in helping them deal with social and emotional isolation. The women talk openly about loneliness and isolation leading to mental health problems, such as depression and anxiety, arguing that, for them, the best solution to help alleviate these issues is not (only) to take medication but to interact with people, talk about their problems and to seek and offer advice to others who have found themselves in the same position. Pamela offered her own very clear assessment:

> The health service will employ psychiatrists, psychologists and all the rest of it, your talking therapy, none of it's the same as coming [to TITP] and talking to people you trust, people that you can relax and really talk to.

All agree that by no means the only solution, coming to TITP has been instrumental in helping them deal with isolation and loneliness and the resultant mental health issues this has caused many members.

On coming to TITP, Tracey thought she was the "only person in the world" suffering from (what she later realised was) depression. She said: "When I came here, I saw there was lots of other people, either in the same position or getting away from that and part of the reason they were getting away from that, was coming here [to TITP]." Pamela reflects the view of many members in saying: "You come [to TITP] for yourself, but after a while you, you're involved with people and you have that sense that . . . it's not all about you. You want to be helping other people." So while on the one level, TITP is a nice meeting place for members to relax, have a cup of tea and a chat, at another level it is very much more. For these women, it is an accessible, friendly, safe and inclusive social space where they are able to alleviate feelings of social and emotional loneliness and isolation, and the concomitant effects this has on health and well-being.

Being part of the wider community

Members of TITP have stressed that being part of the group makes them feel more connected to the wider community. However, this is not simply about 'feeling 'oneself part of the community, it is about active engagement with the concerns of the community. Through this engagement, volunteers and members have, in varying degrees, taken up community-based issues and become involved with local political processes. For example, several group members and volunteers are engaged with organisations dealing with poverty, welfare rights and reforms, mental health, housing and related issues. Geraldine, a one-time volunteer with TITP noted that: "through TITP I have become more socially and community engaged". She sees her role as gatherer of information of relevance to group members and the wider community, and as networking with other agencies in order to seek their engagement with, and support for, TITP. One particularly notable success for the group and indeed for Scotland as a whole was the petition to the Scottish Parliament started by Geraldine to make calls to NHS24 free from mobiles. The petition was successful and this new service has been available since April 2014. Geraldine, along with the volunteers, has been involved in getting members of statutory, non-statutory and third sector organisations to speak to members of TITP about a variety of issues affecting them and the wider community.

Related to this is the increasing number of referrals of women to TITP from other organisations. Although volunteers are committed to supporting all women who come to the group, they have spoken about feeling 'used' by statutory and other referring bodies. Tracey summed up this view: "We just feel that everybody uses us but nobody is prepared to back us . . . You know that . . . it's just getting other agencies to realise the position that we are in. We run on a shoestring here." Here Tracey is highlighting a serious concern about the precarious nature of the groups funding. This is deeply felt by all members and is causing many of them fear and anxiety as to how they would cope should the group be forced to close due to a lack of funding.

Also related to the above, is the idea that TITP are providing a 'social prescription' for women referred to the group by statutory and voluntary organisations. This idea was first mooted when a nurse at one of the local GP practices phoned a volunteer to ask if she could send 'patients' to TITP because 'what the group offered was a social prescription when the doctor could do no more'. However, during the initial research it became clear that the volunteers were unsure as to what a social prescription actually was despite indicating that they provided this service in their promotional material. This lack of clarity led to the second part of this research, which explores the concept of social prescribing and evaluates, based on empirical evidence, whether TITP can be regarded as a social prescription or indeed whether it wants to be. Given that the group prides itself on its informal nature, being used as a social prescribing service would arguably change the very essence of the group, forcing it to be answerable to external agencies and to meet target driven outcomes.

Social prescribing

Kimberlee (2015) has identified four models of social prescribing used by general practice. These range from 'signposting', which does little more than point patients in the direction of community or voluntary services that may help improve their overall sense of well-being, to 'holistic', which encourages individuals to become actively engaged in their own health care and deals with the whole person thus taking into account their socio-economic and psychological needs. Kimberlee (2015) argues that 'holistic' social prescribing only evolves over time and that most social prescribing 'interventions' do not meet the criteria of this model.

While the literature shows that social prescribing is beneficial for a number of people with a variety of issues, there can be challenges and problems in implementing social prescriptions. Kimberlee (2015) argues that the interest in social prescribing throughout the UK is the result of two key factors. The first is the 'increasing burden' of mental health and other long-term health issues and the resultant cost implications and second, the 'crisis' in general practice. Viewed in this context, it could be argued that social prescribing is a form of 'responsibility dumping' by the primary services on the already overburdened voluntary sector. It could also be argued that the very idea of 'social prescribing' is medicalising socio-economic and psycho-social problems.

Drawing on the above, TITP volunteers and representatives of statutory and non-statutory organisations who use the group to either refer or bring women to the group, were interviewed to find out what they understood by 'social prescribing' and if they considered TITP to be a social prescription

What interviewees understand by 'social prescribing' and do they regard TITP as a social prescription?

Possibly because of the lack of a single definition in the literature of what social prescribing is, of the five women interviewed, there was no clear and agreed understanding of what it actually means. While the volunteer who set up TITP notes that the group is considered by volunteers and members alike as a drop in and support service, she notes that: "I didn't know what [social prescription] meant but I understand a wee bit better about it now. [It is] where the medical services can't do anymore for somebody, this is where we step in." However, the other volunteer very strongly felt that the idea of social prescribing is just another "buzz word, like talking therapies". She states that: "Social prescription to me, is when the doctors don't want to give you any more tablets you know, and it's maybe a wee buzz word for them to get away with not doing their job." In terms of the representatives from statutory services utilising the service provided by TITP, there was either a lack of understanding of what a social prescription was or no real agreement as to the benefits of social prescribing. One interviewee who works for the NHS as part of a team dealing with severe and enduring mental health issues notes that:

> To be honest, [social prescription] is not a term that I've heard really, not recently anyway. [But] yes, I think social prescribing is a really good idea because I think what we've all come to learn is you could give someone all the medication in the world but there has got to be a bit of self-promotion as well and wanting to change their whole kind of ethos of the way they're thinking about their illness so yes, I think it's a good idea

She was very keen to point out, however, that what makes TITP 'work' is the informality of the group in that it is not tied to or answerable to any statutory body. This, she feels, gives the women a sense of 'safety' in that what they discuss or share with others in the group will not be 'reported back' to anyone. This fits very well with the ethos of the volunteers in their desire to keep TITP an 'informal' drop-in and support group.

The second interviewee from the statutory services notes that, "The term 'social prescription' is kind of, I don't know why particularly, but it's kind of frowned upon a wee bit [by our] programme." She elaborates on this in saying:

> I think that it's just the social prescribing maybe doesn't really describe the depth of what I would do, which is bringing women along [to TITP] and staying with them and you know, and that kind of buddying, encouraging role.

She also notes that the strengths of TITP is that it is not a 'specialised' service dealing with one particular issue and that it is located at the heart of the community: "So for me, I suppose, that's the biggest thing, that it's a community resource and that it's a community led resource and that the [volunteers] have really built this group up through the years, you know." The interviewee representing the voluntary group which deals with issues surrounding mental health and social isolation, although saying that she thought TITP was like a social prescription, was very unclear as to what the term meant but was very keen to point out that at TITP offered a fantastic service to local women no matter what their 'issues'.

Another very important issue raised by the representative of one of the referring bodies, is that if the group went down the 'social prescription route', it could change the informal nature of the group. She noted that: "I wouldn't want the group to then feel that it had to be changed and it had to become, you know, kind of target driven, business like, or having to do things that they wouldn't necessarily have done before."

TITP: a third place or a social prescription?

Although at TITP all women no matter their histories or background are welcomed by the volunteers and members alike, those interviewed who represent both the statutory and the voluntary sector most often refer or accompany women suffering from social isolation and mental health issues. TITP is regarded by all as a safe and inviting space for women dealing with, at times, very complex issues.

The representative from the NHS mental health service noted that she refers or brings women with mental health problems ranging from schizophrenia to severe depression and anxiety. She points out that these women can

> struggle with their social skills, their interaction with others, their self-esteem, their self-confidence and also they may have some behaviours that perhaps you're trying to change. They might be a bit more chaotic, they might have no structure to their day so having somewhere like [TITP] to come to gives them the impetus to go, to get up, get ready, get dressed, just all the basics and gives them a purpose.

All representatives of the referring bodies interviewed note that those women dealing with issues of depression and anxiety begin to realise, through time, that by coming to TITP and meeting and interacting with group members who are suffering from/have suffered from mental health problems, "it gives them a bit of hope that yes, I can change my life". In terms of those who are suffering from anxiety, the informal nature of the group and the way that the room where the women meet is set out, helps women feel less intimidated because although TITP offers a wide variety of activities for members, there is no pressure to get involved and although the layout of the room encourages social interaction, it does not 'force' it.

The community project worker notes that the "biggest thing [with the women referred] is probably a confidence thing". She points out:

> I think [I] see a change in the women that have maybe been lacking in confidence, or kind of, I don't want to use the word 'meek' because that's not right, but maybe just life has just kind of, battered them about and they're quite kind of, just like, phew, you know and you can see them just getting a wee bit more confident in themselves.

She goes on to say:

> And then, I suppose, when you see people participating in things that you could never have imagined them doing, you know, within the group, you would be kind of like, oh! Do you know what I mean? I never thought that you would speak out loud.

The representative from the mental health voluntary organisation was keen to note that she and other representatives have been using TITP to bring women with problems ranging from depression to psychosis and that all have benefitted from coming to the group. For her, the success of the group can be seen by the fact that "You come in here and see women you have referred to [TITP] four years ago and they are still coming." By this she is raising a very important point that TITP is not simply a group that you attend for a set number of weeks or months (which is often the case with groups provided by statutory services) but is available whenever women want to access it with no time limit placed upon them.

All referring bodies note that they bring/refer women to TITP because 'it works' and is an invaluable community service that, over the ten years it has been running, has helped a countless number of women deal with a variety of problems that negatively impact on their lives and, for many, lead to the onset of or the worsening of mental health problems. Having listened to the members of TITP on what they say the group provides them with and noting that there is confusion as to what a social prescription is, among volunteers and those interviewed from the statutory and voluntary sector, TITP can rightly be viewed as a third place and not a social prescription.

Conclusion

As has been demonstrated through the voices of all the women who either took part in focus groups or individual interviews and provided witness testimonies, the volunteers at TITP have created a safe place for social interaction, which engenders a sense of belonging, helps alleviate feelings of isolation and loneliness and connects members to the wider community, all factors that are known to impact positively on mental health. TITP effectively provides a variety of health and 'social services' to women who come to the group of their own accord as well as those who are 'referred' to the group. No member is asked to provide information other than their name, address and phone number. If referred by other organisations, women are not asked for the reasons behind the referral. However, there is very often a 'self-disclosure' of particularly mental health problems after the women become comfortable in the group and trusting of group members.

In evaluating whether TITP could be considered as a social prescription, especially for women with mental health issues, it is concluded that although it does provide some of the benefits that are found in the 'ideal type' social prescription, it has offered these since its inception and long before the idea of social prescribing had ever been heard of by the volunteers. However, having fully discussed and explored the idea of third place, the women very much recognised themselves in this context – a place beyond the 'first place' of home and the 'second place' of work – which provides a space for women to meet, interact, develop and *feel* a sense of belonging and community. The volunteers at TITP pride themselves on having retained the informal essence of the group arguing that this makes them attractive to all women no matter their background. That said, TITP is not straightforwardly a 'third place' in Oldenburg's terms. Most obviously, it caters solely for women and it is only accessible two days a week. However, it is clearly providing its members with vital aspects of the 'third place experience'. In this respect it seems more appropriate to say that TITP can be seen as an attempt to improvise (creatively and empathetically) something of a third place for all members.

In the final analysis, it is vital that this 'third place' element of the group is retained, protected and nurtured. As has been demonstrated throughout this chapter, a large number of group members have seen highly positive changes in their mental health ranging from helping manage schizophrenia to dealing with the mental health issues resulting from being isolated and lonely. For this the volunteers have to be commended and given immense credit. The very real issue, however, is that in order for TITP to continue to provide the service that it does, they must be properly resourced and not have to 'fight' for what little monies are available to groups such as these. If we want to ensure that mental health and long-term physical health problems are being treated holistically, then we must ensure that voluntary organisations like TITP flourish.

Acknowledgements

Part of this research was adapted from an ongoing collaboration in research and knowledge exchange between Tea in the Pot and the School of Media, Culture and Society of the University of the West of Scotland (UWS). This collaboration is rooted in a broader collaboration between Oxfam Scotland, which counts Tea in the Pot as one of its community partners. Based on a generous contribution from UWS, the UWS–Oxfam Partnership was able to financially support this specific collaboration (see Feeney & Collins, 2015).

References

Brandling, J., & House, W. (2007). *Investigation into the feasibility of a social prescribing service in primary care: A pilot project*. Bath, UK: University of Bath and Bath and NE Somerset NHS.

Cheang, M. (2002). Older adults' frequent visits to a fast-food restaurant: Nonobligatory social interaction and the significance of play in a 'third place'. *Journal of Aging Studies, 16*, 303–321.

Creswell, T. (2004). *Place: A short introduction*. Malden, MA: Blackwell.

Feeney, M., & Collins, C. (2015). *Tea in the Pot: Building 'social capital' or a 'great good place' in Govan?* Paisley: UWS–Oxfam Partnership, Report No. 3.

Friedli, L., & Watson, S. (2004). *Social prescribing for mental health*. Durham, UK: Northern Centre of Mental Health.

Glover, T. D., & Parry, D. C. (2009). A third place in the everyday lives of people living with cancer: Functions of Gilda's Club of Greater Toronto. *Health and Place, 15*(1), 97–106.

Hickman, P. (2013). 'Third places' and social interaction in deprived neighbourhoods in Great Britain. *Journal of Housing and the Built Environment, 28*(2), 221–236.

Kimberlee, R. (2015). What is social prescribing? *Advances in Social Sciences Research Journal, 2*(1), 102–110.

Meshram, K., & O'Cass, A. (2013). Empowering senior citizens via third places: Research-driven model development of seniors' empowerment and social engagement in social places. *Journal of Services Marketing, 27*(2), pp. 141–154.

Oldenburg, R. (1989). *The great good place: Cafes, coffee shops, bookstores, bars, hair salons, and other hangouts at the heart of a community*. New York, NY: Marlowe & Company.

Rosenbaum, M. S. (2006). Exploring the social supportive role of third places in consumers' lives. *Journal of Service Research, 9*(1), 59–72.

Rosenbaum, M. S. (2009). Restorative servicescapes: Restoring directed attention in third places. *Journal of Service Management, 20*(2), 173–191.

Rosenbaum, M. S., & Smallwood, J. A. (2011). Cancer resource centres: Transformational services and restorative servicescapes. *Journal of Marketing Management, 27*(13–14), 1404–1425.

16

INSTITUTIONALISING PEOPLE IN THE COMMUNITY

A reflection on distress

Vimala Uttarkar

In this chapter I aim to show how people mirror their mental distress on to the physical and emotional spaces around them. The distress of service users described in this chapter refers to the chaos and anguish they grapple with as they continue to experience the symptoms of mental illness, and how this turmoil is evidently reflected in their social networks and their physical environments. Previously, when they lived for many years and sometimes for life within the high walls of asylums, service users were stripped of their identities as individuals and isolated from society in the closed systems of psychiatric institutions. Goffman (1961) and Wing (1996) among others, describe the paternalistic attitudes of practitioners who cared for them, pointing out how they too had very little interaction with the outside world themselves. In their dedication to care for and minimise the distress experienced by the service users, they tightly scheduled and strictly monitored the service users' routines and ensured a sterile setting with few stimuli for thinking or imagination. This protected the service users from having to take responsibility for themselves or their actions or, indeed, any past social roles they may have held before being admitted into the asylums. Their mental chaos remained hidden in the clinical environment and the institutionalising effect of these total institutions. The loss of this 'container', however unhelpful it may have been, forces service users to make sense of their internal worlds while struggling to achieve some order in the physical and social spaces they are surrounded by in the community. Hinshelwood and Skogstad (2000) and others pointed out that as service users take responsibility for how they understand and deal with the symptoms of their illness, they often do not share the assumptions of illness or the help they require with the practitioners. With the emphasis on accepting service users as experts in their own situation – who are able to choose how and what help they will accept – practitioners who undertake to work in the community no longer have the comfort of being the expert, or of having colleagues nearby to turn to.

Data source: understanding the effects of community care

Case studies and other material presented here were collected as part of the data for a doctoral thesis in social work that studied the effect on community mental health practitioners of working with service users who were hard to engage — who rejected any attempts of help or care and lived in relative emotional isolation. It was a qualitative study of three different types of community mental health teams, and consisted of using the infant observation method to observe individual practitioners visiting service users and subsequently discussing these visits in their team meetings. These observations of individual visits and team meetings were followed by semi-structured interviews with the practitioners. Practitioners from all the disciplines within a team took part in this study and although the focus of the study was the practitioners, it was harrowing to meet some of the service users and note their abject circumstances. In the interviews, the practitioners from these multidisciplinary teams spoke about the team processes that dictated what areas they should address, and specifically how many times they needed to attempt contact with the service users before they could legitimately give up being actively involved with them and wait for either the police or mental health act assessments to bring them back into the teams' caseloads. Of the three teams, one had recognised the impact on practitioners of working with this perpetual rejection and had set up support systems for them, including spaces to reflect on their practices and feelings. Another team had a very open non-hierarchical structure that enabled them to 'talk' with and draw support from each other. In the third team, there was little facility for reflection or time for discussion. Extracts of work with teams one and three are discussed below.

The role of the worker within these community teams requires forming a relationship with service users who rarely reciprocate. Formal and informal discussions within these teams clearly demonstrated how team processes shielded these practitioners from getting in touch with their service users' distress or developing an emotional empathy that could potentially personalise their contact with service users. Their ever growing caseloads and shrinking resources only facilitated attention to the illness rather than the person behind it, and effectively blocked them from noticing the dismal conditions of their service users' lives. With their restricted responsibility for assessing the risks the service users posed to themselves or others, identifying relapse symptoms and ensuring their compliance with medication, there was little focus on the personhood of the service users. This preoccupation with tasks and the alienation of the practitioners from the 'person' of the service users mirrored the isolation experienced by the service users who were themselves preoccupied with their own chaotic internal processes that they did not seem to even notice the little help that they were offered.

Care in the community

In any type of health service it is easy to envisage that the service user must be at the centre of it. In mental health services the illness envelops the whole life of the service user so that it is not enough to just treat the symptoms of the illness. The universal impact of mental illness affects their very thought processes, their personhood and their ability to acquire or put into practice skills required to live independently. Unlike a failing kidney that requires dialysis a few times a week, during which the patient may still live a relatively normal life, mental illness affects a myriad of life areas and demands interventions both to address the illness and the distress it causes. It affects the ability of the individual to look after themselves, to sustain their accommodation, learn or apply daily living skills, attend to their accommodation, physical health, daytime occupation or social relationships.

As caring for service users with mental illness in the community similar to those with physical illnesses gathered momentum, hospital beds were closed and legislation enacted to facilitate care in the community. Many writers, such as Wood (1994), envisaged the need to focus services on not only the symptoms of the illness but the multiple sources of the disability it created. They pointed out that primary symptoms, individual responses to those symptoms and the societal reactions, such as stigma and discrimination, would render the successful transition of the treatment of mentally ill people into the community impossible without careful planning and substantial investment. Muijen (1996) drew attention to the dilemma of whether the money saved by the drastic reduction of hospital beds should be used to establish community resources to provide alternatives to move service users into or to set up community teams to prevent admissions. Even as these questions were being debated, other major issues surfaced. The most important one – that remains challenging 25 years after 'care in the community' became a key part of our mode of care and treatment for mental illness – is whether the focus should be on providing for the individual's need for care in the least restrictive environment, or on prioritising the community's need for safety through control and the reduction of risk.

There are other equally daunting questions that continue to challenge the provision of adequate care outside the hospital. Do we have the creativity and the resources to address not just the illness but also the person trapped within it? Are the experiences of persons trapped in the illness today different from those who were 'contained' in the Victorian institutions? As new and younger generations of people develop chronicity, what are their expectations and those of the society they live in? Have attitudes to mental illness actually changed enough to facilitate the acceptance of service users living in the community? Many such questions arise as we examine the current situation of hopelessly fragmented services that shunt service users into inadequate, ill-monitored, and ill-funded facilities. This in turn forces them on to the streets, or into accommodation that is so ill-suited that it just increases the depravity experienced by the service users and the helplessness of the practitioners involved in their care. As society fiercely debates these issues, the effects of the current services on both the service users and the practitioners who care for them in the community are examined in this chapter using observations of two visits with practitioners from two different teams.

Working in the community

For many practitioners, working in rehabilitation in the community involves not only the adjustment of their expectations but also a considerable shift of focus, especially for those practitioners whose training and prior experience has been in the health or therapeutic fields. In the community, it is important for practitioners to shift their focus away from placing prime importance on the control of symptoms or the management of behavioural difficulties, and towards giving equal emphasis on developing new skills and the maintenance of social functioning of the service users. The move from being clinical professionals to policing service users and protecting the public greatly affects the morale of care staff. Their struggle with the dilemma of either inappropriately placing unworkable restrictions on service users in the community or allowing them to be homeless or to aimlessly wander the streets takes its toll on practitioners. Practitioners' difficulties are not so much about understanding the science behind the illness, the symptoms and the treatments, but rather with the struggles to get service users to agree with their assumptions of the illness and accept the help they so much want to give. While service users with psychosis may reject the coherent life meanings of the practitioners, those with personality disorders may see the very relationship with their practitioners as exploitative and abusive. Taking into consideration how important they are in supporting service users and ensuring their ongoing care while controlling access to the limited resources, it is surprising how neglected the practitioners themselves are in many community mental health services and how relatively little is done, in the normal course of setting up these teams, to protect them from an accelerated pathway to apathy and burnout.

As people with different professional backgrounds work together on a team activity, more pressures are placed on them by destructive psychodynamic forces that work below the surface, such as splitting, scapegoating and the development of subcultures among professional groups or individual team members. My research findings were in agreement with those of several authors — indicating that, despite practitioners drawing on their own sources of sustainment, such as their innate need for reparative work, their previous experience, their professional and personal values and motivations, their personal support networks and how these networks view and value their work, they also required some organisational structures, such as clarity of purpose and roles, policies and procedures to help them to maintain the boundaries of their involvement with both the service users and other providers. More importantly they need processes such as team meetings and reflective spaces/staff support groups and other informal peer discussions, which they can experience as providing support and sustenance for their day-to-day work. The re-ablement of a person with mental illness requires both a variety of support services and the continuity of the care and support they receive for many years. Despite a number of other agencies providing a wide spectrum of services, the core containment for the service users comes from a group of different professionals working as a team to re-able them to become independent of mental health services and ultimately re-integrate as a person in their community.

Focus on the service user

The 2007 Amendment to the Mental Health Act introduced the Community Treatment Order (CTO), to facilitate treatment of service users outside the hospital. The aim was to discharge service users from expensive hospital beds into the community and prevent relapse and the need for readmission, by making them subject to some compulsory conditions, such as compliance with medication. In order to get away from the incarceration in hospital, service users frequently agree to comply with these conditions, irrespective of whether they agree that they are mentally ill and need medication, or that these medicines actually help them. It also facilitates mental health practitioners to act as social police – using medication to keep service users out of hospital while ensuring that they do not pose a risk to the public through a relapse in their symptoms. The CTO conditions do not require meaningful involvement with the service users' day to day lives or address their harrowing experiences in the community or even the distressing side effects of medication, such as weight gain, loss of libido, diminished sexual potency and reduced general energy levels. Service users' experience of their practitioners as impermeable objects having the power of taking away their liberty may drive them to despair, apathy or even violence. Community care is supposed to provide a new kind of patient-focused service geared to service users' views and needs. However, critics such as Laurance (2003) claim that this has merely exported the coercive nature of hospital-based services into the community and has not done anything to address the exclusion of the personhood from the person. The role of mental health practitioners has shifted from being a positive source of care and support to one where they have a supervisory role 'focussing on the control of service users' illness and the protection of others and, less upon the needs of service users themselves' (Pritchard, 2006). Studies have shown that the psychiatric recidivism caused by isolation and dis-engagement is more expensive than providing personalised care and helping service users to 'become more in touch with themselves and less violent through skilled, sympathetic attention to helping people understand their own behaviour and its effect on others' (Cigman, 1995). As society moves towards policing the quality of public life with zero tolerance of anomalies in behaviours, service users get arrested for behaviours caused by their symptoms such as disturbing the peace or even simply loitering (Richardson, 2009). Hospitalising service users for posing a risk rather than being 'at risk', or arresting them for begging or being inappropriately dressed in public, often results in an intense feeling of failure, de-stabilising their already fragile existence in the community.

Mentally ill people are more likely to have frequent contact with the police than with professionals. This could be both as the victim of crime, or more rarely for perpetrating an offence, which may be an expression of their symptoms. Studies continue to find that service users do not have the opportunity to talk with anyone about the things that matter to them, current practices in psychiatry paying little if any attention to the practical, social or leisure-time needs of its service users. Proper care in the community is time consuming, hard work and involves taking risks.

It requires understanding that 'home' is where one needs to belong, love and share, in addition to resting, eating and sleeping. Being provided with just a roof and four walls could be like drifting aimlessly in an alien world. Foster (2001) points out, that as service users try to make sense of their chaotic inner lives, having to organise their exterior spaces may seem more burdensome than it is worth, especially if they are so preoccupied with these internal struggles that they are oblivious to their external environment. For a number of service users who have either had negative experiences in their parental homes or have never developed a secure sense of home, independent living and setting up a home may be beyond their grasp. Is this a skill one is able to learn beyond the formative years of adolescence and early adulthood? Poor living skills, a lack of social networks and high emotional support needs do not constitute an appropriate mix for successful independent living in the community. Care in the community involves working with carers and helping significant members of the service users' network to understand the extant of the illnesses, the intensity of their symptoms and the limits these place on the service users. Although not as expensive as running a hospital ward, an adequately staffed resource in the community, with appropriately skilled practitioners, does not come cheap. Moreover, these types of services have clearly evidenced the positive effects they can have on the lives of even the most difficult service users placed with them, as can be seen below.

The following extracts from two case studies describe the effects of two different kinds of environments that these service users were placed in.

Martyn

As we drove to meet Martyn, his CPN Eleanor told me about him. He was 40 years old and of Caribbean origin. He was diagnosed with chronic schizophrenia in addition to a personality disorder. His mother had a recurrent depressive illness and was often admitted to hospital. His father, who left while Martyn was still a child, used to severely physically beat him. His mother's subsequent boyfriends plied him with drugs before sexually abusing him. This kind of abuse seemed to have continued after he was removed into foster care, resulting in his own addictions, violence and convictions. He entered the mental health system as a teenager. He spent many years in and out of hospital, with short periods in independent accommodation, sometimes with marginal staff support, but with frequent readmissions to hospital due to tenancy breakdown or following arrest for drug-related offences. This time he had been in hospital for a number of years before it was decided to place him in a supported flat, where he had been for four months at the time of our visit.

He lived on a large housing estate with identical buildings with only the identifying letters on their sides to distinguish them from one another. We went to the front door of building D-IV and rang the buzzer to his flat several times with no response. As we continued to ring, an older man came out of the main entry doors and we managed to get into the building before the door could shut behind him. We went up a flight of stairs and along a long grimy balcony with many doors and windows that were either shut or had drawn curtains behind them. When we arrived in front of a heavily stained door, Eleanor knocked on it. It swung open freely and she called out to Martyn and announced us as we entered his studio flat. The first thing that hit us was the strong odour in the flat – the dank smell of unwashed bodies, stale cigarette smoke and the reek of human waste emanating from the tiny bathroom. The flat consisted of a room with a bed in one corner with a dirty stained mattress and no linen on it. There was an array of broken musical equipment strewn around the room. There was an old faded sofa covered with dirty clothes in another corner. On the floor were several mugs encrusted with dark stains and cigarette butts. There were a number of large liquor bottles and dirty plates with dried remnants of food on them strewn around. Martyn was a thin wiry man dressed in a hat and an old threadbare suit. He sat on a box with his chin resting in the palm of his hands staring into space. He seemed unaware of us until Eleanor touched him as she greeted him again. He slowly turned his eyes towards her and continued to mutely gaze at her. Ignoring the many questions asking about his welfare and circumstances, he muttered, 'I don't want me [sic] injection'. When asked if he had eaten anything, he said he could not remember. She offered to make him a cup of tea and, picking up some of the cups and plates, went into the kitchen. In the kitchen, the counter along the wall was strewn with silver foil and syringes, and some more used cups. The sink had some wrappers, bits of paper and empty boxes of mind-altering substances that were not (then) illegal and so were cheaply and openly available in small local shops. She came back into the bedroom and pushed the clothes to one side of the sofa so we could sit down. She said 'there is no milk, why don't we go to the cafe and have a cuppa? You really must eat something!' He looked away before turning back to ask if she could give him some money as he owed a 'friend' who was demanding it back. She persisted about going for a coffee but he declined, saying he just wanted some money to clear his loan so he could get another fix. Eleanor asked when he had received his benefits and he said that they were not due for another two days. She sat on the edge of the sofa and implored him to take his depot, stressing that he would be recalled back to hospital if he continued to refuse his medication. At last, he agreed to take his injection and she said that she would ask his housing support worker to bring him some food later that afternoon and that he must let her in. He looked at her blankly, seemingly uninterested in her offer.

As we left him, we encountered a group of children calling to each other as they cycled in the passage. Two women, who were talking to each other from the first floor flats across the passageway shouted, 'he's a psycho, why don't you take him away?'

Discussion

Eleanor explained to me that Martyn did not really have a social life and that the only contacts he had were with his housing support worker, who was supposed to see him weekly, and practitioners from her team who visited him fortnightly to give him his depot injections. She suspected that he was being preyed upon by drug dealers. He was on a CTO, with the conditions that he should take his medication and maintain contact with his care team. He was also barred from visiting his mother, as he had assaulted her a few months earlier, when he had visited her during a period of leave from the ward. She had refused to give him money and he had severely beaten her. His brother and sister had supported his mother to take out an injunction against him visiting her. Eleanor hoped that despite his desperation for some immediate cash, he would not break the conditions of that injunction and assault his mother again.

She wistfully admitted that he had lost a lot of weight and it was difficult to monitor if he regularly ate or did anything meaningful with his time, but as long as he remained in his flat and took his medication they would leave him alone. He was placed in supported housing, which meant that he had help to retain his tenancy from housing practitioners who were not skilled in getting involved in his mental health needs. She said that the police could force a Mental Health Act assessment for admission if his flat was taken over by drug dealers and turned into a drug den or if he became aggressive as a result of taking drugs or because of withdrawal due to a lack of them. She said that her team had tried to reason with him about his drug taking, but he insisted that it was 'normal' for people of his age to take drugs, arguing that even high achievers like bankers and lawyers took them routinely. She said how helpless she and her team felt to discover that recently he had also started taking other more available but highly addictive substances. The next day, when she discussed her visit in the team meeting, her colleagues agreed how difficult it was to support him as he refused to take his medication or would not be in his flat at the time of the appointments. She reminded them that this was her fourth visit to give him his depot injection and expressed relief that they did not need to recall him back to hospital now. She said that he again asked for money, which evoked disparaging laughter from the team. There seemed little recognition for his concern that he owed money and so may be vulnerable to being assaulted by drug dealers. Her colleagues agreed that his drug dependence was a behavioural problem rather than a symptom of his illness, and as long as he continued to take his medication, the symptoms of his illness would remain under control. This meant that if he got into trouble, he might be arrested and sent to prison rather than be admitted to hospital. Although this indicates an extremely narrow view of his care with the focus on his medication compliance and tenancy maintenance, the team did spend a lot of time getting him to co-operate with these issues so that there was little time or energy left to address his quality of life concerns.

Martyn himself did not seem too concerned with the quality of his life – it was difficult to gauge whether the isolation and loneliness concerned him. He seemed oblivious to the mess around him, as if he had deliberately emptied the clutter from his mind on to the physical space around him and found it easier to keep it there rather than in his mind. He seemed to be striving for some respite from his inner turmoil and a quest for peace and quiet. When we were with him, he seemed very quiet and preoccupied with sorting something out in his mind or afraid to disturb the fragile mental equilibrium he seemed to have achieved, perhaps with the use of illicit drugs. More than the medication that was offered by his care team, the illicit drugs seemed to either empty his mind of the difficulties or dull his affect so he experienced some relief from having to grapple with the pain of his internal experiences. Questions remained whether he had turned to mind-altering substances to calm the internal chaos created by his symptoms or the distress caused by an inner world populated with his experiences of abuse and even the images of his abusers. The stillness he had strived to achieve was almost tangible both in the decay surrounding his physical space and in his minimal verbal and non-verbal communications with us.

Carl

The next visit was with Pamela, a social worker from a different team. Carl had been known to psychiatric services since his childhood. For many years he was constantly moved around the various staffed rehabilitation units of the local NHS Trust and privately run supported accommodation, both in his home borough and in the surrounding areas. Each time he was evicted within three or four months due to sexually inappropriate behaviours or threats of or actual violence to on-site staff, following the use of illicit drugs. These were seen as behavioural issues that could not be addressed by therapeutic interventions in hospital or in the community, and so each time an eviction order would be made, he would be moved into another supported accommodation. Eventually he was moved into an intensive support hostel with 24-hour staff.

We arrived at a large house with a garden and a communal lounge, buzzing with activities. We were shown into the meeting room where the annual placement review was held. The care home practitioners read their report, which said that he had come to this hostel with a large ulcer in his leg. He had been registered with the local GP services and was prescribed antibiotics, which he took erratically and refused to have his wound dressed. Between periods of treatment on antibiotics, he would violently tear the dressing and puncture the wound to drain the pus on to the floor of the communal lounge. With persistence, the staff had gradually encouraged him to start clearing up the mess with help from them. In recent weeks, when he was informed about his room being cleaned, he sometimes stayed back and got involved in cleaning it. Carl did not trust anyone else with his medication and took tablets in handfuls when he remembered, rather than as prescribed. Even when he was taken to the GP for his ulcer, he would grab the prescription, rush to the pharmacy, get the painkillers and the antibiotics and take a handful of them immediately. Working with the GP and his psychiatrist, the hostel staff had gradually taken control of his medication. Now they were able to give him the right dose at the right intervals, although sometimes this still provoked verbal aggression from him.

When he was first accepted into that hostel, he had agreed for staff to help him buy food every week, as long as they did not dictate what he could do with the rest of his benefits. He spent all his money on illicit drugs and alcohol. Because of the variable quality and nature of these substances, his health was often seriously affected by them resulting in staff needing to call an ambulance. If he was conscious he would refuse their help or, if taken to the Accident and Emergency Department in a state of delirium, he would discharge himself from the hospital once he regained consciousness. When he ran out of money, he would sell his food items and anything else he could find for a fraction of their price to support his cravings. Staff would provide food from their supplies when he ran out, but had eventually got him to agree for them to hold his weekly food shopping securely, allowing him access to choose the meals he wanted at a given time, so that he now ate regularly.

The report said that soon after moving in, he had become friendly with another young man with similar behaviours. Together they would persistently harangue older and more subdued residents to 'lend' them large sums of money. When his key worker became aware of this, the home put in place close observations of the two perpetrators, so that their communications with the more vulnerable residents were monitored. He then tried to supplement his income by aggressive begging in the neighbourhood, until staff started to intervene. He changed his location to the nearby train stations and shopping areas and was brought back by police several times. However, the police declined to charge him as he was 'mentally ill'. Practitioners in the care home had prevailed upon the police to charge him. Three months prior to this meeting, he had been charged and kept in the local police cells for a few days. He was produced in court and had been handed a suspended sentence and barred from begging in public places. He had refrained from begging since then. The report concluded that the care home staff felt they had achieved as much as they could with him by regulating his food and medicine intake and reducing incidents of violence. They recommended that his care manager should look for a specialist drug rehabilitation place for him.

Carl's father visited him regularly and sometimes took him out on short breaks. Lately these breaks were more successful as they could go away for a few days without getting into conflict with each other. He was present at this review and tearfully acknowledged that after many years he could actually see that his son was being adequately cared for. He said that he had struggled for a long time to look after his son who had become increasingly violent towards him and so he had decided that he was unable to continue caring for him. He expressed disappointment that his son had not continued his education despite having shown good academic promise as a child. He was distressed that Carl lived in a hostel and did not have a job or the prospect of settling down to a 'normal' life in his own accommodation. However, he acknowledged that his son seemed more stable than he had been in many years. He expressed concern at the suggestion of moving him on and thought that he could be helped in his current placement to give up drugs. Carl himself said that he liked the hostel and wanted to stay on. He wanted help with maybe accessing a course of study that might distract him and reduce the amount of drugs he took.

As we prepared to leave, Carl rushed up to us and asked if he would be made to leave the hostel – he feared that he may be evicted as he did not let staff attend to the ulcer in his leg. Pamela encouraged him to let them attend to it or he may lose his leg altogether and said that she would look for a specialist drug rehabilitation service for him in the next six months unless he gave up the habit before then. Pamela sighed with relief as she said that for the first time in several years she had attended a meeting about Carl that was not about eviction. He had lasted for over 18 months in this intensively staffed hostel. She said that in all the years as his care manager, she had never seen him actively engage in a care review. She said that the staff in this home were doing really good work with him and seemed to be succeeding in preparing him for an eventual move back into less supported accommodation.

Discussion

There is considerable evidence that an important factor in psychiatric breakdown is the absence of meaningful key relationships, of not being adequately supported to overcome the challenges of life in the community, and of being isolated and not feeling engaged with the world. 'Services that work with, rather than for, users and which provide a sense of purposefulness, constantly checking users' motivations and aspirations, are essential if people are to recognise their potential and avoid being warehoused' (Pritchard, 2006, p. 227).

The 2007 amendment to the Mental Health Act also recognised personality disorders and granted the same provision of care and treatment for people diagnosed with them, as well as for people with mental illness. As he had been diagnosed with a borderline personality disorder, it had taken many years and much effort and negotiation on Pamela's part to gain funding for the expensive accommodation that could offer the support and care he required in order to address his complex needs.

Carl's functioning seemed to alternate between the paranoid schizoid position and the depressive position as described by Klein. This switch in behaviour seemed to be without any apparent external stimulus or perhaps he unconsciously perceived certain people and their behaviours as the stimulus that switched on either mode of functioning depending on his interpretation. His response to the world around him was that of feeling persecuted, afraid that he will be either manipulated or abused. Even his apparently caring father could not escape this treatment nor could his body, which he constantly needed to attack in order to feel in control. He had learnt that when he behaved in certain ways, the people around him were distressed, so he used these behaviours when he felt himself cornered and helpless or when he wanted something. His ability to function in a depressive position was evidenced when he accosted us to express his unhappiness about being moved on. The staff in the hostel seemed to have hung on to his depressive position despite his constant paranoid behaviours. This unconscious confusion between feeling persecuted and feeling remorseful was reflected in his inability to settle down in a place where he may be helped to grasp the reality of his situation and to learn the skills of independent living.

The teams' responses

Following these visits, I attended the team meetings where these practitioners discussed their visits. They were from two different teams, with two different philosophies of care and vastly different practices; In one team, practitioners had direct responsibility for up to 15 very high-needs service users, but each practitioner had to be aware of the up-to-date circumstances of all the service users on the team's caseload, as they had to respond to and resolve the difficulties of any patient allocated to the team as a whole. In the other team, each practitioner worked individually with up to 35 service users whose needs ranged from simple monitoring visits to arranging very complex packages of care. In addition to occasionally visiting the service users, practitioners' main responsibility in the second team, was to co-ordinate the services of the network of providers who were involved in supporting the service user to remain in the community.

Both teams had a number of service users with whom they felt emotionally attuned, as well as others who caused much anxiety due to the risk they posed or the demands they made. A third type of service user, who were severely ill but had quietly disengaged from services and only occasionally became seriously unwell, were often left in a very poor state in the community. Both the teams had rules and regulations with clear primary tasks and roles. These included rules for the conduct and expectations of their practitioners. Their written policies and procedures and unwritten communications manifested in creating defences against getting too emotionally involved with service users. These structures that the teams had erected in the spaces between their practitioners and their service users, worked reasonably well as social defences against the onslaught of the unbearable pain that service users presented. These structures may be needed to maintain their own sanity but did not promote emotionally intelligent practice. As described by Morris (2000), they did not facilitate the reception of the unconscious communications desperately sent by the patient or enable them to hold in mind the patient as a whole person.

Although the workload was different, the amount of responsibility and the actual work itself did not differ substantially between practitioners in the two teams. Both teams were made up of practitioners from a number of disciplines. However, in the first team where a team approach was used there seemed to be less stress experienced by individual practitioners despite working with very hard-to-reach service users. They said that appointments with their allocated service users were carried out irrespective of whether they were at work or on leave. They also felt that, since everyone knew all the service users, they could support each other when they experienced difficulties with any service user. They acknowledged that they were less affected by the projections of service users and could openly discuss with the team when service users tried to split and scapegoat any of them. They especially valued their joint training events, frequent team meetings and reflective practice meetings with an external supervisor. They had built on these and developed other informal spaces and practices that facilitated a trust in each other and the confidence that they could depend on their colleagues. However, practitioners in the second team said they just did not have the time for luxuries like reflective discussions, nor did their managers acknowledge that they needed such supportive structures to deal with their own emotional responses to the work they did or the harrowing demands made on them by their service users.

Considering the impact of working with very difficult-to-engage service users, who were too preoccupied with their own internal conflicts and so frequently rejected any help offered by practitioners, teams need to work cohesively with shared values and beliefs. To achieve more as a team than as individuals, teams must allow reflective spaces and ensure respect for the individual autonomy of the practitioners while sharing the belief in their primary task and the knowledge of their service users' needs and how they should respond to those.

In contrast, a group of disparate professionals loosely working together with similar understanding of their tasks but no meaningful communication or opportunities to understand the thoughts and experiences of their colleagues or to offer significant support to each other to reduce internalising the projections of service users in order to continue to work effectively with them, is neither helpful to service users nor the practitioners.

Impact on the practitioners

Inevitably practitioners develop emotional responses to their service users and their behaviours. The problem here is to remain in touch with these subjective emotions while objectively assessing the situation, being alert to the unconscious communications of the service users, relating their behaviours to their state of minds and responding resourcefully to all these. Despite all the systems available to defend them against the harmful projections of service users, their own emotional responses to their day-to-day experiences with the service users and constant exposure to their shattered worlds are deeply disturbing.

I accompanied practitioners from both teams as they made a number of visits where they experienced traumatic events. We visited service users who were extremely abusive, sometimes verging on physical violence or those who posed a threat by, for example, precariously holding a ferociously barking dog while talking to the practitioner, or repeatedly not being available for appointments or not answering the door. Practitioners from the first team were aware of their colleagues' difficult encounters with that particular service user and so felt prepared for these experiences. They said that since they knew they could talk to their team early next morning, they did not dwell on the impact of these experiences. Their ability to distance themselves from the responses of the service users and not personalise these attacks, clearly contributed to their confidence in their own worth and the effectiveness of their team. However, practitioners from the second team seemed very tense or dejected. They often talked about the effects of these threats or rejections pushing them to the edge of their tolerance. There seemed to be no forum to talk about these experiences or the effects on themselves. Although individual practitioners expressed these feelings as I visited with them, they were largely unaware that their colleagues in the team had similar feelings. Even though they had monthly supervision with a sympathetic manager, because of the large number of cases they had to discuss, they felt that it was difficult to dwell upon the trauma of their own day-to-day experiences.

To work effectively, practitioners need to build relationships with service users who are rarely able to reciprocate or even agree with their view of the world. Service users with psychosis may not be capable of constructing a world that is meaningful to the worker. On the other hand, a service user with personality disorder may view any attempts to help by the worker as being manipulative and eventually abusive in line with their early experiences or other significant relationships. As service users alternate between expressing their persecutory anxieties with threats followed by intense remorse through attempting to self harm, it is extremely confusing for practitioners visiting on their own, to respond reasonably to these projections and restrain from retaliating in harmful ways. If things do go wrong, the possibility of an official enquiry would confer failure on the practitioner placing their career at risk. It is inevitable that practitioners withdraw from personal interactions and resort to the social defences created by the teams and build impenetrable walls in the already tiny spaces between themselves and the service users. To avoid any personal involvement, practitioners will apply the objectivity of targeting the illness, thus treating the service users as symptoms rather than as persons requiring help. The human significance is lost on both sides as the service users' internal struggles engulf their external world and the practitioners reject the prospect of understanding them and retreat behind the barrier of their professional world.

Conclusion

As hospital beds close due to government cuts and it has become inevitable that service users are increasingly cared for and treated in the community, it is important to recognise that mental health support is not a simplistic procedural activity; it is a complex and emotionally charged reality of the messiness of working through relationships with people who are alienated from their own mental processes and thus have difficulty interacting with their environment. There is sufficient evidence that working in groups can enhance the performance of individual practitioners if the team is thoughtfully set up with consideration to improve cohesiveness and inter-relatedness. For effective multi-professional teamwork, it is essential to minimise the detrimental effects of role blurring and the loss of professional identity. One way forward is to have a team that requires each professional practitioner to split their work roles to carry out both the generic functions of the primary task of the team and the more specific tasks of practising their particular professional skills.

Both Martyn and Carl had been designated as service users with severe and enduring mental illness for many years, during which time they had been too preoccupied with their struggle to make sense of their internal worlds and find meaning within the confusion in their minds to be concerned about how they presented themselves to the external world. Their verbal communication was coloured by this confusion, so their expressions of their perceptions or thoughts were not understandable to the people around them. Their priority was to get rid of the unwanted contamination in their minds by projecting it on to anything that might receive these projections, such as the physical spaces around them and their conscious and unconscious communications. Their strong unconscious communications makes it impossible for them to have a reasonable conscious interaction with the world. Too afraid to make sense of the internal commotion, they may disengage or display psychotic symptoms or appear very needy, by projecting their chaos into their physical and relational environments. We label their attempts to communicate with us as being perceptual disorders or thought disorders and when they do not agree with our assumptions about life and how to live it, we declare that they 'lack insight'. Thus, even their small external world, confined mainly to their professional practitioners, finds it difficult to interact with them in any meaningful way.

Service users spill their internal chaos and meaninglessness into their physical and relational spaces making them humanly impossible to live with. Similarly, practitioners reflect their own struggles of working with these service users by erecting emotional barriers and defensive systems to avoid human contact that could possibly have the mutual benefit of, on the one hand, making service users feel heard and, on the other hand, giving practitioners a sense of real achievement in their work.

Large asylums had provided practitioners with containment in the form of the proximity of colleagues who had a range of professional skills to instantly deal with crises, such as serious physical illness or the sudden display of violence or relapse in symptoms. There were always informal spaces for catharsis when practitioners had soul-destroying experiences of ongoing rejection by service users who refused to engage or became hurtfully abusive. The systems within the walls of a hospital with their strict regimes and rigid policies and procedures provided implicit leadership in the care and treatment of service users so that individual professionals did not have the sole responsibility for any disasters that occurred. Routines and rotas meant that practitioners did not need to develop a personal relationship with service users and the clear distinction between 'staff' and 'patient' groups provided a containing boundary for the practitioners. Despite destroying the personhood of the service users and making them institutionalised, these social defences provided a safety net for practitioners. In contrast, visiting service users in the community in an attempt to 'normalise' them, can potentially promote involuntary identification with the service users as persons just like themselves rather than as 'objects' requiring confinement away from society. In focusing entirely on the objective medical solution to the treatment of service users, the opportunity to help them re-integrate as a person is often lost. In the pursuit of scientific objectivity, practitioners lose the subjective inquiry and understanding of their own response and the ability to relate to service users as people.

Setting up a service in the community without the containing structures could result in creating a system where other unhelpful social defences are constructed in the form of viewing service users within two dimensional frameworks as consumers of medicine and poor quality, minimally supported housing and of monitoring a few aspects of their life in the community, such as medication compliance and prevention of relapse in symptoms and risky behaviours, rather than paying attention to the service users' experiences, thoughts and wishes. These defences allow practitioners to avoid the powerful emotional demands of acknowledging the intense psychic pain experienced and sometimes expressed by the service users. They reduce the impact of the unbearable experiences they have when they visit service users in isolation with no provision for easy access to relief in the form of support from colleagues. Rules and procedures provide a necessary structure to ensure consistency, accountability and help for practitioners to remain on task. However, an outcomes and efficiency focused, resource-shrinking, risk-averse system does not easily balance with the less measurable emotional and relationship based practices that are required for effective mental health work in the community. As we recognise the expressed and unconscious discomfort of practitioners and put in place the facilities required to sustain and even enhance their ability to adequately support people struggling with the alienating experiences brought about by mental illness, we could finally begin to expand our imagination and creativity to rise to the challenges of effectively responding to the needs of mentally ill people in the community.

References

Cigman, R. (1995). Schizophrenia and the freedom to be irresponsible. In J. H. Berke, C. Masoliver, & T. J. Ryan (Eds.), *Sanctuary: The Arbour's experience of alternative community care*. London: Process Press.

Foster, A. (2001). The duty to care and the need to split. *Journal of Social Work. Practice*, *15*(1), 81–90.

Goffman, E. (1961). *Asylums: Essays on the social situation of mental patients and other inmates*. New York, NY: Anchor Books

Hinshelwood, R. D., & Skogstad, W. (Eds.). (2000). *Observing organisations*. London: Routledge.

Laurance, J. (2003). *Taking care to the community in pure madness: How fear drives the mental health system*. London and New York, NY: Routledge.

Morris, M. (2000). Tyrannical equality in observing organisations. In R. D. Hinshelwood & W. Skogstad (Eds.), *Observing organisations*. London: Routledge.

Muijen, M. (1996). Scare in the community: Britain in moral panic. In T. Heller, G. Reynolds, R. Gomm, R. Muston, & S. Pattison (Eds.), *Mental health matters: A reader*. London: Macmillan.

Pritchard, R. (2006). The accommodation dimension: Housing and mental disorder. In C. Pritchard, *Mental health and social work: Evidence-based practice*. London and New York, NY: Routledge.

Richardson, T. H. (2009). Conceptual and methodological challenges in examining the relationship between mental illness and violent behaviour and crime on the internet. *Journal of Criminology*. www.internetjournalofcriminology.com.

Wing, J. K. (1996). Research designs for the evaluation of services. In H. C. Knudsen, & G. Thornicroft (Eds.), *Mental health service evaluation*. Cambridge: Cambridge University Press.

Wood, H. (1994). What do service users want from mental health services? Unpublished report to the Audit Commission.

17
INCORPORATING SERVICE USER PERSPECTIVES AND THE ROLE OF THE HOME ENVIRONMENT IN MENTAL HEALTH DESIGN

Stephanie Liddicoat and Joe Forster

In this chapter we consider space and the built environment[1] in relation to mental health and therapeutic practice, with a particular focus on the environment of the home. A discussion of literature evaluating the influence of good design practice on therapeutic efficacy and delivery is first examined. Following this, a discussion of the research design and methods undertaken by Liddicoat is outlined, which was informed by the emerging discourse on practice research. Subsequently, following the fieldwork data collection and analysis, the role of the environment of the home,[2] its significance to service users[3] and therapeutic outcomes, are discussed. When considering the significance of the home environment, three key themes are presented that are predominant in the fieldwork undertaken, and in studies examining mental distress and the crossover into architectural discourse: the fostering of communication, the quelling of dissociation, and the evolving sense of self. The home is analysed as a contributor to therapeutic processes, improved service user outcomes and experience. Therapeutic implications are analysed, and future research avenues suggested, including the development of self-help materials related to the home, for use in therapy. This exploratory research thread illustrates the significance of the built environment in relation to mental health, and the importance of incorporating service user perspectives into mental health design, in order to understand how best to design these environments and deliver mental health care.

There is a considerable body of literature affirming links between mental wellbeing and good design practice (Ulrich, Zimring, Quan, & Joseph, 2006; Ulrich et al., 2008). Evaluations of specific design interventions have shown that good design of clinical and treatment environments leads to better clinical outcomes and less stress for the users; both patients and staff (Marberry, 2006; Ulrich, Zimring, Quan, & Joseph, 2004). When considering environments for therapy and counselling specifically, research illustrates how design can affect therapeutic delivery and suggests that the incorporation of spatial and built elements should form a part of therapeutic techniques (Sivadon, 1970) and that many techniques utilised in psychiatry have spatial implications (Carlson, Speca, Patel, & Goodey, 2003). The counselling environment is regarded within clinical literature as having an effect on a service user's sense of well-being (Gross, Sasson, Zarhy, & Zohar, 1998; Ulrich et al., 2008). Service users' experience of such spaces can have a highly emotional dimension (Pressly & Heesacker, 2001), which is suggestive that design aspects of environments are a potential means to influence therapeutic efficacy (Liddicoat, 2015).

Methods

The above discussion serves to emphasise the importance of spatial encounters within counselling and therapeutic practice, as defined in the literature. A formal empirical study was undertaken by Liddicoat with the aim of understanding the spatial constructs and perceptions of individuals who self-harm,[4] with the view to analysing ways or approaches in which architecture and the built environment might contribute to the success and efficacy of treatment. A limited number of existing studies have focused on this area of research, however these studies are limited in several key ways. Studies predominantly considered therapist perspectives of the issue, rather than interviewing patients/service users (Pearson & Wilson, 2012), studies claimed straightforward connections between design aspects and service outcomes without acknowledging the complexity of influential factors and studies often broadly consolidated all service users together in a research focus, which was noted as problematic due to the variance between mental health conditions and the related needs of service users. In order to mitigate these limitations, the discourse on practice research was examined to inform the research design and methods employed within this chapter.

Practice research is an emergent notion in social work fields, whereby theory is built not only from academia but from practice also (Julkunen, 2011). Practice research begins with a curiosity about practice and processes, critically examining these with the aims of developing new ideas through experience and collaboration (Epstein et al., 2015). This approach privileges the generation of knowledge with close affective ties to the professional practice itself. To meaningfully develop this knowledge, practice research "recognises that this is best done by practitioners in partnership with researchers, where researchers have as much, if not more, to learn from practitioners as practitioners have to learn from researchers. It is an inclusive approach" (Epstein et al., 2015, p. 711). Practice research may capture practitioners, researchers, service users and educators collectively to engage in processes of inquiry, where each party "become partners in research instead of only consumers of it" (Uggerhoj, 2011, p. 46). In this manner, social work practitioners, and other collaborating parties, can meaningfully and enthusiastically engage in research that has implications for their own practice, and impacts for service user outcomes and experience (Epstein & Blumenfield, 2001).

Throughout the past decade, social work practice has been confronted with increased expectations to measure outcomes of service delivery (Osborne, 2002). This is also seen in architectural discourse, where measurable outcomes of built environments in relation to well-being are increasingly sought (Ulrich, 2006). Terms such as 'evidence-based practice' (Uggerhoj, 2011) and 'empirical research' have become commonplace in research seeking to understand health and social work services, and their associated built environments. This "age of accountability" (Austin, Dal Santo, & Lee, 2012, p. 175) has placed increased pressures on managers and practitioners at human service organisations to specify service objectives, and quantify outcomes of these objectives, involving significant investment of time and resources. This focus has led to an emphasis on developing new knowledge in a scientific approach (Uggerhoj, 2011) that is also closely related to local needs (Julkunen, 2011). However, researchers have noted how reports from such research have focused predominantly on outputs, such as how many clients served in a given timeframe, and less on outcomes, such as level of improvement of service user experience (Austin et al., 2012). Further, "even when outcome data is available, it is rarely presented in a form that practitioners can either understand or utilise to improve their practice" (Austin et al., 2012, p. 175).

Alongside the emphasis on measurement of outcomes, practitioners are increasingly expected to demonstrate how knowledge from their organisation or research centres is being meaningfully incorporated into the services provided (Epstein et al., 2015). This has led to explorations of new ways in which practice may be assessed, and new practices developed. There is growing interest to incorporate the service user voice, alongside those of carers, into the research process, and the development of evidence-based strategies that can improve service user outcomes and experience (Epstein & Blumenfield, 2001).

Fieldwork undertaken involved a series of focused interviews with five respondent groups: service users of mental health services, practicing therapists/counsellors, carers of a loved one with a mental illness, architects/designers who practice in the field of designing for mental health and design experts/researchers who work and research in the field of design for mental health. This fieldwork was undertaken in order to understand service user experience of built environments delivering therapy. The collected data was analysed through a thematic network (Attride-Stirling, 2001) and was re-interpreted to draw conclusions on spatial perception and implications for how built environments relate to the function of therapy. Open-ended questions were asked in order to facilitate participants expressing their views on the issues being investigated (Creswell, 2003). The interviews lasted from 40–90 minutes depending on interviewees' responses to interview questions. This exploratory qualitative analysis (Attride-Stirling, 2001) was undertaken with the data from the five respondent groups noted above.

Through this fieldwork undertaken by Liddicoat, a key exploratory research thread emerged relative to the influence of the built environment on therapeutic outcomes and service user experience: the significance of the home environment and its relationship to therapeutic processes. This research thread is discussed below, as it was reflected upon by interview participants. This analysis is also presented with reference to clinical literature to better enable an understanding of why these specific spatial environments/perceptions and their particular design is significant. Following this is a discussion on how the home environment might be utilised to inform therapeutic processes through self-help materials.

The home

The notion of home and its relationship to human experience and potential therapeutic application is discussed within this chapter. There have been many phenomenological studies examining the relationship between an individual's constructs of self and experience in relation to home (Bachelard, 1969; Cooper Marcus, 2006). Experience of the home has been linked to creativity (Buttimer, 1983) and to therapeutic effect (Peled, 1976). Peled and Ayalon (1988, p. 87) note how the "re-designing [of] an existing dwelling may play a role in . . . disintegration processes . . . [and] may reactivate previous conflicts". They also explain that "dealing with these conflicts therapeutically and probing their spatial implications at an early stage" (p. 87) is closely related to therapeutic affect. Particularly, the spatial configuration of the home is important, the relationship of the home and its territories may be a manifestation of other interpersonal or intrapersonal relationships (Altman, 1975; Cooper Marcus, 2006), and spatial conditions of the home may create avenues for improved dialogue and communication (Golembiewski, 2012; Joseph, Keller, & Gulwadi, 2009).

There is also a body of literature examining person and environment fit, exploring how characteristics of individuals and their environments affect well-being (Caplan, 1983; Evans & Cohen, 1987). Person and environment fit is also examined in terms of the perceived supportiveness of the environment in connection with personal goals, as environments may offer facilitation and motivation for action in the world, and thus influence an individual's image of their environment and themselves (Canter, 1991; Kaplan, 1983). Within such studies, the role of the home environment is seen as significant, with up to 100 per cent of respondents citing the home as an influential environment in their lives (Wallenius, 1997). This is suggestive that interaction and engagement with the home may have significant effects relative to mental well-being and individual images of the world. The spatial organisation of a home may provide insight into the self and individual identity, perhaps the spatial organisation of a home may become a platform for therapy to unfold and be explored. This was examined, with service users who self-harm, and is discussed below across three themes: communication, dissociation and evolving sense of self.

Communication

Individuals who self-harm commonly find an inability to communicate through conventional language means (Simpson, 2006). In the therapeutic literature, it is acknowledged that perhaps the increasing incidence rates of self-harm and the poor success rates of therapy processes are due to their reliance on words for communication (Nathan, 2004). Therapies "encourage patients to examine their inner conflicts, their interpersonal functioning and the meaning of symptoms" (Lammers, Exerkate, & DeJong, 2007, p. 101). Here the patient is forced to voice their innermost sensitivities in a situation where they may not feel comfortable or do not feel they have the means to express themselves without communication via the body, as occurs in self-harming (Huband & Tantam, 2009). This instead is a kind of "communicate[ion] through . . . [a] body language, not in . . . verbally articulated terms" (Palasmaa, 1998, p. 29).

Communication can also be afforded via engagement with physical environments, such as through personalisation (Cooper Marcus, 2006; Golembiewski, 2012). Professor Clare Cooper Marcus explores how the home environment can be a signifier for aspects of ourselves, and the personalisation of space speaks of the self to others. This is also supported in literature on designing for mental health, where affording personalisation and communication is important to therapeutic outcomes (Golembiewski, 2012). This is reinforced by fieldwork conducted by Liddicoat. Service users speak of physical environments in relation to communication:

> If I am in a contained room, you can't talk to me, no! I am in my head, I need to escape somehow, and then you can't because there is nowhere to look! There is nowhere to feel safe [and to express] . . . if I could move the furniture around the room, that flexibility would be good.
> *(Service user, 2015, personal communication)*

Conversely, when a space is not supportive in this way, communication shuts down: "I found that very confrontational, it was a very small room . . . I just felt that I wanted to get out of there, it was just like too full on . . . I just wanted to run out" (Service user, 2015, personal communication). The home may also be used as a communicative tool by the individual, via engagement and personalisation, which may have therapeutic relevance. The home may consciously express aspects of the inhabitant through the possessions within the dwelling, the symbols of self, functioning as representations of conscious decisions about personal expression (Cooper Marcus, 2006). Reflecting upon the meaning of these communications contributes to psychological development. Carolyn Verheyen (1990) and Cooper Marcus (2006) suggest allowing the service user to assess what they have been consciously and unconsciously expressing about themselves through the home, and also how this communication may be adjusted as an increasing awareness of self and identity is developed through this process. This is closely aligned with aims of therapeutic processes, enabled by an engagement with, and consideration of, the home environment.

Dissociation

The notion of dissociation is one correlated with individuals who self-harm. Self-harm is an act that removes the 'numbness' described by the service users

(Huband & Tantam, 2009) and allows them to be present again in the environment, to reconnect with their body and wider spaces. The physical environment relates closely to dissociation: "Having things we can touch and stuff . . . it should be in the whole environment . . . it helps bring you back to the present, but also gives you access to memories and things, in a safe way" (Service user, 2015, personal communication). As another service user explains, of her time in an inpatient care environment:

> Engaging with the senses can also be an escapism, and be fully present but also to escape from the overbearing nature of the psychiatric unit and the intensity of that, so it allows you to be present and in your own body, but also to escape from the physical environment which is so intense . . . when I become triggered or stressed, I need something to hold, so that brings me back to the present.
> *(Service user, 2015, personal communication)*

Dissociation may be relieved through sensorial engagement with meaningful environments, such as the home. Service users describe how they use the built environment to try and derive sensory encounter in order to try and remain present. Cooper Marcus discusses how engagement with the home may bring about a stronger sense of mindfulness and presence. The aim of this is to uncover lost parts of the self through a consideration of the senses, first psychologically, then physically. This is in line with the notion of dissociation, where individuals who self-harm explain how they feel as though something is missing, and they are detached from reality and sensory encounter (Aiken, 2000). This illustrates how an engagement with the home environment may be supportive of aims of therapy.

Evolving sense of self

Alongside the dissociation behavior noted above, individuals who injure themselves may also experience unstable self-image or sense of self (American Psychiatric Association, 2000). There is architectural discourse discussing linkages between the architectural environments, skins, exposure and the self (Colomina, 1992). Environments are discussed in literature in relation to self-harm and identity,[5] through concepts of territories (Goffman, 1971). This is linked to identity through the notion that each individual has a territory within an environment, a space to exist (Huband & Tantam, 2009). Evolving sense of self is also alluded to through notions of identity in relation to physical space:

> From a therapeutic perspective, I think it's important to be able to put your identity on space, because then you are an individual, that you are somebody, that you are not just a number, that you can make a difference, that you feel validated and listened to, all of those reasons. If I could have a space to adjust and make it mine, that would absolutely make me feel more validated.
> *(Service user, 2015, personal communication)*

As another service user remarks of her time in inpatient care:

> I would never want to go back to a psychiatric unit. The space can be just, so, traumatising. Because, there is no identity, it's like it has no heart. It would be helpful if you [the service user] could give the space identity.
> *(Service user, 2015, personal communication)*

Further, Goffman notes how territories can be marked or delineated by the placement of the body, bodily gestures and the glance (Goffman, 1971). These each have design and spatial connotations, including proxemics, spatial layouts, surveillance and placement of glazing. As the home environment is closely experienced and understood, the territories of the home may have particular significance relative to mental boundaries and identities.

Cooper Marcus (2006) explains that the home, and an individual's relationship with the home, can have profound effects in transforming a crisis into an opportunity for change. She suggests a consideration of the home environment in conjunction with therapeutic treatment. During therapy "ensues an almost agonising conflict between security and movement, between feelings of comfort and the yearning need for expansion and change . . . [the home] may be safe, but it may also be constricting" (Cooper Marcus, 2006, p. 113). Further, evolving self-image often centres on moving beyond spaces that feel particularly alienating; these spaces may offer clues to uncovering hidden aspects of the self. This is in line with research supporting the ability to personalise hospital environments as conducive to therapeutic effect (Golembiewski, 2010). This further reinforces the potential inclusion of personalisation of spaces of the home as useful in identity production alongside therapeutic interventions.

Therapeutic implications and self-help materials

The above discussions of communication, dissociation and evolving sense of self enabled by a therapeutic consideration and exploration of home may be relevant in treatment of individuals who self-harm, with the view to improving service user outcomes and service user experience in mental health. One service user responded to the idea of involving their home in therapy practice:

> Yes, adjusting their home environments would be great! Taking ownership and control which is empowering, I think that would be really helpful . . . Because that person might feel safe while they are with their counsellor, or whatever, but then they have still got to go home . . . it would be empowering to re-adjust your home space, because again it gives that identity, and makes it your own, you're safe, some control over your environment. You would have to confront some of the things you are dealing

with . . . that can be a mindfulness thing as well, you know, looking around . . . [thinking about] how they feel about being in that space

(Service user, 2015, personal communication)

This chapter suggests the development of a self-help guide to be employed by service users, as part of therapeutic processes. This may be in the form of a series of tasks, to be undertaken by the service user in their own home, between therapy sessions. This can then be usefully employed as points for discussion and elaboration in therapy sessions. A series of example exercises from existing literature have been selected and analysed with relevance to the service user perceptions discussed in this chapter. These are presented below, as a potential means to integrate the home environment with therapeutic practice and improve service user outcomes and experience. These exercises explore relationships based on physicality/location, relationships based on personalisation/identity, and exploring the home as a space for the development of agency through the control and manipulation of space to meet individual needs (Liddicoat, 2015).

Peled's Location Task was developed as a means of eliciting an individual's constructs of important spatial regions of a space (Peled, 1976), which was used in subsequent therapy sessions as a platform for discussion. By making explicit the individual's desired position, portioning and orientation of spatial regions, a consideration of the meanings imbued within this division of space may be developed and explored. Individuals may use two boards to locate the inside and outside places of an ideal spatial entity, such as a home (see Figure 17.1).

All regions, as well as inside versus outside and the interrelationships of the system as a whole, must be considered by the individual. This resultant layout is a representation of the interaction and balance of integrative and self-assertive forces (Koestler, 1967), or a representation of "the multiple relations that are eventually constructed as its identity, as this place" (Peled & Ayalon, 1988, p. 100). This location task is essentially a tool linking the design of a home, and the associated

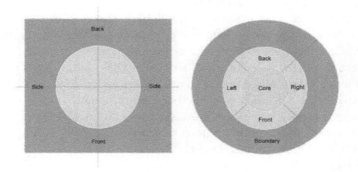

FIGURE 17.1 Location task.

Source: image based on those found in Peled and Ayalon (1988).

perceptions of spatiality, to the identity of a home. Further, this tool may serve as an exploratory platform to examine aspects of an individual's own identity as manifest through the meanings imbued in the resultant spatial configuration.

The home may also be used as a communicative tool by the service user via engagement and personalisation, which may have therapeutic relevance. The home may consciously express aspects of the inhabitant through the possessions within the dwelling, the symbols of self, functioning as representations of conscious decisions about personal expression. Carolyn Verheyen suggests an exercise involving an inventory and categorisation of the visible material contents of the home in order to understand what is consciously or unconsciously disclosed about oneself in a private home environment (Verheyen, 1990). Cooper Marcus suggests another exercise, whereby one draws a symbol of what the home means, noticing one's emotions and sensations while doing so, A dialogue is then begun, where one might ask questions of the house, and listen to what it may have to reply. "Continue these dialogues with the house, objects, images, rooms . . . [consider] what is it that you communicate about me? What is in store for you in the future?" (Cooper Marcus, 2006, p. 76). This exercise is rich in communicative skills, allowing the service user to assess what they have been consciously and unconsciously expressing about themselves through the home, and also how this communication may be adjusted as an increasing awareness of self and identity is developed through this process. This is closely aligned with aims of therapeutic processes, enabled by an engagement with, and consideration of, the home.

The development of sense of self and personal agency may also be afforded through an engagement with meaningful physical environments (Liddicoat, 2015), such as those found in the home. This may at first be confronting, by disrupting the familiar and provoking hitherto dormant issues or unresolved conflicts, but is ultimately a means to develop empowerment (Liddicoat, 2016). Cooper Marcus suggests an exercise whereby a service user might recall an environment where they felt safe and at home, and then adjust a space in their home environment to become a kind of sanctuary, to evoke comfort, control and empowerment (Cooper Marcus, 2006). This physical adjustment of space to meet individual needs creates a supportive space and simultaneously develops a sense of ownership and empowerment (Seamon, 1979). This may then be used to prompt discussion and self-reflection in therapy sessions. Cooper Marcus (2006) also suggests the assemblage of found objects to create a sacred space, a space for the individual, to reflect and de-stress. This is in line with research supporting the ability to personalise hospital environments as conducive to therapeutic effect (Golembiewski, 2010). This further reinforces the potential inclusion of personalisation of spaces of the home as useful in identity production alongside therapeutic interventions.

The exercises described in this chapter may also be relevant to the evolving sense of self. These exercises unfold to offer clues as to what parts of the self and identity may no longer be manifest, and what may be brought to the fore and developed through a physical interaction with, and modification of, the current environment, such as the home. This emphasises both the notion of an adjustable environment that can be personalised, and the therapeutic links between psychological development and the home. Further research is needed to explore other potential means for the significant home environment to be integrated into therapy, and the format of associated self-help materials. The nature of the interaction between the service user and the home environment is a unique research thread, which is worthy of further investigation to unpack the significant elements of this interaction.

This chapter has confirmed, through a review of the literature, key connections between design of built environments and mental well-being. By exploring the role of the home in therapy, this chapter has investigated the relationship between mental health and spatial encounter. The fieldwork conducted demonstrated that for these service users, environmental encounter and spatial engagement with the home is significant and meaningful. A focus on this, together with consideration and a physicality of activities being privileged, may be usefully employed as points for discussion and elaboration in therapy sessions. As suggested by this chapter, such integration of the home environment with therapeutic practice may improve service user outcomes and service user experience, and increase the service users' sense of empowerment and agency through the articulation of physical space (Liddicoat, 2015). Further research directions are also identified, including further developing the understanding of the role of the home in therapeutic processes, to advance comprehension of the nature of these interactions and how this may be gainfully utilised in a self-help guide to integrate the home into therapeutic practice. This chapter confirms, through a literature review and fieldwork with service users, therapists and carers, strong links between space and service user outcomes and service user experience. This chapter emphasises the importance of the service user placed at the centre of future research to understand these individuals' perceptions of spatiality and the self, and to enable their participation as co-designers to be understood within that context.

Notes

1 The built environment can be conceptualised as the human-made space in which people live, work and recreate. Within this research, the focus was the environment of the counselling workspace (the space where a therapeutic/counselling session occurs), but this extended to a broader discussion of the wider facility of a therapy/counselling practice, an inpatient hospital and similar and the home environment, which was noted by service users as significant.
2 Within this chapter, the term 'home' is considered as inclusive of physical items, such as furniture and similar; physical aspects such as ceiling height, colours, lighting levels and similar; and other aspects such as control, personalisation, territories, interpersonal distances and similar.
3 The term 'service user' is used within this chapter referring to the individuals who are clients of mental health service delivery. The terms patients and service users are used interchangeably.
4 Self-harm is defined within this research as the physical harming of the body without suicidal intent. This self-harm usually involves self-cutting or burning of the skin, but may include other methods of injuring the body tissues. More broad definitions of what may

constitute self-harm, such as eating disorders, tobacco smoking, alcohol abuse or some forms of tattooing are correlated by clinically separate conditions, also conditions such as depression are not included in this research.
5 The term 'identity' is used within this chapter as it is used by Altman (1975), Goffman (1971) and Cooper Marcus (2006).

References

Aiken, C. (2000). *At home, no one hears you scream*. London: Jessica Kingsley.
Altman, I. (1975). *The environment and social behaviour: Privacy, personal space, territory, crowding*. Monterey, CA: Brooks/Cole.
American Psychiatric Association. (2000). *Diagnostic and statistical manual (DSM-IV-TR)* (4th ed.). Arlington, TX: American Psychiatric Association.
Attride-Stirling, J. (2001). Thematic networks: An analytic tool for qualitative research. *Qualitative Research*, 1(3), 385–405.
Austin, M. J., Dal Santo, T. S., & Lee, C. (2012). Building organizational supports for research-minded practitioners. *Journal of Evidence-Based Social Work*, 9, 174–211.
Bachelard, G. (1969). *The poetics of space*. Boston, MA: Beacon.
Buttimer, A. (1983). *Creativity and context*. Lund, Sweden: Royal University of Lund.
Canter, D. V. (1991). Understanding, assessing and acting in places: Is an integrative framework possible? In T. Garling & G. W. Evans (Eds.), *Environment, cognition and action* (pp. 191–209). New York, NY: Oxford University Press.
Caplan, R. D. (1983). Person-environment fit: Past, present and future. In C. L. Cooper (Ed.), *Stress research* (pp. 35–78). New York, NY: Wiley.
Carlson, L. E., Speca, M., Patel, K. D., & Goodey, E. (2003). Mindfulness-based stress-reduction in relation to quality of life, mood, symptoms of stress, and immune parameters in breast and prostate cancer outpatients. *Psychosomatic Medicine*, 65, 571–581.
Colomina, B. (1992). The split wall: Domestic voyeurism. In B. Colomina (Ed.), *Sexuality and space* (pp. 73–130). New York, NY: Princeton Architectural Press.
Cooper Marcus, C. (2006). *House as a mirror of self: Exploring the deeper meaning of home*. Berwick: Hicolas-Hayes.
Creswell, J. W. (2003). *Research design: Qualitative, quantitative and mixed method approaches*. London: Sage.
Epstein, I., & Blumenfield, S. (Eds.). (2001). *Clinical data-mining in practice-based research: Social work in hospital settings*. New York, NY: Haworth Social Work Practice Press.
Epstein, I., Fisher, M., Julkunen, I., Uggerhoj, L., Austin, M. J., & Sim, T. (2015). The New York statement on the evolving definition of practice research designed for continuing dialogue: A bulletin from the 3rd International Conference on Practice Research (2014). *Research on Social Work Practice*, 25(6), 711–714.
Evans, G. W., & Cohen, S. (1987). Environmental Stress. In D. Stokols & I. Altman (Eds.), *Handbook of environmental psychology* (vol. 2, pp. 571–610). New York, NY: John Wiley.
Goffman, E. (1971). The territories of the self. In E. Goffman (Ed.), *Relations in public: Microstudies of the public order* (pp. 28–62). London: Penguin.
Golembiewski, J. (2010). Start making sense: Applying a salutogenic model to architectural design for psychiatric care. *Facilities*, 28(3/4), 100–117.
Golembiewski, J. (2012). *There's something in my head (but its not me). The complex relationship between the built environment and schizophrenia: From aetiology to recovery* (Doctorate of Philosophy) Sydney University, Sydney.
Gross, R., Sasson, Y., Zarhy, M., & Zohar, J. (1998). Healing environment in psychiatric hospital design. *General Hospital Psychiatry*, 20, 108–114.

Huband, N., & Tantam, D. (2009). *Understanding repeated self-injury: A multidisciplinary approach*. Basingstoke: Palgrave Macmillan.
Joseph, A., Keller, A., & Gulwadi, G. B. (2009). Improving the patient experience: Best practices for safety-net clinic redesign. Retrieved from www.chcf.org/~/media/Files/PDF/S/SafetyNetDesign.pdf.
Julkunen, I. (2011). Knowledge-production processes in practice research: Outcomes and critical elements. *Social Work & Society, 9*(1), 60–75.
Kaplan, S. (1983). A model of person–environment compatibility. *Environment & Behaviour, 15*, 311–332.
Koestler, A. (1967). *The ghost in the machine*. Michigan: Macmillan.
Lammers, M., Exerkate, C. C., & DeJong, C. A. J. (2007). A Dutch day treatment program for anorexia and bulimia nervosa in comparison with internationally described programs. *European Eating Disorders Review, 15*(2), 98–111.
Liddicoat, S. (2015). Exploring relations between body, communication and agency in therapeutic space. Paper presented at the Living and Learning: Research for a Better Built Environment: 49th International Conference of the Architectural Science Association 2015, Melbourne.
Liddicoat, S. (2016). *Counselling workspace design and therapeutic practice*. Paper presented at the Fifty Years Later: Revisiting the Role of Architectural Science in Design and Practice: 50th International Conference of the Architectural Science Association 2015, Adelaide, Australia.
Marberry, S. (Ed.) (2006). *Improving healthcare with better building design*. Chicago, IL: Health Administration Press.
Nathan, J. (2004). In-depth work with patients who self-harm: Doing the impossible? *Psychoanalytic Psychotherapy, 18*, 167–181.
Osborne, S. (2002). *Public management: A critical perspective*. London: Routledge.
Palasmaa, J. (1998). *Encounters: Architectural essays*. Finland: Rakennusteito Oy.
Pearson, M., & Wilson, H. (2012). Soothing spaces and healing places: Is there an ideal counselling room design? *Psychotherapy in Australia, 18*(3), 46–53.
Peled, A. (1976). The Strathclyde location test: A projective technique for eliciting the constructs of spatial division of an experienced environmental event. In P. Suefeld & J. A. Russel (Eds.), *The behavioural basis of design. Book II* (pp. 107–119). Stroudsburg: Dowden, Hutchinson, & Ross.
Peled, A., & Ayalon, O. (1988). The role of the spatial organisation of the home in family therapy: A case study. *Journal of Environmental Psychology, 8*, 87–106.
Pressly, P. K., & Heesacker, M. (2001). The physical environment and counselling: A review of theory and research. *Journal of Counselling and Development, 79*(2), 148–160.
Seamon, D. (1979). *The geography of the lifeworld*. New York, NY: St Martin's Press.
Simpson, A. (2006). Can mainstream health services provide meaningful care for people who self-harm? A critical reflection. *Journal of Psychiatric and Mental Health Nursing, 13*, 429–436.
Sivadon, B. (1970). Space as experienced: Therapeutic implications. In H. M. Proshansky, W. H. Ittelson, & L. G. Rivlin (Eds.), *Environmental psychology* (pp. 409–419). New York, NY: Holt, Rinehardt & Winston.
Uggerhoj, L. (2011). What is practice research in social work: Definitions, barriers and possibilities. *Social Work & Society, 9*(1), 45–59.
Ulrich, R. S. (2006). Essay: Evidence-based health-care architecture. *Medicine and Creativity, 368*(December), 538–539.
Ulrich, R. S., Zimring, C., Quan, X., & Joseph, A. (2004). *The role of the physical environment in the hospital of the 21st century*. Retrieved from www.healthdesign.org.

Ulrich, R. S., Zimring, C., Quan, X., & Joseph, A. (2006). The environment's impact on stress. In S. Marberry (Ed.), *Improving healthcare with better building design* (pp. 37–61). Chicago, IL: Health Administration Press.

Ulrich, R. S., Zimring, C., Zhu, X., DuBose, J., Seo, H., Choi, Y., . . . Joseph, A. (2008). A review of the research literature on evidence-based healthcare design (Part I). *Health Environments Research and Design, 1,* 61–125.

Verheyen, C. (1990). *The therapeutic function of the home and personal objects*. San Francisco, CA: San Francisco State University.

Wallenius, M. (1997). Personal projects in everyday places: Perceived supportiveness of the environment and psychological wellbeing. *Journal of Environmental Psychology, 19,* 131–143.

18

THE OUTSIDER GALLERY

Using art and music to open up mental health spaces

Ben Wakeling and Jon Hall

Introduction

The Outsider Gallery is situated in Clarendon Recovery College in Haringey, London. The idea grew out of collaboration between artist Ben Wakeling and music therapist, Jon Hall. Working together with people in psychiatric wards, they developed a model for extending this work into the community. One part of the project is the gallery, which displays work created by people with experiences of mental health problems. Some of this work is for sale, and some is not. Some has been created during the therapeutic process and some by people who are no longer using mental health services. In the same space, Jon and Ben run art and music therapy 'modules' that last for ten weeks and end with a showcase or exhibition open to friends, family and the public. This part of the project is known as Creativity and Recovery for Wellbeing, or CREW. CREW was funded for 2016/2017 by the local mental health trust.

Interview and tour of the gallery with Ben Wakeling, artist and co-founder

The gallery and therapy rooms are spread over two floors. Downstairs are three interlinked rooms, two gallery/therapy rooms and the café. Upstairs are the art room and recording studio. Artwork is also displayed in corridors and on the stairs.

Downstairs: room 1

Ben: We've got three rooms that we use as the gallery and this first room is for people who are based in the community who previously have had issues, been under section and been in services. So there's a variety of work, we've got international people as well.

Laura: So these works weren't created here, they've been brought here?

Ben: We have works here from Belgium and West London, and a gentleman who is now in the peer support part of our peer support programme. We met him on the ward and over the two years he's progressed to the point where he hasn't gone back to the ward since working with us. Which is really great story, a victory for him. And now he's at the point where in our sessions he's working with us as a peer support individual. He's got a lot of experience of what the wards are like and dealing with bipolar so his experience comes in very valuable.

The great thing about having someone who's been through the system themselves is that they can relate to someone who's struggling on the day and it's an approach where it's non-clinical. And it means that someone who's struggling or on our programme can find that less daunting to talk to. It opens up more avenues for them to build a stronger relationship within our project. And it just offers another avenue. I just really believe that mental health is such a variety. An individual might have the same diagnosis but their reaction in dealing with it or coping with it is always different. So having that in our sessions is a great tool to draw upon. It's why peer support, or working with individuals who know that system, know what it feels like to be in that head space is so valuable. I do believe that you need to be cautious as well. So with this specific individual it got to the point where we didn't want to keep dragging him back to the point of being a service user, we wanted him to be able to move on. So giving him this job role is another major step in his development. And understanding how to maintain a healthy relationship with his mental health.

This is a very non-clinical setting. That was our very first objective to make a therapy room non-clinical. We've painted the walls. We've hung amazing art works, because there were no images at all here. And this is used as a therapy room. And I think letting people surround themselves in an environment where there's other likeminded individuals puts people at ease a bit more. I mean everything's got its own place. Clinical rooms are just as important but I think our aim was to make it less threatening.

Laura: What was the aim in having the artwork up here, how do you think that changes the experience of being here for people?

Ben: I think it can show it can inspire an individual to think 'oh so this person's got a diagnosis' or 'there's people out there like myself who are struggling' so perhaps this might inspire people to go on to use other services. So hopefully having a well-dressed room inspires other people who use it.

Laura: I notice you have very much made it like a gallery, rather than a therapy room. So you've got the text about the artists, the prices. So why have you made that decision?

Ben: This is the community part, so everyone was comfortable with having their names on show, and perhaps a price tag. With our therapy work that we do here we don't go as far as that. So we might hang their work and certainly not a price tag because it's a different part of what's happening. Having it in a safe place, for people to see. Our results show that it's empowering for someone, because they hear the compliments and they can see the reactions of the public or other service users.

Laura: So who would come in and view these?

Ben: So it's open to the public as well. But we take care to look after people who are attending the sessions so we don't put the names up, or the prices until further on down the line. Because they're not necessarily wanting to be artists or wanting to go further afield than their therapy programme.

Laura: So they are concurrent streams of work. This seems like a good time to ask you to describe the overall project. What are the different bits of work you're doing here?

Ben: So we have a music therapist, Jon Hall. I'm an artist, and I manage the gallery side as well as the expressive arts sessions. We're working with yourselves, UEL, who are delivering an evaluation that hopefully we can take forward to funders and generate stability. So there's two sides of what the Outsider Gallery does. We have the gallery, commercial art, where we invite the public in to see what the mental health world looks like from our point of view and the work that we're trying to deliver. The other arm is the therapeutic side, so working in hospitals or out in the community. And that part of Outsiders, our idea is to work with patients in hospital up until their release date and once they are back in the community we pick them up in this building, which is open to the community, and carry on that work. Because what we saw was that once someone was discharged they are likely to go back into hospital so we want to stop that conveyor belt. And I think that idea of building a relationship on the ward and then allowing that to continue in the community has stopped that. That's what we've seen in our pilot programme. Everyone we've worked with, except one, hasn't returned to hospital. So I think that's a massive achievement. And those numbers supposedly its £360 odd per night and if you got back into hospital you're there for weeks or months. So stopping that saves the NHS money as well. For the fraction of money to fund us. It's good for the individual, but also for the NHS as well.

Laura: I know that you are in the NHS but also not as well. Do you think it's possible to create a space like this within usual mental health services?

Ben: Yeah we just need to be given rooms or a building. I think it's as simple as that. It would be amazing to perhaps take over a building that's not being used and really create a flagship for what we're trying to do. How to do that I don't know. But I don't see it as us solving problems for the NHS or other services. It's more adding to their skillset. Because everything's valuable, from CBT, to medication, they're all important. But I think what we're doing adds to those approaches. We're not approaching it as 'oh look at us we can solve your problems'. We just want to help because there is a problem. We just want to be one of the options rather than saying we're going to ride in on a white horse and solve all your problems. We just need to band together because you know society is hard at the moment money is tight and we're just a group of people that want to help, along with people already doing great work.

Downstairs: room 2

Ben: So this is our second room, which is works that have been made by people in our sessions. And because they're still very vulnerable, we take each person case by case. So we might not list their names unless they are very adamant that we do, because they might be proud. So this is a room to show what's happening within our therapy sessions. We have speakers as well so the music side can play in here. And these are some of the images from our sessions.

Laura: So can you explain what you and Jon do during the sessions and how you work with people?

Ben: At the moment we are only able to deliver a ten-week session. Personally I would like longer. All the data that UEL are picking up shows that people want it to go on for longer. We work upstairs, we've got an art studio and a music studio upstairs. And our approach is to build that relationship and eventually start teasing out their personal story. Through them telling a personal story I believe it to generate awareness within themselves and for them to begin to understand some issues or life moments. And through that self-awareness I think there's various possibilities and directions that they can go towards. We try to engage with them through art specifically. So it's all about, well perhaps it's not all about a self-portrait but it is definitely about trying to engage with them and tell their personal story, to create their self-portrait. Which has positive knock-on effects I think.

Laura: And have you had any feedback from people, say, whose pictures are here and how they feel about them being displayed like this?

Ben: We wouldn't show anything unless we are very confident that that's what they want. The gallery is always secondary to the work that we're doing. So we might not introduce that idea of them showing their work to the gallery until later on. And because of their trust with us, we don't want to persuade them to show in the gallery as well. So that process is constantly shifting with each individual. There are a couple of people who don't want them on show. That's not an issue at all. Our CREW programme has to take priority over the gallery. I'll give you an example. At our last show, this person here was so excited to have his work. He's never seen himself as an artist or perhaps doesn't but he was so proud of what he was creating. So during our private view he was going up to complete strangers and bringing them over to show his work, and to discuss his work and what he's been doing. That happens quite often. Obviously there's always individuals who are nervous about that. And I suppose that's when I need to put on my gallery hat and manage them through expectations or some of the pitfalls that might happen to showing your work to the public. And some of the possibilities as well. But there are individuals who do eventually want to try and sell their work. So it's always different. Each individual is different. And I think because we're in a bit of a niche and our team's quite small we're able to man manage, and work with everyone as an individual as well as a group. I think we've got the space here to accommodate all scenarios. If someone doesn't want to show it, that's fine. If someone wants to sell it, that's fine too. If someone wants to be anonymous, that's fine.

Laura: So you mentioned there the private view. So you do a showcase at the end of each ten weeks. Can you just explain a bit about what that is and why you decided to include that in the programme?

Ben: Part of our idea with helping with recovery was as simple as let's find a private space just for everyone who's attended therapy to hang up our work or show our music that we've created, as a way of acknowledging the end of the programme. A way of sharing within the group what's been happening and where they are, a kind of check-in. And it was a way, we felt, was quite a positive way to end the programme. And that naturally lead to some people wanting to invite their families and friends and the organic process of inviting the public came about as well. So we would always discuss it as a group if we wanted to do an exhibition. And we leave it as entirely their decision. Jon and I whatever their decision is, we try and make it happen. And it's also a great way for them to get involved as well so they can help with perhaps some of the writing, which goes up if we are having an exhibition, or perhaps the layout. So it gives them a bit of purpose as well and it's just really good closure. It's a really nice way to end the programme.

Laura: So how have those gone, have you had two?

Ben: We've had three. So we opened the gallery last September and we had about 250 people come. Again everyone was comfortable with opening it up to the public. We made sure over a number of weeks because again minds can get changed. You can be in one place at one point and then change. And everything was given the green light. And the numbers were amazing. And the press picked it up, and UEL got involved. And then we've gone on to have two other exhibitions, and our last one will be in September. And that will show everything we've done over the past year. So I think it will be a very moving experience to be a part of. And I think it's a great way for people who attend our programmes to bring people who are close to them in their lives. It's a great way for them to understand their journey in perhaps a different way. I think it's a very sharing process.

One father of a person we were working with really struggles with managing his son. When he attended the exhibition he was in tears, he found a new way of understanding what his son was going through. So those connections or understanding and more learning that goes into it is so important. And the father was given a fresh lease of life, and it gave him a bit more energy to deal with what his son goes through. So it was amazing to be a part of that and to help facilitate it.

Laura: So it strikes me that normally, or often, family and friends are quite excluded from people's mental health care and journey. We tend to take people away and put them in therapy. So was that a conscious decision?

Ben: Yeah a little bit, yeah for sure. This is speaking from experience, as I'm diagnosed with bipolar. I think when I was in a bad way, and for years afterwards, people just walked on eggshells around me, or wouldn't even ask. It's easier to just change the conversation, or perhaps that's what they felt was the best thing to do. And I've sort of seen that from other people with the patient and their family in a room together. Because it's such a taboo, people don't know how to start that conversation. So what we do is completely break down that barrier, that awkwardness. We want to ignite that conversation between the family. And it happens. It's great we can get mental health awareness out there from the gallery side, but I think it's more important to acknowledge that we're helping start these conversations. It's helping a family member bring up the subject of what's going on.

Laura: And it seems like that's quite multi-layered isn't it. Because it's the work itself, it's having art or music to say this is me, I don't have to tell you directly because I've produced this thing. But then it's also doing it in quite a normative context as well. 'Come to my art show' is different to 'come to family therapy'.

Ben: Again, that's really important. But our way of helping that subject is to help start that conversation. That seems to be happening. Hopefully it's helping. But that seems to be happening, and that's worth noting.

Downstairs: room 3

Ben: So then there's the café. Which again is for patients in the system, or in our programme.

Laura: So these are people who've made the stuff here again?

Ben: Yes that's right.

Laura: So why did you decide to put them in the café as well?

Ben: We're just taking over the entire building. Because this building's all dealing with mental health, so we have service users running workshops, we have private services delivering some of their programmes, we've got us here. The café is a relaxed environment obviously for people to have teas and coffees so it makes sense to put up a bit of work as well. And it's just all of us in this building finding a bit of rhythm together to carry on. We've got the corridors as well.

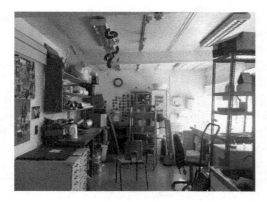

FIGURE 18.1 Art room at the Outsider Gallery.

Downstairs corridor

Ben: Here, because it's wheelchair accessible, one thing I've never seen in a gallery is if you're in a wheelchair is art at the height for a wheelchair. And I've never seen it in a museum or gallery before, and I thought in the corridor we could lower all the work so if you're in a wheelchair it would be the correct height for you. So again it's putting service users first and making sure that they're part of the conversation as well, that everyone's part of the conversation. So we've got staff as well to start creating work and putting their work up. So making everyone part of the conversation or being part of the ecosystem of mental health. So that's why the work is quite low.

Laura: It's great. So this is stuff that's been made here again?

Ben: Yes, these ones have been made here.

Art room

Ben: This is our art room where we cause loads of trouble. As you can see we draw on the walls, on canvasses. Anything that I can get my hands on I bring in. I think having a proper studio, which, we're not there yet, but for people to really let go is really important. A lot of the situations I've been in or witnessed is that you might have a desk, and A4 sheet of paper and a few colouring pencils. And I don't think that's enough. You need to be able to drop paint on the floor, it's ok. If you wanna throw paint at a wall. A room where anything can happen is quite a powerful thing to have. And once that individual understands that, what they create is just endless, and so moving.

Laura: And how do you communicate that to people, that this is a different kind of space where you can do anything.

Ben: A conversation's really important to have. I might be able to say it all in one go but for them to understand and believe me takes a bit longer. My way of engaging most of the time is that I create my own artwork with them. Which a lot of the time sparks an idea for them, and then they're up and running. And then I'm just their personal assistant.

Laura: And if you come into a room and people have drawn all over the walls you know it's a bit different, that this is a bit more of an open space.

Ben: Yeah for me I think that drawing on walls is a great tool that people should implement a lot more. Because there's a sense of rebelliousness in there. It's a great way to build trust and release that inner child that we all have and we all grow out of. So it's good to return to that sometimes. As he would say, get some shit off your chest.

Laura: Yes, so this looks like an art room, rather than a mental health room. So that was a deliberate choice?

Ben: Yes, because I think my position is now that we all have a mind, and we all have mental health. We're taught how to eat right, go to the gym and look after our body. But that conversation about looking after our mind, which we all have, needs to happen. So having a non-clinical room helps with that conversation of understanding that we all have a mind. And again it's not to say that clinical, that there's anything wrong with that. But having an option of somewhere like this only adds to helping people recover I think.

Laura: So what's the future looking like here?

Ben: So these guys are really happy with us here, we can stay here as long as possible. We just need funding to keep the therapies going. I'm mean the team's great, so hopefully we can find a bit of funding to continue the work and get more projects going, more variations. So it's a great starting point where we are, a lot of directions we can go into. We just need decision makers who look after money to look at us and help. So what the future holds I don't know, but there's a few of us who really want this to keep going.

Music room: interview with Jon Hall, music therapist

Laura: So, we are sat here in the music studio. Can you just talk me through what you do here, and how you work with people?

Jon: Well I think music plays an active role in getting people going. Often people come in and they might be isolated, they might be anxious, they

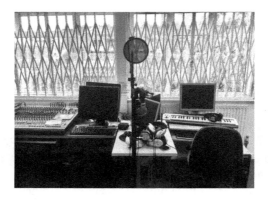

FIGURE 18.2 Music room and recording studio.

might not even have wanted to come. They might not trust that it's something that they want to do. So I usually begin with music therapy improvisation. And I think the great thing about improvisation is that through people singing, or playing or pitch and rhythm, that becomes the scaffolding through which people can start to communicate again. I think a lot of the time some people can be very complex. They don't want to talk, or they don't find it easy to connect. I think music improvisation can be a great way of building that trust.

And then what I do is I build on that. I encourage people to share their stories, so things that have happened to them. And I think music is a great container for those stories. I think that sometimes if put someone's harrowing stories of what's happened to them in the medium of music, it acts as a benign way of containing it. So it's a lot easier to express, even through it's quite uncomfortable. And another thing that I've been discovering more and more is that through the process of recording. Because you have to do it over and over again to get it right, and people do want to get it right, and I think it becomes almost like a physical exercise machine. It's a motivating force for people who may normally be quite resistant to the idea of doing anything. If you give them an opportunity – 'here's a song and it's sounding pretty good, let's try it again'. And I think that's cultivating resilience. Once they have been through with this kind of programme, they can use some of the skills they've learnt in other services. I think the creation of the song is great. It doesn't always work for everybody.

Sometimes it's a bridge too far for some people, and they are happy just to take part in the group, improvising and things like that. But I think that if somebody has written a song, what works really well is introducing the idea of it being on a CD. And then what I normally say to them is 'well what would the song suggest to you visually?' And then they might go next door and paint a record cover with Ben, which we can then print out the CD for them. So that gives them again an opportunity to think about their stories, through music and art.

And I think the final thing that I've really come to is performance. Sometimes I feel like it's a bridge too far for people, but it always seems to work. I remember with the young person's cohort, one girl I worked with was very scared about performing. Very scared about revealing her singing and her song. But she is an excellent singer, and she'd written an excellent song. In the live performance she was shaking so much, her body was going backwards and forwards. And I did think 'oh I hope this is ok'. But then afterwards someone came up out of the audience and said 'I love that song, can I buy it?' And I said, 'oh I just so happen to have a CD here!' And we sold it, the lady got the money out of her purse and I gave the money to the young person. She was very excited and I don't think she could quite believe it. She's gone on to do a psychology course.

So sometimes I do worry that the live performance is a bit too much. I think though that's for everybody. I was telling you about Michael downstairs [a member of staff at the Clarendon Centre]. Performing for him was so terrifying, and the fact that he did it just feels great. And of course he's not a service user, but it works for everybody actually. If you ask someone to step up to a microphone, if you ask someone to perform, it can be terrifying. But something happens through that process of taking on a different identity. And I think for people who can perhaps be stuck with complex issues, to have that opportunity to experience that, is powerful.

One lady, actually who I met in the hospital. I was working with her right from there. She came up to the group and she couldn't believe that we were going to be doing singing or videoing. She was very frightened of the camera. I showed her some of the work I'd done with previous groups and she was happy to then go ahead with the camera. I ended up working a lot with her in hospital, and then she came here. That often works quite well, if I've met someone in hospital, then rather than when they come out they might go back round again into the hospital, they come and meet me here. They know me and it's a great way of getting them to feel comfortable. Anyway, what happened to her is that she got asked to go on one of these TV shows where you win things. And she was saying to me that her sister was saying 'I don't know how you can possibly be up there in front of the camera, I don't know what's happened to you!' And she was telling me it was this process of having gone through having been filmed and recorded, she's built this kind of resilience inside her. To the point that she was winning a holiday to Ibiza! I mean that's a kind of top of the range story. A lot of people have enduring mental health issues and music's great but it can only do so much.

Laura: So what are the differences in working in those kind of environments and working here?

Jon: I think some of the things I learnt in hospital, I didn't really anticipate. How it works is I'll go into the hospital and I'll say I'm upstairs, I'm going to be doing some music, I'm going to be recording, if you fancy doing it come along. We're going to play, we'll have fun. I showed them some videos of people I've worked with before, and a bunch of people come up. Then a couple of weeks later I'd go to the morning meeting and I'll show them the video. And I think the biggest realisation I had was the impact on the staff. They were like 'Oh my God is that these people?' Because I think what happens to people when they're singing and when they are excited and they're happy and they're recoding, is that they become very animated. And it's almost like people get an opportunity to see them as they really are. So that's been a really powerful thing in a hospital setting. There's other things as well because people are often on anti-psychotic drugs, and they're in a treatment zone. My experience of people in the hospital is that they are very open to being creative. Not everybody. Some people can be seriously resistant. But generally I've found that people have been very open to being creative.

Working in the community here. I think there's much more of a feeling of it being a more normalised environment. People come here, they use the cafeteria downstairs, they use the building. There's a sense that it just feels a lot more natural. Almost as if I was working in a studio and doing much with a band. It feels a lot more natural here. Of course some people come along and they are very complex characters. And they're at the point in their journey where they need a lot of support. So that can be a bit tricky sometimes. Whereas in the hospital I'm dealing with people who are very complex, who are at that point in their journey where anything can happen. I think it's down to the referrals as well. In terms of the way the project was set up, I think the referrals have come through the doctors and the care coordinators who in some ways are mindful who can come on to the programme and benefit the most from working with music or art. It's more supported. In a way though, in the hospital you have an audience, you've gone to the ward and they are there. They come upstairs and think 'great, I'm coming off the ward, this is amazing'. Whereas here there's the added difficulty with people suffering from anxiety, depression, stuff like that, they will need to be rung up, talked to cajoled, reminded. They might be feeling awful that day. That's where UEL's been great in getting in touch with people, talking to them, and encouraging them to come. So I think that's one of the differences.

Laura: So you said that here is more normalised. I've always been struck by how – this room looks like a music place, next door looks like an art studio. Neither of them look like a mental health place. Can you talk a bit about why you made the decision to set them up in this way?

Jon: I think for me it wasn't conscious, from the music side. This is all my gear. I was working as a record producer and I had a studio in Tottenham Court Road. So then when I left college I started integrating being a record producer and being a music therapist. Part of my dissertation was about what are the values in recording that can give additional benefits in music therapy. I'm not totally pleased with it in here. I'd like it to feel a lot more like a recording studio with sofas. And I have discussed with Gavin that we get rid of the cupboard. It's horrible. I'd change these bars. Those to me are awful – like what's that saying to someone that you're locked in.

So, I would change that so it looks like a recording studio, change the carpet a bit. Make it more that someone can come in here and feel like they are in a studio. A lot of the sessions that I've done with bands in a studio will be sitting round on sofas trying to write a song chilling out. Whereas this room. I don't think it's quite there. I mean I really try to make it feel like a recording studio. When people come in I make sure there are instruments out. I just want them to feel comfortable that it's fine to just hang out and let's come up with some tunes and be creative. But there's still work to be done. I worked at this other centre when I left my training over in Seven Sisters. And there the guy that was running it gave me carte blanche. So I had a massive room with sofas, with carpet. And it was really nice. There were points where you could have a load of people in there. Some very complex clients would like to be in there as well.

You know the Vygotsky idea of zone of proximal learning. If you got somebody in there who's very complex, who might not find it that easy to take part, but you've also got some people who are very able, it's easier for that person to then create on that level. So yeah I'm not totally happy with this room yet. You know like this [indicating mixing desk] is good but it's really old and really unnecessary, but it does mean that when people come in here they feel like they're in a real studio.

Laura: It's very impressive looking. It does look like the real deal. So the recording element of your practice, is that quite an unusual element?

Jon: Yeah. With music therapy, you're looking at people, at how they present and you're using the tools of music to look at what musical things you can do. If I play on the piano with someone and I speed up and they don't speed up. You're looking at what the interaction is and you analyse it through music. So generally I think that process is very beneficial. And generally improvising together with people with instruments is also beneficial to build those bonds of trust. Where I brought the recording in, is I noticed that if I was running a group people would kind of start to lose interest after about 40 minutes. Whereas if I was recording, people just want to go on all day. So in terms of motivating people with mental health it's a really great thing. And also I've seen people actually getting quite sweaty. They're basically having a workout, singing, doing chorus vocals together, you're really exercising the body. That's just something I've found myself that I've integrated that can add additional benefits. The other thing I do that music therapists don't often is videoing clients. You might do that to take to supervision to show your supervisor how you're working with clients and if you need to change anything, or feedback.

Laura: Yeah. And also I suppose it means that something that normally stays in the room, instead they have a product that they can take out into the world and show people. Is that part of the purpose?

Jon: Yeah, I think it's important to be able to show friends and family. It can be a bit tricky sometimes when people then start to see themselves as X Factor and they want to put it on YouTube. I worked with one girl who had learning disabilities. And we'd done this great Bangra track. And that was the first time that we were confronted with this problem. Every week she would come to the sessions and say 'I want it on YouTube'. And we had to talk with the organisation about how that would work, because I think people can be quite horrible online. So in the end what we did was we put it up and we took off the possibility of people making comments. And it worked fine. And she was really overjoyed. She shared it with all her family in India. So it can work really well but I think sometimes you have to be careful. Because sometimes the people you're working with are very vulnerable as well.

Laura: So how do you make the transition, or the decision, about who is going to perform and what they are going to perform. I'm thinking of the transition from being in here, making stuff in here together, to a public performance.

Jon: Well what I normally do is I find out the people who want to perform and then usually the people who don't want to perform want to take part supporting. So we may have written a group song together, which I try and do. And if it's difficult to write a group song, because the group aren't really coalescing, then sometimes we do famous songs. So for one of the events we did quite a lot of famous songs. I don't know why, there was just an appetite for singing famous songs. And sometimes that can be the most healing thing. You get a group of people together and they just want to sing famous songs. So part of that process of performing those songs is also, I think, just sharing together, being in it together. It's a good feeling. Almost like choirs, which now are a big thing, it brings people together. So what I usually do is I try and find out who wants to do a song individually, is happy to do experience that, and then everybody else I get them to take part. Either supporting somebody, doing their own song, or the group song. I think it's really important to have everybody taking part. I think that's the thing I've found people talk about, this shared experience.

Laura: So I was really struck at the performance event, what an amazing atmosphere it was, and you could really feel that sense of community. Can you just talk a bit about the impact of that event?

Jon: I think some of the people were hanging out outside when we were clearing up, and just the sense I got from them was 'wow!' 'This was just an amazing experience'. And I think it was a lot more amazing than we could have envisaged. Perhaps it is that thing of bringing the generations together. And the transparency of some of the performers, and the hearts that they wanted to share with the audience. It was very moving. And so the feedback that we've got from the audience was that 'this was just incredible – we loved it!' I don't think it could have gone any better. I don't think anyone really knew what was going to happen. I think the performance itself, like the event, everything seemed to conspire to make it a wonderful feeling for everybody. Which is why I think it's worth thinking about that for a yearly thing for this place. Because there's a lot of people who come here who don't come to our programme, who come to do other things. And I think the chance to take part in something like this would be really exciting for everybody. So I think we've started something and we want to carry it on.

For me, the best moment was just as we started, as the first person came on, my daughter and her friends who are all about 8, came right to the front and started dancing. And I thought 'yeah, it's happening, it's ok, this is gonna be good!' And I was thinking ok there's a lot of really different types of styles and performances, and sometimes hard things to listen to. But I think there were definitely moments where the audience was able to feel some of the discomfort that happens when trying to get everyone to coalesce. And I think sometimes in therapy sessions I do have to sit through what can be an uncomfortable place, where noone knows if it is happening. And I think there's elements of that in the event. We thought – what is going to happen now? Is this person going to completely take over, or is it all going to be fine? So some of those moments I was really glad that they were played out in the performance.

Laura: It really did feel like a gig, rather than a 'mental health event'. Which I think is also true of the art that is set up like a gallery, not like a mental health thing. So there's something really un-patronising about the whole approach. It's about showing things at their best. Getting people together in a way that doesn't look like . . .

Jon: An apology?

Laura: Yeah – is that part of what you've tried to achieve, or is that just the way it's worked out?

Jon: Not really sure about that. Because I know that there was an appetite for this project for it to include people from the music industry. I think both Ben and I thought that was a bad idea. People would just have freaked out, they wouldn't have felt happy, perhaps would have felt undermined performing. And I know sometimes people have said when they've come to some of our events that there were too many posh, public people there, and there weren't enough mental health people. I think in terms of the appetite to include people from the music industry, I think the fact we didn't do that was good. It's interesting that you say it was like a proper gig. I wanted people to feel confident in their performances. I didn't want them to feel that anyone could turn round and say 'well that's shit, that's no good'. But I didn't want to pump it up too much. I think Ben and I are both really aware of that with the art and with the music, it's not making it alienating for people but trying to work with them. So we've asked a lot of the participants, 'how would you like this to be'. And different cohorts have responded differently. But with this last performance the sense I got from everyone was that they were really excited, they really wanted it to be public, they wanted loads of people to be there. That was the general consensus. So we worked with them in a co-production way. Often I feel unsure about including staff in the events. But every time I do it really seems to be very powerful.

Laura: So do you think that is because in mental health services there often is this binary between staff and service users, especially on psychiatric wards. And that can filter through services, probably least somewhere like this, but it can still filter through. So is what you're saying that if you include both people in the production of the same thing, it dissolves some of those boundaries?

Jon: I think so. And I think music is a great way of doing that. I've often been working in hospital and I've said to staff come on, come and sing this now, you come and help. And they've gone 'oh no I can't sing, I can't sing'. And that's the thing, once they do, and take part – the service user feels better because the hierarchy has changed –we're all in this together

	we're all on one level and that bleeds out into the whole vibe of the community. So when they're back on the ward – rather than it being a staff member, we're all mates in making this stuff together.
Laura:	And do you think your work will change the way they set things up here at the Clarendon?
Jon:	Well I think it's had a big impact on the staff, I think the events have been great but I also think they've been a big of upheaval for the staff as well because we have to get it all out and then quickly put it all back together again. But I think including the staff in the musical performance, getting them to sing, is a really great way to get them to feel like they are participants. They go through the anxieties and the nerves and I think it's a really great bonding mechanism for the whole place. And I think what we're probably going to do now is look at trying to do a yearly 'Clarendon Festival'. You know we've already had people saying 'when's the next one?' 'Can I join in?' I was in the café the other day and there was a lady on the computer, and me and Simon, who sang at the event, started singing. She joined in and we started doing a kind of gospel jam in the cafeteria. And she said 'I've got to be at the next event'. I think we've brought a lot of life to this place, which can be a bit sort of doomy. The space of it. I think it's a good feeling for people to celebrate themselves with music and art and have the public here. I think it really works for everybody.
Laura:	And what do you think it is about those performance events that manages to do that, that has such a positive atmosphere?
Jon:	Well I think to get to the point where you've written a song by yourself and you're going to perform it, I think that takes a lot of doing. And I think the same happens for a group. If a group's going to be performing a song together, there's something about that performance. I suppose it's asking people to step into a different identity, for that moment. And I think one of the significant things that has come out of this project is the shift in perspective of the carers and the professionals, who see people's hidden talents as assets rather than a diagnosis.
	I think it's a range of people, it's friends of the people who are performing. It's friends and family who are excited for people to come and see them perform their songs. I think it's clinicians and care coordinators who come to marvel at their clients who seem to have changed into these performers. It's quite amazing what people are able to do once they are given a bit of help and guidance and support.

INDEX

abuse 12, 58, 135, 151–152, 268
accountability 278, 282
acculturation 239
ACT *see* assertive community treatment
action research 27, 91, 237
admission 106, 113
adolescents 74–84, 104–105; discourse of adolescence 74–75; outpatient services 65–66; sensory spaces 103, 107–115
adventure based therapy 215
aesthetics 89
agency 3, 11–12, 16, 19; community meals 129; homeless people 136; life-space 24; 'primacy of technology' 203; Psy models of distress 149, 153; sensory spaces 26; service user perspective 288, 289; topological approach 204; young people 83
aggression 15, 16, 57, 108
agoraphobia 5
Akhurst, Jacqueline 27, 214–233
alcohol use 168–169, 170–171, 272
alienation 2, 120
alliances 81–82
Altman, I. 176
Amaze 151
anchoring 12
antidepressants 151, 152
anxiety: anxiety disorders 5; austerity 119; danger 12; entrapment 11; everyday experiences of 3; homes 26–27; nature experiences 215, 218, 219, 229, 231; sensory approaches 102, 108, 110; social media 212; Tea in the Pot 255, 259
art 54, 293–300
ASD *see* Autism Spectrum Disorder
Ashon, W. 144
assertive community treatment (ACT) 181
asylums 1–2, 77, 263; closure of 2–3; institutional control 89; legacy of sequestration 6; Madlove project 50–54; practitioners in 277; private 76; risk discourse 58; *see also* institutional spaces
atmospheres 16–18, 90; CAMHS 61; digital spaces 201; parent support groups 158
attitudes 197, 265
austerity 26, 119, 135
Austin, M. J. 282
Australia 18
Autism Spectrum Disorder (ASD) 102, 107
autonomy: CAMHS 26; community mental health practitioners 275; hospital design 106; nature experiences 230; sensory spaces 110, 114, 115
Ayalon, O. 283, 287

Bantebya-Kyomuhendo, G. 9
Bauman, S. 200
'being in place' 157
Bell, M. 14
belonging 10–11; community integration 181, 184, 195, 196, 197; community meals 26, 120, 121, 127, 128, 129;

parent support groups 156; 'sense of duty' 158; Tea in the Pot 27, 250, 253, 254, 260; 'third places' 252, 254
Berg, M. 149
Bergson, H. 203
Bhabha, Homi 247
Bike Minded 154, 158
Bilfulco, A. 12
bipolar affective disorder 170, 172, 183, 298
Boden, Zoë 26, 88–101
bodies: digital spaces 201; embodied relations with 204; smoking room 41, 43, 45–47, 48; territories 286
borderline personality disorder 168, 273
boredom 9, 150, 194
Bowers, L. 16
Boydell, J. 8
Brandling, J. 250
Braun, V. 168
Brighton Unemployed Families Centre Project 156
Brown, George 9, 11, 12
Brown, Steven D. 26, 135–148, 203, 204, 209
Building Bridges 240, 241, 243, 248
built environment 7, 10, 280, 282; CAMHS 57, 59, 60; expansion of the 229–230; impact on the physical and the psychological 55–56; institutional spaces 14–16; service user perspective 282–283, 289

calmness 218, 221, 222, 225
CAMHS *see* child and adolescent mental health services
camping 217, 220
capability approach 7–8
capitalism 21–22, 44, 136
care: care practices and space 156–160; children 68; enclaves of 120–130; ethics of 152, 159
Carling, Paul 182
Cedar House 19
Chalmers, A. 106–107
Chamberlain, Kerry 5, 26, 119–134, 135–136
Champagne, T. 114
Chase, E. 9
child and adolescent mental health services (CAMHS): adolescent mental health wards 26, 74, 78–84; outpatient services 25–26, 55–70

children 25–26, 55–70; acculturation of migrants 239; constructions of childhood 58, 65–67, 69; sensory spaces 26; Somali culture 238
choice 3, 14, 16; sensory spaces 107, 110–111, 113, 115; walking and solo experience 230
churches 145–146
CICI *see* Community Integration Census Index
Cigman, R. 267
citizenship 124, 157
civic participation 7
Clarke, V. 168
class 84, 151
cleanliness 165–166, 176
Cloutier-Fisher, D. 165
co-design 26, 89–99
coercive practices 88, 98; *see also* restraint; seclusion
Colaizzi, P. 78
collaboration 92–93, 95–96, 114, 138
colour 57, 62, 63
'common notions' 204, 208, 209, 212
'the commons' 150
communication 197, 277, 280, 283–284, 288
community attitudes 197
community care 2, 4, 19, 263–278; case studies 268–274; community mental health teams 264, 266, 274–276, 277–278; day services 4; focus on the service user 264–265, 267–268; risk discourse 58; shift to 3, 9, 167–168; shrunken spaces of 6; social prescribing 153–160
community centres 242, 245
community, feeling part of the 252, 256, 260
community integration 19, 180–199; barriers to 191–195, 196; data collection and analysis 183–186; facilitators of 186–190, 196; factors affecting 180–181
Community Integration Census Index (CICI) 184–186, 196
community meals 26, 120–130
community psychology 20, 181, 240, 248
community spaces 26–27, 163, 176
Community Treatment Orders (CTOs) 267, 270
confidence 27, 227, 228, 250, 259
confidentiality 96
confinement 79, 141–142, 277
connection 10
Connellan, K. 15
contact hypothesis 94–95

control: adolescent mental health wards 26, 78, 80; institutional 89; lack of 57; walking and solo experience 230
Cooper Marcus, Clare 284, 285, 286, 288
Corker, E. 9
counselling 281
Coventry and Warwickshire Mental Health Trust (CWMHT) 92, 96–97
Crafter, Sarah 25–26, 56–73
Crawley, H. 58
Creativity and Recovery for Wellbeing (CREW) 293, 296
Creswell, T. 250
crime 8, 10, 12, 267
Crisp, N. 91
critical-developmental psychology 58, 65
Cromby, J. 10
cross-generational learning 240, 246–247
CTOs *see* Community Treatment Orders
cultural hybridity 247
culture 20, 242–243, 244–245, 247
Cummins, S. 104
Curtis, S. 14, 17, 104, 105, 106, 108, 114
cycling 154, 156

Dailey-O'Cain, J. 238
Dal Santo, T. S. 282
danger 12; CAMHS 57, 58, 61; homeless people 136, 146
data analysis 60, 139–140, 168, 186, 206–207, 218
Davidson, L. 180
day services 3, 4
debt 119
Deegan, P. E. 19
DeJong, C. A. J. 284
Denmark 8, 39, 40, 48n2
dependency 4
depression: clinical 155; community integration 183, 192; entrapment 11; everyday experiences of 3; humiliation 9; lack of green space 13; loss 12; moves to the suburbs 10; nature experiences 215, 218, 219, 231; parental 151; sensory approaches 102–103; Tea in the Pot 255, 259
depressive position 273
deprivation 7, 8, 119, 151, 165, 252
design 57, 89, 105, 280–281; *see also* experience-based co-design
despair 120, 124–125, 126, 129–130
detention 75, 76, 83, 84, 88
developmental psychology 65, 66, 144
diagnoses 149, 154–155, 159

Diez-Roux, A. V. 104
digital spaces 27, 200–201, 203, 210–212; *see also* social media
dignity 15, 120, 149; community meals 26, 122, 124–125, 128, 129; smoking room 39
disability 151, 180
disciplinary power 13, 41, 47
discipline 40, 41, 44, 45, 48
discourse 206
discrimination 9, 120, 245, 265; *see also* exclusion
disease 152
dislocation 120
dissociation 280, 284–285
distress 2, 14, 28, 88–89, 263–278; adolescents 76; austerity 119; containment 16; eco-therapy 215; experience-based co-design 97; fluidity 154–155, 156, 160; gardens 167; hidden nature of 136; home spaces 163, 164, 175–176; homeless people 137, 138, 140–141; housing 181; internalised distress of poverty 129–130; isolation 10–11; mess of 152, 154–155; political, social and economic forces 152; Psy models of 149, 153; public space 5; social experiences 151; social materialist models of 160; social media 200, 205–206, 209, 211, 212; topological approach 212; walking and solo experience 218
Dixon, J. 5, 136
domestic violence 12, 254
Douglas, Mary 5–6
Duff, C. 157
Dunham, H. W. 8
'dwelling' 23, 24

EBCD *see* experience-based co-design
eco-therapy 167, 214, 215, 228, 231
ecological approaches 22–23
educational spaces 66
Edwards, C. 164
Einstein, Albert 22
electro-convulsive therapy 88
Elefriends 200, 204–212
embodiment 20, 164, 204, 209, 229
emotions 14; community mental health practitioners 275–276; homeless people 142; sensory spaces 26; service design 89; social status 9; touchpoints 90
emplacement 127
employment 9, 12

empowerment 105, 106; homeless people 138; Outsider Gallery 295; sensory spaces 26, 107, 110, 113, 114, 115; 'service places' 252; service user perspective 288, 289; walking and solo experience 228
enclaves of care 120–130
engineering 89
Enhancing the Healing Environment 15, 89
entrapment 11, 12
environmental psychology 20
Epstein, I. 281
equality 7
Erikson, E. 66
ethics: of care 152, 159; experience-based co-design 96
ethnic minorities 11
ethnicity 83, 84; *see also* race
everyday life 164
evidence-based practice 90–91, 98, 103, 282
exclusion 5, 119, 126, 151; CAMHS 68; homeless people 135–136; neurological changes 152; precariat 120; shared space 138; Somali men 245; young people 75
Exerkate, C. C. 284
expectations 98
experience-based co-design (EBCD) 26, 89–99
experts, service users as 263
expressed emotion (EE) 10

family: acculturation of migrants 239; community integration 197; educational interventions 197; Fathers and Sons Project 240–248; living arrangements 182; resilience 239–240; Somali culture 238; *see also* parents
Faris, R. E. L. 8
Farnworth, L. 18
Fathers and Sons Project 240–248
Fatimilehin, Iyabo 27, 237–249
fear 8, 12, 197
Feeney, Maria 27–28, 250–262
feminist geography 21
Fenner, P. 90
films 96–97
finances 190, 191, 194–195, 196
Finland 130
Finlay-Jones, R. 12
flexibility 106, 111, 113, 114
fluidity 154–155, 156, 160
Fogel, B. S. 172
Ford, R. 17
forests 143, 144–145, 219

Forster, Joe 28, 280–292
Fossey, E. 18
Foster, A. 268
Foucault, Michel 13, 41, 44, 46, 47, 89
Frame, Janet 1–2
Francis, S. 14, 104
freedom 3, 107, 220–221, 222, 228
Freeman, Elizabeth 27, 214–233
Friedli, L. 7–8, 251
Furedi, F. 150

gardening 167, 215
gardens 52, 166–167, 169–170, 175
Geedka Shirka 27, 246
gender 84, 151, 186; *see also* women
Geographic Information Systems (GIS) 183, 184
Gesler, W. 14, 104, 105, 114
Glasgow 27, 250, 251
Goffman, E. 263, 285
'Going Local' project 153
Golembiewski, J. A. 70
Goodings, Lewis 27, 200–213
Graham, Rebekah 26, 119–134
green space 12–13, 52, 144, 219, 230; *see also* gardens
group walking 230

Hall, Jon 28, 293, 300–307
hallucinations 151, 189–190
Hanna, Paul 26, 149–162
Harper, D. 10
Harris, T. O. 11
Harvey, D. 237
Harvey, J. 165
Hassan, Amira 27, 237–249
health barriers to community integration 191, 192–193, 196
Heidegger, M. 127
Hickman, P. 252
Hinshelwood, R. D. 263
Hodgetts, A. 5, 135–136
Hodgetts, Darrin 5, 26, 119–134, 135–136
Holen, Mari 25, 39–49
'holistic' social prescribing 257
homeless people 26, 135–146
homeliness 15, 57, 62–63, 64–65, 69, 70
homes 5, 11–12, 26–27, 163–176, 280; community care 268; crisis of 141; 'dwelling' 24; home spaces as an ideology 164; institutional spaces designed like 15; ordering of home and garden spaces 165–167; Peled's Location Task 287–288; service user perspective

28, 283–286, 287, 288–289; *see also* housing; supported accommodation
hospitals 1–2, 6, 13–14, 19, 25–26, 104–105; built environment 14–16; challenges in acute mental health services 88–90; children 57; cost of hospital stays 295; experience-based co-design 89–99; Madlove project 50–54; music therapy 302, 303, 306–307; practitioners in 277; smoking room 39–48; ward atmosphere 16–18; *see also* institutional spaces; psychiatric wards
House, W. 250
housing 8, 27, 119; community integration 181–183, 185–186, 187–188, 191, 195, 196, 197; housing models for individuals with psychiatric disabilities 181–182; single rooms 141; *see also* homes; supported accommodation
How Clean Is Your House? (television show) 165
Hubbard, P. 14, 21, 104
Hull, Hannah 25, 50, 52
human geography 5, 20–21
humiliation 9, 142
hybridity 247

IAPT *see* Increasing Access to Psychological Therapies
identity 106, 111, 237, 285; 'being in place' 157; cultural 248; home spaces 164, 165, 175, 176, 286; musical performance 307; Peled's Location Task 287–288; professional 276; *see also* self
ideology 164
Ilyas, S. 152
immunology 137–138
improvisation 300–301, 304
Imrie, R. 164
'in-between' status 25, 40, 47, 48
inclusion 5; community integration 180, 181, 196; community meals 26, 122, 125, 129; food poverty 129
incomes 185, 190; *see also* finances
Increasing Access to Psychological Therapies (IAPT) 152–153, 159
independent living 168–171, 182, 268
individualisation: psychiatric wards 47; of responsibility 4
individualism 10
industrialisation 2, 74
inequalities 4, 7, 74; contact hypothesis 94–95; distrust 10; power 19, 68, 84; risk factors for mental illness 76; urban environments 8

infantilisation 76–77
informal community spaces 153, 156–160
Ingold, T. 23–24
inner city areas 8
inpatient services *see* psychiatric wards
instability 12
institutional spaces 1–2, 13–18, 19, 25–26; adolescent mental health wards 74, 77–84; CAMHS 60–61; challenges in acute mental health services 88–90; experience-based co-design 89–99; homeless people 145; Madlove project 50–54; older people 167–168; smoking room 39–48; *see also* asylums; hospitals; psychiatric wards
integration *see* community integration
intergenerational tensions 237, 239, 240
interiority 138, 141, 144–146
intimacy 47, 141
invisibility 142, 143, 146
isolation 10–11, 273; community integration 192; food poverty 129; gardening 167; homes 26–27; migrants 239; precariat 120; psychiatric recidivism 267; 'service places' 252; Tea in the Pot 27, 250, 253, 255, 260, 261; 'third places' 252
Italy 9–10

job insecurity 12
Jungian approaches 215, 216, 228

Kagan, Carolyn 27, 237–249
Kimberlee, R. 257
Klein, Orly 26, 149–162
Kloos, B. 181
knowledge 157–158, 281, 282
Knowles, C. 5, 136
Kuo, F. E. 12–13

LAC *see* Liverpool Arabic Centre
Laing, R. D. 18
Lammers, M. 284
language 111, 113–114, 239
Larkin, Michael 26, 88–101
Latour, Bruno 20, 40, 141, 201
Laurance, J. 267
Law, J. 154
Lawson, B. 15
Leadbitter, James 25, 50, 52
Lee, C. 282
Lefebvre, H. 21, 120, 166, 237
Lelliott, P. 3
Lemyre, L. 12
Levine, M. 5

Lewin, Kurt 22, 23, 24, 202–203, 204
Liddicoat, Stephanie 28, 280–292
Liebscher, G. 238
life-space 23, 24, 202–203, 204, 207–211, 212
lighting 15, 16, 57, 112–113
Liverpool Arabic Centre (LAC) 241, 246, 247
Location Task 287–288
locus of control 11
London 13, 135, 143, 146
loneliness: gardening 167; 'service places' 252; Tea in the Pot 27, 250, 253, 255, 260, 261; 'therapeutic culture' 150; 'third places' 252
Loopstra, R. 135
low incomes 119
Lupton, D. 201

McAuley, R. 5
McGrath, Laura 26, 56, 70, 135–148, 163
McIntosh, D. N. 102
Macintyre, S. 104
McKenzie, K. 8
Madlove project 25, 50–54
madness 2, 3, 25, 41
mainstreaming 3
Marks, Nick 26, 149–162
Marmot, M. 7
Marres, N. 203
Martin, W. T. 10
Marxism 20, 21
Massey, Doreen 21–22
material objects 40–41, 127, 141, 173–174, 175
materiality: CAMHS 25–26, 56–57, 61–62, 67–69, 70; educational spaces 66; home spaces 164, 165; risky 56–57, 61, 67–68, 69, 70; service user experiences 55
May, D. 15
meals 26, 27, 120–130, 237–238, 243–244
meaning-making 204, 214, 217, 229, 237
medical profession 149–151, 159
medication 3, 152–153, 302; antidepressants 151, 152; case studies 271; collective capacity for meaning 204; compliance 267, 278; social media 208, 209
meditation 215
Mental Health Act 88, 98, 267, 270, 273
mental health services 189–190, 191, 193–194
Merleau-Ponty, M. 20
'meshwork' 23–24
migrants 58, 237, 238–239
Miller, D. D. 163, 164

Miller, L. J. 102
Mind 167, 205
mindfulness 285, 287
Mol, Annemarie 149, 154
Moncrieff, J. 152
monitoring 41
Moos, R. H. 16
Morag, B. 104
moral management 2
moral panic 58
morale 266
Morris, M. 274
Mosher, Lauren 18–19
movement 23
Muijen, M. 265
Musarò, P. 129
music 53, 102, 110, 123, 293, 296, 300–307

narratives 240–245, 248
National Health Service (NHS) 88, 89–90, 103, 108, 295; experience-based co-design 92, 93; nature experiences 231; social prescribing 153
National Institute for Health and Clinical Excellence (NICE) 159
Natural England 214–215
nature 12–13, 27, 52, 144, 214–231
neglect 61, 62, 65, 70
negotiation 45, 74, 77
neighbour relationships 181
neighbourhoods 181, 187–188, 191, 195, 196, 197
neoliberalism 119–120, 123, 124, 130
Networks of Community Support (NoCS) 183
new social settings 238, 248
New Urban Agenda 6
Newnes, C. 149, 150
Newtonian physics 22
NHS *see* National Health Service
NICE *see* National Institute for Health and Clinical Excellence
Nicholls, D. 18
Nicholls, V. E. 230
Nikitin, L. 18
NoCS *see* Networks of Community Support
noise 57
Nussbaum, M. 7

objectification 2
observation 41
Oldenburg, R. 250, 251–252, 255, 260
older people 26–27, 163–176; independent living 168–171; supported accommodation 168, 171–175, 176; 'third places' 252, 255

oppression 4, 11, 124, 130
order 6, 165–166, 176
othering 2; children 58, 66, 68; smoking room 41, 46, 48
outpatient services 55, 57, 59–69, 70
Outsider Gallery 28, 293–307
Outsider Witness 243–244
Oxleas Mental Health Trust 92, 93, 94, 95, 97
Oxley, D. 176

Palasmaa, J. 284
panoptic power 74, 80
Papoulias C. 15
paranoia 10, 96, 192, 273
parents: acculturation of migrants 239; Fathers and Sons Project 240–248; parenting skills 241, 245, 246, 247; support groups 151, 155–156, 158; *see also* family
Parks, Rosa 46
Parnell, Nathan 26, 102–116
Parr, H. 5, 6, 41, 60
participation 26, 28, 129, 248
Payne, H. 15
peer support 4, 155–156, 158, 205–206, 207, 208–209, 211
Peled, A. 283, 287–288
performance: adolescent mental health wards 82–83; musical 301–302, 304–306, 307; service design 89; social performance of behaviours 175
personal space 80–81
personalisation 53, 284, 286, 288–289
personality disorders 168, 266, 268, 273, 276
Pescosolido, B. 9
pharmacological treatment 88; *see also* medication
Phelan, J. 9
Phiri, M. 15
photo booth 111–112
photographs: CAMHS study 78; community integration 186; homeless people 138–139; personal photographs in the home 165, 173; walking and solo experience 229
physical activity 53–54
physics 22
Pinfold, V. 5
place 20, 104, 217, 239, 250
Planetree 15–16
police 272
policies 3–4, 6–7, 231
political participation 7, 76
Pols, J. 152, 159

Poole, Jason 26, 74–87
Porter, Roy 2, 3
Postle, Denis 150–151
poverty 4, 7, 8, 151; food poverty 129; internalised distress of 129–130; lack of agency 11; precariat 120; shame 9; substandard housing 182
power 11, 14, 93; adolescent mental health wards 26, 79; adult institutional 74, 75. 81; community psychology 20; disciplinary 13, 41, 47; home spaces 164; inequalities 19, 68, 84; organisational structures 95; panoptic 74, 80
practice research 281
practitioners *see* staff
precariat 119–130
pressures 218–220, 222, 228
prevention 153
Prigogine, I. 22
Prince, C. R. 181
Prince, P. N. 181
Pritchard, R. 267, 273
privacy 15, 18, 105; agency and entrapment 12; Madlove project 53; smoking room 39; Tea in the Pot 254
private space 6, 163; home spaces 174, 175, 176; Madlove project 53; smoking room 42; *see also* homes
projections 274–275, 276, 277
Psy disciplines 149–151, 152, 153, 158, 159, 160
psychiatric wards 3; adolescent mental health wards 26, 77–84, 104–105; built environment 14–16; challenges in acute mental health services 88–90; sensory spaces 103, 106–115; smoking room 39–48; staff/service user binary 306; ward atmosphere 16–18; *see also* hospitals; institutional spaces
psychiatry 149–151, 159, 267, 281
psychodynamic forces 266
psychology 20, 159; community 20, 181, 240, 248; developmental 65, 66, 144; 'Psycommons' 150–151; 'therapeutic culture' 150; topological 201–204, 206–207, 210–211, 212
psychosis: adolescents 83; community mental health teams 266, 276; everyday experiences of 3; evidence-based practice 91; Soteria project 18
psychosocial environment 90
psychotherapy 152–153
'Psycommons' 26, 150–151
public/private dichotomy 136

public space 5, 6; homeless people 135–136, 138, 142, 143, 144–146; young people 75
purity metaphors 5–6, 136

quantum physics 22
Quirk, A. 3

race 151, 183, 185, 186; *see also* ethnicity
racism 4
Radley, A. 5, 135–136
Rapley, M. 150
Reavey, Paula 26, 56, 70, 74–87, 135–148, 163, 203, 204, 209
reception areas 67–68
recidivism 267
recovery 19, 107; anchoring 12; 'everyday work of' 157; focus on the individual 103; inpatient wards 104; models of 3
reflective listeners 243–244, 245–246
regulation 39–40, 41, 42, 43, 45, 77
rehabilitation 182, 197
Reisman, J. E. 102
relapse prevention 278
relationships 14, 15–16, 18; absence of 273; adolescent mental health wards 81–82; community integration 181, 187, 195, 197; community mental health teams 276; community psychology 248; Fathers and Sons Project 247; home spaces 164, 283; lack of interaction 17; life-space 24; reciprocal 120; social media 208, 211; in space 21–22, 237; topological psychology 202–203; *see also* social relations
relaxation 110, 113, 166, 222, 223
residential continuum model 182
resilience 6, 7, 239–240, 302
resistance: adolescent mental health wards 26, 74, 78, 79–81, 82, 83, 84; community meals 130; sitting down 46; smoking room 25, 39, 41, 46–47, 48; victim-blaming narratives 126
resources 7–8, 76
respect 105, 106, 110, 122, 125, 128
responsibility: accepting 19; escaping responsibilities 218, 221, 225, 228; individualisation of 4; social prescribing 257
restraint 19, 48n2, 81, 88, 98, 108
Ridgeway, Priscilla 182
Ringer, Agnes 25, 39–49
risk 14, 16, 17, 18, 41; adolescent mental health wards 80–81, 83; CAMHS 56–57, 58, 67, 68–69, 70; children 25; risk management 13–14, 104–105, 110–111, 113, 114, 136; service user fears 93
risky materiality 56–57, 61, 67–68, 69, 70
Rivers, I. 200
Rooney, Bernice 26, 102–116
Rosenbaum, M. S. 253
Rosenheck, R. A. 182
rumination 226–227

safety 12, 17, 18, 56–57, 137; adolescent mental health wards 83; CAMHS 69; community integration 181, 195; home 164; homeless people 26, 136, 146; informal spaces 157; Madlove project 53, 54; Tea in the Pot 258
schizophrenia: community care 268; community integration 183, 189–190, 192; expressed emotion families 10; living arrangements 182; Tea in the Pot 259, 261; urban environments 8
Scotland 27, 250, 251, 256
Seale, C. 3
seclusion 19, 88; adolescent mental health wards 79, 80; reduction of 15; sensory spaces 106–107, 108
sectioning 6, 175
security 12, 26–27, 56–57, 105
Segal, S. P. 181
self 280, 283, 285–286, 288; *see also* identity
self-awareness 228, 296
self-determination 41
self-esteem 229, 259
self-harm 15, 16, 28, 168–169, 276, 281, 283–286, 289n4
self-help 27, 287, 289
self-reflection 26, 28, 288
self-respect 19
self-worth 120, 156, 252
Sen, A. 7
'sense of duty' 158
sensory spaces 26, 102–103, 106–115
separation 2
Serres, Michel 201
service design 89, 91
'service places' 252
service user perspective 28, 106, 280–289
sexual minorities 11
shame 9, 142–143, 146, 192
shared activity structures 120
Sibley, D. 136
Silverman, C. J. 181
Simon, J. 102
Skogstad, W. 263
Skorpen, A. 39

Sloterdijk, P. 26, 137–138, 141, 143, 144
Smail, David 11
Smith, Barbara 149
Smith, Lesley-Ann 26–27, 163–179
smoking room 25, 39–48
social anxiety 96
social capital 7
social cohesion 7, 8
social constructionism 40
social defences 274, 276, 277, 278
social determinants of health 119
social disorganisation 8
social exclusion *see* exclusion
social experiences 151
social inclusion 3, 4, 129
social interaction: community meals 122, 127, 128, 129; discourse 206; hospital design 105; 'service places' 252; Tea in the Pot 253–254, 259, 260; 'third places' 252
social media 27, 200–201, 203, 204–212
social practices 120, 157, 163, 208
social prescribing 26, 150, 153–160, 250–251; models of 257; Tea in the Pot 27, 253, 256, 257–258, 260
social relations 22, 120, 157; *see also* relationships
social status 9
social support 150, 180, 187, 196; *see also* support
social welfare 130
societal disenfranchisement 75
Soja, E. W. 248
solidarity 126, 128, 129, 155
Somali men 27, 237–248
Soteria project 18–19
South Africa 8
space: art room 299–300; CAMHS 25–26, 55, 56–57, 61–65, 67, 69–70; care practices 156–160; contemporary contexts 3–6; educational spaces 66; experience of distress 28; fluid 154–155, 156, 160; inpatient wards 104–105; mental health practice 40–41; migrants 239; music therapy 303–304; Peled's Location Task 287–288; personalisation of 284, 286, 288; psychosocial environment 90; relational 104, 115, 237; sensory spaces 6, 26, 103, 106–115; service user perspective 289; shared 137–138; smoking room 39–40, 43, 45, 48; spatial order 6; spheres 137; theorising 19–25; therapeutic 103–104; topological psychology 202–203, 212; walking and solo experience 217; *see also* homes; institutional spaces; public space

space-time 4–5, 22, 237
Spandler, H. 4
spatial imaginaries 237, 238
spheres 137
Springham, Neil 26, 88–101
staff 15, 17; adolescent mental health wards 79, 82; CAMHS outpatient services 63, 64, 70; community mental health teams 264, 266, 274–276, 277–278; demoralised 88; experience-based co-design 91, 93; music therapy 306–307; relationships with service users 16, 97, 276; safety and security 57; sensory spaces 111; smoking room 42–43, 45, 46
Standing, G. 12
status anxiety 9
Stengers, S. 22
Steuve, A. 9
Stichler, J. F. 15–16
stigma 9, 95; CAMHS 57, 60; community care 265; community integration 181, 191–192, 196; cultural-level 98; educational interventions 197; precariat 120; young people 76
stillness 223–224
Stolte, Ottilie 26, 119–134
stores and services, proximity to 184, 196, 197
stories 208, 301
storytelling 27, 237–238, 241, 243, 247
strengths 240, 241, 248
stress 12, 119, 215, 218, 231
Stromberg, N. 114
Stroup, T. S. 182
struggle 39, 43, 48
substance misuse: austerity 119; case studies 168–169, 170, 268, 270–271, 272; walking and solo experience 218, 225
suburbs 10
suicide 119, 130
supervision 113
support 126, 128, 150; community integration 180, 187, 196, 197; emotional 95, 268; lack of 273; parent support groups 151, 155–156, 158; practitioner support networks 266; 'service places' 252; social media 200–201, 205–206, 207, 208–209, 210, 211; social prescribing 153, 157
supported accommodation: case studies 270, 271–273; community integration 181, 183, 185–186, 187–188, 189, 191, 196, 197; older people 168, 171–175, 176; rehabilitation 182

surveillance 41, 105, 286; adolescent mental health wards 79, 80, 83–84; children 58; gardens 167; young people 75
Sweden 8, 130
symbolism 105
Symonds, A. 4

Tea in the Pot (TITP) 27–28, 250–261
temperature 57
territories 285, 286
'therapeutic culture' 150
'therapeutic landscapes' 55, 74, 90, 104, 159, 215
therapeutic relationship 90
'therapeutic space' 158
therapy 152–153, 159
'third places' 27, 238, 250–252, 253–255, 260–261
'third spaces' 247, 248
time 4–5; home spaces 176; life-spaces 203; smoking room 43–45, 46, 48
topological psychology 201–204, 206–207, 210–211, 212
touchpoints 90, 91, 92, 94
Townley, Greg 27, 180–199
transportation 188–189, 191, 193, 196
trauma 12, 58, 102–103, 135
treatment 43, 45–46, 197
trust 10; eco-therapy 215; experience-based co-design 92–93; music therapy 304; social media 210; Tea in the Pot 253–254
Tsai, J. 182
Tuan, Y. F. 217
Tucker, Ian 27, 200–213
Twigg, Julia 12

Uggerhoj, L. 281
unemployment 151, 156, 239
United Kingdom: cost of mental illness 230; experience-based co-design 92; homeless people 135; mental health care 2–3; nature experiences 214–215, 216–231; social media 200, 204–212; social prescribing 153, 257; Somali men in the 237–248; young people 75; *see also* National Health Service
United States: community integration 183–197; community psychology 181; homeless people 135; housing 27; inner city areas 8; low quality of life 9–10
urban environments 8, 135, 143, 146
Uttarkar, Vimala 28, 263–279

value 9, 125
vandalism 12
Verheyen, Carolyn 284, 288
victim-blaming narratives 126
violence: community mental health teams 275; domestic 12, 254; homeless people 136; precariat 120; psychiatric wards 16, 47
virtual communities 27; *see also* social media
voice hearing 11, 151–152
volunteers: community meals 122–123, 124; Tea in the Pot 250, 255, 256, 257–258, 260, 261; therapeutic nature of volunteering 158
vulnerability 142, 239
Vygotsky, L. 304

waiting rooms 63–64, 67
Wakeling, Ben 28, 293–300
Walker, Carl 26, 149–162
walking 215
walking and solo experience (WSE) 214, 216–231
Wardhaugh, J. 12
Warner, Richard 9, 19
water 224
Watson, S. 251
Watters, J. 238
Weaver, Tassie 26, 135–148
well-being 18, 76, 90; community meals 128; experience-based co-design 99; gardening 167; good design practice 280; nature experiences 214–216, 224, 225, 229, 230; person-environment fit 283; sensory approaches 102; space and place 217; 'therapeutic landscapes' 104
Wells-Thorpe, J. 15
Werner, C. 176
wheelchair users 299
wild spaces 215, 216–231
wilderness therapy 215
Wing, J. K. 263
Wise, M. J. 165
women: green space 12–13; homeless people 136; moves to the suburbs 10–11; oppression of 11; Somali 238, 240, 248; Tea in the Pot 27–28, 250–261
Wood, H. 265
WSE *see* walking and solo experience

Yanos, P. T. 180
Young, I. M. 152
YouTube 304

Zorwaska, Anna 25, 50–54

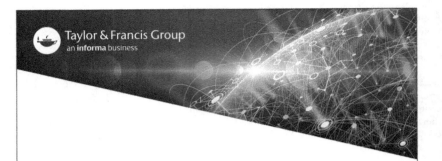